PALEO: 12 WEEKS TO CHANGE YOUR LIFE

Achieve the Ultimate Transformation

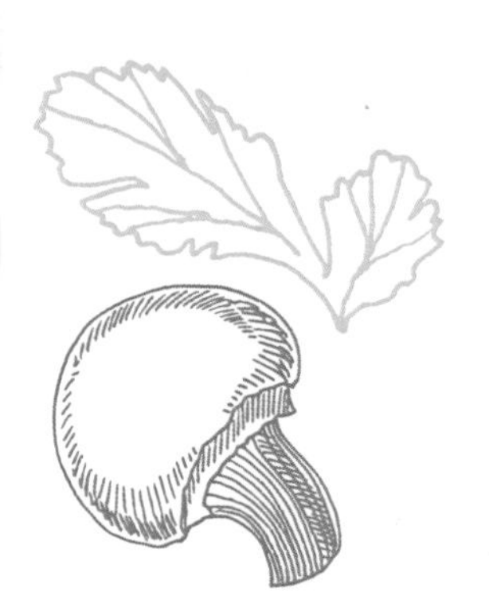

REBECCA FIELD

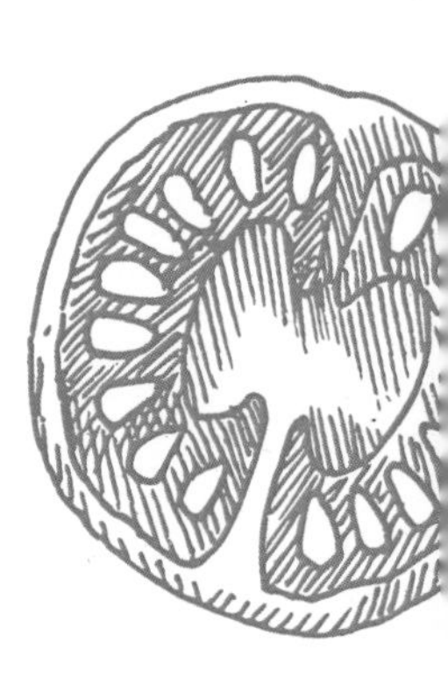

Published by Starfish Publishing UK

Printed and bound in the UK by CMP (UK) Limited
First published in the UK in 2015
A catalogue reference for this book is available at the British Library

ISBN 978-0-9932593-3-3

This book is intended as a reference volume only. The information given here is designed to help you make informed decisions about your health. It is not intended as a substitute for any medical advice or treatment that you may have been provided with or prescribed by your doctor or health care professional. It is advisable to seek professional medical attention before changing your diet and lifestyle especially if you have a known medical condition.

CONTENTS

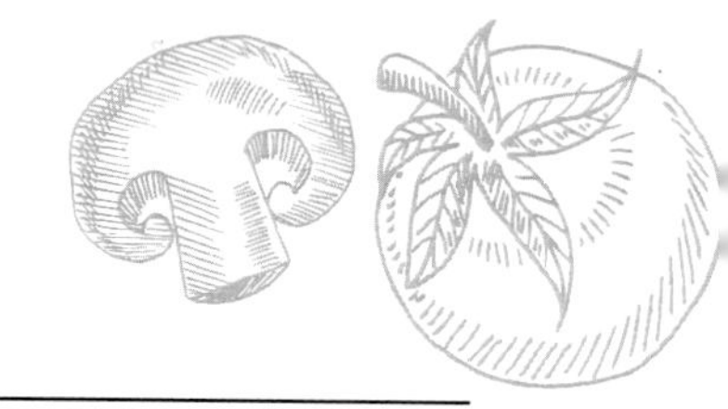

INTRODUCTION

Welcome to Your Paleo Journey

The Paleo Diet and Fitness Plan has been designed to help you transform every aspect of your health and wellbeing to achieve a sustainable and healthy lifestyle. This goes much further than just changing your diet. We believe in adopting a holistic approach which includes focusing on exercise and your overall wellbeing as an important part of your transformation. Not only will this approach greatly assist with weight loss and toning, it will help you to identify and manage stress triggers and will provide a feeling of self-confidence and self-belief that will change your whole outlook on life.

Many of you will already have kick-started your Paleo journey with *Introduction to Paleo* which provides a 7 day introduction plan. *Introduction to Paleo* sets out the basics of the Paleo diet providing information on Paleo foods and why it is that Paleo can help where other diets have failed. You will also have been provided with a wealth of information on the Paleo lifestyle including tips on exercise and wellbeing. If you have not yet read *Introduction to Paleo* we would suggest that you do this as it provides a great pre-cursor to the information that you will be provided with in *Paleo: 12 Weeks to Change Your Life.*

Introduction to Paleo took you through the biochemistry that lies beneath eating and you learnt that it defines practically all of the food choices that you make. You discovered how biochemistry affects your behaviour and how food interacts with your body to produce the chemicals necessary for life as well as the health benefits of choosing to follow a Paleo lifestyle. We looked at the foods that you should and should not be eating for optimal Paleo nutrition and how a holistic approach is essential in any healthy approach to weight loss.

We believe that the better informed you are, the more likely you are to succeed with permanent and ongoing change. *Paleo: 12 Weeks to Change your Life* has been designed to consolidate the information that you learned from *Introduction to Paleo* and will guide you through everything that you need to know to make your Paleo journey a success. Using an easy to follow approach that encourages understanding alongside a real life case study, it will set you up for life and answer all of the questions that may arise, helping you along every step of the way.

You will learn about the benefits of nutrient dense food and will gain an understanding of how to make good food choices and how to shop effectively for Paleo foods. You will gain a deeper understanding of what foods can be toxic to the human body and why they have been eliminated from the Paleo lifestyle. To complete the holistic approach to your transformation we will take you through the importance of exercise along with stress management and self-awareness techniques.

Throughout *Paleo: 12 Weeks to Change Your Life* you will receive input from our detailed case study. In her own words, our willing guinea pig will tell you about her own Paleo journey and offer real life advice from someone who has been there and completed the Paleo Diet and Fitness Plan. Keep an eye out for these comments throughout each section. They will give you a useful and honest insight into what you can expect throughout the 12 week programme.

Remember that this is your body and it is a gift. You have the opportunity to learn how to give your body everything that it needs for you to lead a full and energetic life with confidence and self-belief. These opportunities do not come along often. Grab it with both hands and make a commitment to yourself. You can do this.

Are you ready
to start your
Paleo journey?

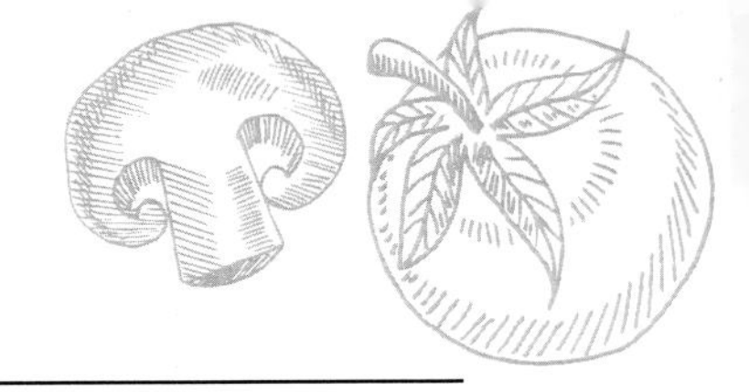

SECTION 1

A Few Thoughts Before You Start

We have provided a 12 week programme in relation to both the diet and fitness aspects of our plan. There is a reason for this. It is the time that is needed in order to make an effective change and for those changes to become habit forming. You will start to see and feel results after a couple of weeks and by the time you have completed *Paleo: 12 Weeks to Change Your Life* you will feel like a new person.

Health Concerns

If you have any concerns in relation to a medical condition or treatment, you should consult with your doctor or health care professional before starting the Paleo Diet and Fitness Plan. It is always advisable to consult a doctor or health care professional before making any changes to your diet and exercise regime.

How does the Paleo 12 week programme work?

The Paleo programme is based on three healthy and nutritious meals a day, plus snacks if needed. We have even included dessert a few nights a week. We have done all the hard work for you and set out your meals for each day. These have been combined into weekly meal planners so that you have a useful quick reference guide to see what you will be eating on a daily basis. We have also provided a shopping list to accompany each weekly meal planner so it really couldn't be simpler to get started. All of the ingredients can be found in your local supermarket or your local butcher, greengrocer and fishmonger. In Section 6 we will be providing you with the information that you need in order to get the most out of your shopping.

We have provided over 200 recipes for you to follow. The Paleo kitchen is not a stressful place; when you cook with fresh natural ingredients there is no need for complicated techniques or long lists of ingredients. Everything that you need has been provided for you in the weekly meal planners and shopping lists.

Flexibility

The recipes have been developed with flexibility in mind. We are conscious that most people will be eating lunch away from home during the week and this has been taken into consideration. We have therefore provided lunches which are easy to prepare and often incorporate the leftovers from the night before to make things as easy as possible for you. None of the recipes are overly complicated and all are within the capabilities of every one of you. If you are a beginner in the kitchen then please do not worry. You will soon learn how easy it is to make simple yet delicious recipes.

We also realise that people enjoy treats so we have incorporated desserts into the meal plans to satisfy those with a sweet tooth. You will be surprised at how much you enjoy these treats and they will become firm favourites along the way quickly replacing the sugar filled treats that you will be used to.

You may wish to stick to the weekly meal plans quite rigidly or you may wish to change things around a bit – it is completely up to you how you want to approach it. This is about you and your lifestyle and you are in control. If you want to experiment with our recipes or use them as a spring board for your own ideas then please do so. We encourage you to take time to find what ingredients you like and finding your own style and tastes in the kitchen can be fun and entertaining and often has delicious results.

By the end of the 12 week programme we would like everyone to feel that they have progressed in their cookery skills and learnt a thing or two along the way. You will be encouraged to use ingredients in new and exciting ways and will learn a whole host of new tastes and textures.

What snacks can I have between meals?

In the first few weeks you will probably find that you eat a lot more than you will once your body has adjusted. Eat when you feel hungry but take on board what you have already learned in *Introduction to Paleo* about biochemical behaviour and learn to question if it is hunger you are feeling or merely cravings. If you have had very little in the way of nutrients over the past few months (or even years) then your body will continue to crave food until its reserves have been topped up.

Choose nutrient dense snacks such as cooked meats, hard boiled eggs, avocado (delicious with a pinch of salt and a touch of lemon), a handful of nuts or some fruit; although bananas have a high GI and are eschewed by the mainstream diet crowd, they are actually a great source of vital potassium and can be a lifesaver when hunger strikes between meals. You can also treat yourself to a bit of dark chocolate occasionally.

To keep things varied we have provided some snack recipes for you. These can be found in the recipe section. These will hopefully help to give you some inspiration to start creating your own snack recipes. We have also provided some dessert recipes that can be eaten as a treat during the week to satisfy any sweet cravings. You are of course free to devise your own desserts or to simply just have a piece of fruit if you want something light.

If you are out and about you can also buy snacks from health food shops (but make sure you check the label to ensure they are Paleo friendly). Learning to limit snacks is the best way forward for long term weight loss, but in these early weeks they could mean the difference between success and failure.

Will there be any side effects?

For most, the transition to a diet of Paleo foods is smooth and symptom free; for some it can be a bumpy ride. The first few days are the ones most likely to pose certain challenges. For those who have completed *Introduction to Paleo* you will hopefully have made it through your 7 day plan without any symptoms. For those of you who did find that the transition was not as smooth, you should now be through the worst and feeling the energising effects of Paleo. You will be able to see the side-effects that our case study faced in the first entry below.

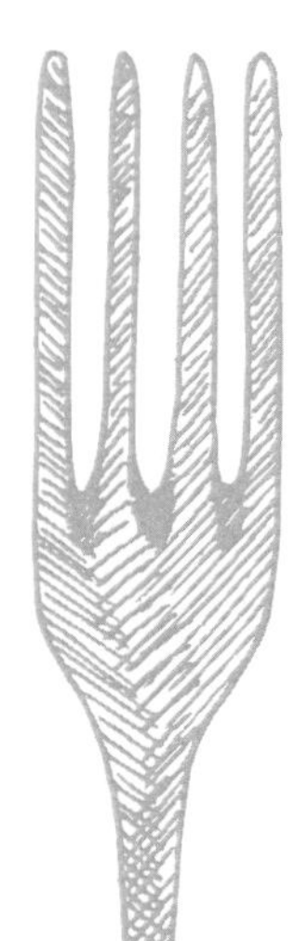

Case Study

Hi, my name is Jenny and I am your case study. Throughout the course of *Paleo: 12 Weeks to Change your Life* I will provide you with my thoughts and insights as to how I found my Paleo journey. Just like you, I found Paleo Diet and Fitness and made a commitment to follow the 12 week programme. I hope you find my comments useful. Good luck on your journey it is a fun and interesting road of discovery. I have set you off with my first entry below which takes you through my first 7 days of Paleo.

"When I first began with Paleo I was looking forward to feeling instantly energised and alive. At 43, four stone overweight, and with some appalling eating habits, I was long overdue a change. I gained most of the weight during pregnancy and scoffed at

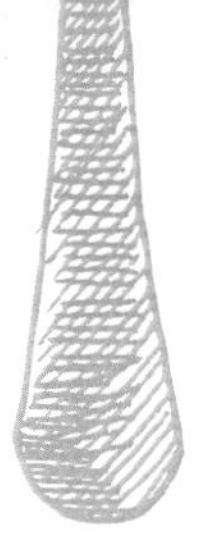

the health visitor who told me that 80 percent of mothers never lose the weight they gain. Not me...

12 years later I had lost and regained the lot; twice. Each time I had lost the weight through reducing my intake and upping the exercise; energy drinks and chocolate bars were my daily sustenance of choice and cycling like a maniac my preferred activity. Each time I stopped paying attention the weight went back up but I chose not to notice until reaching the extra 3 stone mark. The worst thing? Knowing that my terrible food choices have affected the way I feed my family.

I began with "Introduction to Paleo". Day one was fine, nothing to report but a day of satisfaction at eating the right foods. The main turning point for me was learning about the biochemical mechanisms underlying it all: BIOCHEMISTRY DRIVES BEHAVIOUR was what it said. EVERYTHING made sense from that moment on.

By day two I was nauseous, tired and had a headache. I was drinking litres of water and needing the toilet every fifteen minutes. Day three brought much of the same followed by a restless night's sleep. It was uncomfortable but it also felt strangely right and good.

On day four I awoke with a low-level headache but yet an oddly exhilarating feeling pushing closer to the surface. The day was slightly easier but I knew that I could do little but rest. Day five brought hope to the horizon. I awoke, still with the headache but I packed my breakfast and headed outdoors. Once I got moving with the wind on my face and the green of trees around me I felt energised and alive.

I learnt that movement and fresh air help, but that you need to listen to your body too. If Paleo is about one thing, it is about learning to listen to your body and understand what it is telling you.

By the end of the week I had a weight loss of over half a stone. I was tired and exhausted but I didn't crave anything; not once. A definite silver lining for a lifelong scoffer of empty carbs!

Did the side-effects make me give up? No way. I knew that these feelings were a reaction and that this was a really important thing to do for myself; as a wife and a mother there hadn't been too much of that for over a decade. Exactly because of the severity of the reaction I knew that I couldn't give up but what kept me going the most was the underlying feeling of vitality that was pushing stronger each day; like something way below my skin, my flesh even, right at the cellular level. Change was on its way..."

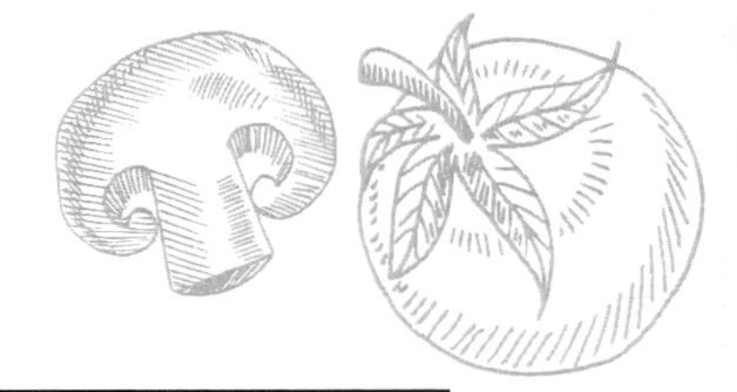

SECTION 2

The Paleo Store Cupboard

First things first; you are going to need some ingredients. Depending on the kind of person you are (and trust us, if you know that then you are one step ahead of the game. If not, then don't worry; we are here to help you become self-aware savvy) and how many non-Paleo eaters you share your domain with, you may want to completely clear out all the pre-Paleo foods, or you may just wish to add in the new ones.

We have provided a general guide below as to the food you should be clearing out and the food you should be replacing it with. *This is by no means comprehensive and is simply to give you an overview of what adjustments you will need to make.* The general rule to use is that anything processed should be removed. Watch out for many ingredients such as wheat, sugar, and soya on labels too; even though your shopping will now consist of real whole food there may often be occasion to check a label. You never know where a completely unnecessary additive or filler may crop up next.

We know that this can be a lot to take in but do not worry; there is a comprehensive shopping list provided for each week which includes all of the ingredients that you will need for the recipes. Remember that *Introduction to Paleo* contains a colour coded food chart that is handy to keep with you to make good food choices when out and about.

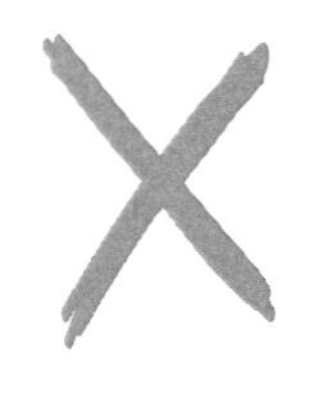

These things must go...

DRINKS	Normal/Diet Soft Drinks Normal/Diet Squash Milk	Flavoured Waters Fruit Juice (from concentrate)	Energy Drinks
BAKING	Baking Powder Cornflour	Grain Flours Sugars	Yeast

CONDIMENTS	Ketchup Brown Sauce Mayonnaise	Bottled Dressings Soy Sauce Stir Fry Sauce	Jam Marmalade Marmite
FATS & OILS	Sunflower Oil Vegetable Oil Trex	Margarine Spreads	Oil Sprays Corn Oil
DAIRY	Butter Milk Yoghurt	Cheese Ice Cream Cream Cheese	Cottage Cheese Cheese Spread
GRAINS	Breakfast Cereals Popcorn Oats	Rice Couscous Polenta	Bread Products Barley Crackers
LEGUMES	Lentils Chickpeas Peanuts	Peanut Butter Canned Beans Dried Beans	Tofu Soya
MEAT	Processed Cold Meats Processed Sausages Processed Burgers	Canned Meat Products Ready Meals	Nitrate-treated meats (such as hot dogs, salami etc)
SNACKS	Biscuits Crisps Sweets	Chocolate Bars Chewing Gum Granola Bars	Tortilla Chips Fruit Leathers

Fill your basket with these lovely foods instead

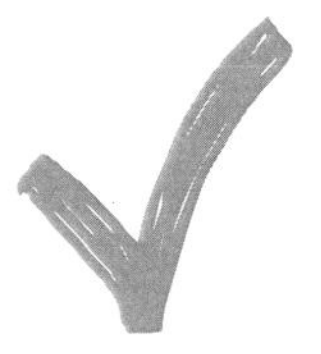

VEGETABLES

ALL VEGETABLES INCLUDING (BUT NOT LIMITED TO)

Artichoke
Asparagus
Avocado
Beetroot
Aubergine
Bok Choy
Broccoli
Brussels sprouts
Cabbage
Carrot
Cauliflower
Celeriac
Celery
Chicory
Cucumber
Endive
Fennel
Green beans
Kale
Kohlrabi
Leek
Lettuce
Mushroom
Okra
Onion
Parsnip
Peas
Pepper
Sweet potato
Pumpkin
Radicchio
Radish
Rocket
Romaine Lettuce
Salsify
Shallot
Spinach
Squash
Swiss Chard
Tomatillo
Tomato
Turnip
Water chestnut
Watercress

HERBS

ALL HERBS INCLUDING (BUT NOT LIMITED TO)

Chives
Coriander
Dill
Garlic
Ginger
Parsley
Chilli
Mint
Basil
Tarragon
Lemongrass

FRUITS

ALL FRUITS INCLUDING (BUT NOT LIMITED TO)

Apple
Banana
Blackberry
Blueberry
Grape
Fig
Guava
Lychee
Mango
Melon
Passion Fruit
Peach
Plum
Nectarine
Pear
Persimmon
Pineapple
Pomegranate
Raspberry
Rhubarb
Strawberries
Watermelon

MEAT **ALL UNPROCESSED MEATS INCLUDING (BUT NOT LIMITED TO)**	Bacon Beef Gluten free sausages	Goat Lamb Nitrate free salamis	Organ meats (offal) Pork Veal
POULTRY AND GAME **ALL POULTRY AND GAME INCLUDING (BUT NOT LIMITED TO)**	Chicken Duck Pheasant	Pigeon Quail Rabbit	Turkey Venison
EGGS **ALL EGGS INCLUDING (BUT NOT LIMITED TO)**	Hen	Duck	Quail
SEAFOOD **ALL SEAFOOD INCLUDING (BUT NOT LIMITED TO)**	Mackerel Prawns Salmon	Sardines Shellfish Tuna	White fish (cod/haddock/sea-bass/monk fish etc)
NUTS AND SEEDS **ALL NUTS AND SEEDS INCLUDING**	Almonds Brazil Cashews Chestnuts	Hazelnuts Macadamias Nut butters Pine nuts	Pistachios Sesame seeds Sunflower seeds
FATS AND OILS	Beef dripping Coconut oil Duck fat Olive oil	Goose Fat Hazelnut oil Lard Macadamia oil	Walnut oil Ghee

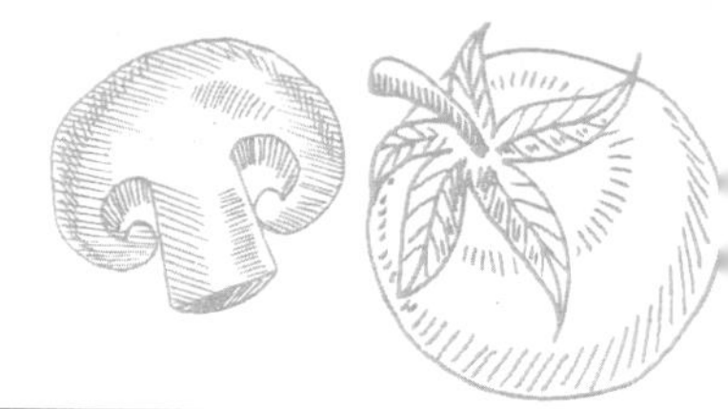

SECTION 3

Getting Started

We appreciate that it can be quite daunting at the start of the 12 week programme. For many the transition to a Paleo lifestyle involves a completely new way of thinking about food and involves a huge change to their overall lifestyle. This can take some getting used to and the first couple of weeks are all about getting into a routine. Once you have achieved this you will be surprised at how easy it becomes and how natural it feels. Not to mention you will be feeling great and full of energy.

To make a smooth transition into the Paleo lifestyle you will need to get organised. Taking steps to prepare for the journey ahead will mean that you eliminate any surprises along the way and will be prepared for any change in situation that would normally throw your eating habits off balance.

For those of you who live with non-Paleo eaters the first couple of weeks can be tough as you watch others eat the foods you would previously have enjoyed. Being organised will help you to stay on track and will mean that you are not caught out without any Paleo friendly foods at mealtimes. It is often the case that we revert to old eating habits when we are hungry and need to eat something quickly but there is nothing available as we have not planned ahead. It takes only a small amount of your time to plan ahead and it will make sure that you do not fall at the first hurdle. You will find that after a few weeks others will be jealous of your food as it looks and tastes so good!

There will be things to think about, some of which we covered in *Introduction to Paleo*, such as shopping, advance preparation and clearing the decks. This week is an important week and where at all possible needs to take precedence above all else. By committing to the Paleo lifestyle for the next 12 weeks you are prioritising your own health and taking back control. This is your time now.

"Failing to plan is planning to fail"

Planning is of paramount importance; not only when it comes to fitting good food into your life but in every aspect. If you want to live life to the full then you need to get efficient. We realise that for some planning is not a natural way of life. There are many of us who will happily go from one day to the next without making any preparation or plans for the week ahead, whereas there are others who have to apply military style planning to every aspect of their life. You will be pleased to know that there is a happy medium to be found.

There is a huge difference between being obsessive and being organised. Obsessive is rigid and often just a form of procrastination, whilst being organised just enough to be effective can be truly liberating plus we have done the hard work for you.

Planning ahead for a week of food solves several issues all at once. How many of these scenarios are you familiar with?

- Skipping breakfast because there is just no time
- Grabbing a cereal bar and a skinny latte on the way to work
- Facing only unhealthy choices at lunchtime; however good your intention
- Eating the contents of the fridge (standing at the fridge) because you are too hungry not to
- Having toast for dinner, again, because you didn't make it to the shops

If you can nod in understanding at any of these scenarios then you seriously need to start thinking ahead. It may seem like extra work but eventually it will become second nature and make life an absolute breeze. Not to mention being able to button up your skinny jeans.

Make Planning a Priority

1. Make planning a part of your plan; stand or sit in the kitchen with a nice cup of tea and make it a weekly priority
2. The best laid plans are absolutely no good if not written down; digitally or on actual paper
3. Think about the week ahead; does each week follow a pattern or is each one different? What does the week in question bring; lots of long days and late home-times or a quieter week with a rare bit of space?
4. Plan your meal ideas taking the week's schedule into account. Think about doubling up on recipes, even making enough to freeze. Think about good use of leftovers and how a decent breakfast will fit in for you. Whilst we have done menu plans and recipes for you, with finely tuned ideas to maximise time and budget, you may need to tweak it a little to suit your lifestyle

5 When is a good time to go shopping and will you need to change where you shop to make it more Paleo friendly? We look at shopping realistically within your individual restraints in Section 6. Will you do one big shop, or is it more convenient to do a little every few days? Perhaps you need to build in time for an online delivery?

6 Are you already fairly competent in the kitchen or a complete newbie? It may take some of you longer to prepare ingredients than others

Once you start asking yourself these questions you will be able to identify the areas you need to work on and how you can make planning a part of your weekly routine. The more organised you become the more you will realise that your downfall in previous weight loss attempts more than likely lay with a lack of organisation. You really should give it a try and see what a difference it makes.

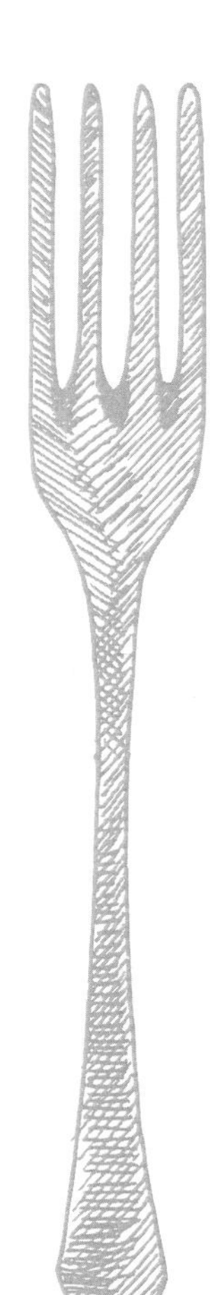

Case Study

"Living with two non-Paleo eaters and being in charge of all the cooking I naturally had some concerns about how it was going to work. I have a demanding job with long hours and have little time to focus on myself at the best of times. To make things more complicated I usually end up cooking a different meal to please each member of the family as they all have different tastes and requirements.

When I started the 12 week programme I made a conscious effort to ensure that the cupboards and fridge would always be stocked with Paleo friendly foods to stop me being tempted by old habits. I am often guilty of picking at food when it is cooking for the rest of the family and then just having toast or cereal for dinner for myself as it is quick and easy. If I was still hungry it would be followed by some chocolate for dessert.

By making sure that I planned head and did a big shop to include Paleo friendly snacks it meant that I never had an excuse to stray back into old habits. Being able to head to the cupboards knowing that I would be able to find something that I could eat without feeling guilty was great.

I have no doubt that being organised meant the difference between success and failure to me. The first couple of weeks it does feel like a chore but then the more I made it part of my routine the quicker and easier it became until it ended up being second nature. Having the weekly meal plans and shopping lists worked fantastically for me as it meant I just needed to tweak according to what my hours would be that week."

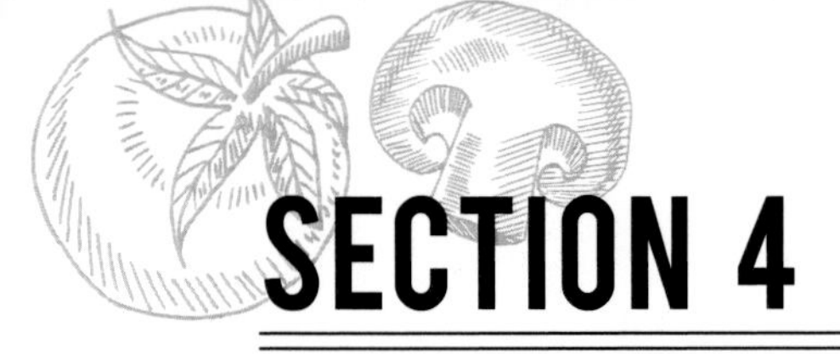

SECTION 4

Incorporating Exercise

Exercise is an important part of the Paleo lifestyle and focuses on functional fitness and improving your health by working with your body, not against it. This is very much in line with the Paleo approach to food and lifestyle in general.

Just as conventional dietary wisdom has been focused on one thing for the past several decades, mainstream exercise theory seemed to follow the same route. Namely promoting the idea that the more hours you put in, the better with some people attending the gym at least once a day and putting themselves through painfully long cardio sessions, often resulting in injury. Modern science will now tell us that this is not the most efficient approach and nor does it provide the best results. Yet people continue to inflict this punishing routine on their bodies.

The Paleo approach to exercise emphasises structured exercise combined with brief, but intense, strength and resistance training workouts as opposed to extended sessions of cardio. It also encourages perpetual movement as opposed to long periods of inactivity. You were encouraged to include perpetual movement into your daily routine during *Introduction to Paleo* by ensuring that you moved around every 30 minutes.

Why should I exercise?

Anyone who has ever embarked on an exercise programme will tell you that the benefits of exercise are far reaching and are most likely way beyond their expectations when they started out. Let's start with the main reason why people start an exercise programme. This is simply to lose weight and look better. Creating a lean and toned body is something that many people desire but all too often it gets lost under the label of "too busy" or any other excuse that people come up with to avoid being active. The result is that two thirds of the UK adult population are now classed as overweight or obese.

Exercise can also help to reduce stress, prevent depression, improve memory, and create better sleep patterns. It can improve your immune system, lower your risk of diabetes, heart disease and stroke to name but a few. It keeps your body strong and healthy and allows you to enjoy your life unencumbered by preventable illness and feelings of fatigue and lethargy. It is an essential part of your transition to a truly sustainable and healthy lifestyle.

When should I start exercising?

We would recommend that you start to incorporate exercise into your weekly regime from the beginning. The benefits that you will obtain are overwhelming. The sooner you make it part of your weekly routine the sooner you will feel these benefits and realise how powerful it can be, not only for your weight loss goals but to raise your confidence and improve your overall wellbeing. It will help you to think clearer and approach life with a new bounce in your step.

What exercise should I be doing?

The Paleo Diet and Fitness approach to exercise is about flexibility and it being adaptable to each person's individual needs. This is the ethos that permeates throughout our entire approach to the Paleo lifestyle. We believe that it is the only approach that will work to create a truly sustainable and healthy lifestyle that can be maintained forever.

With this in mind we have created *Tabata Transformation* and *Introduction to Yoga* to compliment the Paleo diet and to help you achieve the most out of your Paleo journey. The programmes are flexible to meet your needs and provide a variety of movement and exercises. The work outs can be completed in as little as 20 minutes and can be carried out at the gym or at home making it easy to slot into your hectic schedule.

Tabata Transformation is based upon high intensity interval training which has been shown to burn fat and improve your overall fitness much faster than traditional cardio exercise. The best part is it only requires a 20 minute work out. It is exhilarating and provides fantastic results in a short period of time. It includes compound, plyometric and bodyweight exercises along with resistance training to build strength and stamina. The Tabata programme encompasses all aspects of Paleo thinking when it comes to exercise and is the perfect accompaniment to your Paleo lifestyle.

Introduction to Yoga will teach you how to identify stress triggers and how to develop a mechanism for controlling stress and the impact that it can have on your everyday life. You will learn how to tackle the curve balls that life throws at us and how important relaxation is to achieving a healthy body and mind. The fact that it will also help you to lose weight and tone up makes Yoga essential for every hectic lifestyle.

Each of the exercise programmes is based on a 12 week programme to complement *Paleo: 12 Weeks to Change Your Life*. Incorporating exercise into your regime may seem quite daunting for those who have been inactive for a while. Do not worry; it will soon become second nature and you will be amazed at how good it makes you feel. Not only will it greatly assist in your weight loss goals but it will provide you with increased energy and a feeling of self-confidence and self-belief.

The important thing is to stop making excuses.
Why not give it a go today?

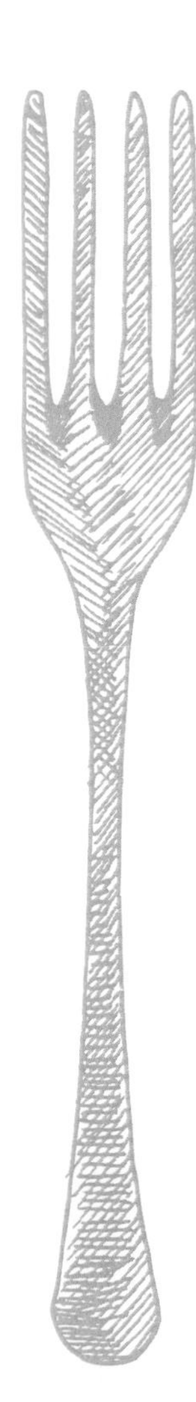

Case Study

"Exercise for me has always been a mode of transport; to do exercise for any reason other than getting from A to B has just never made any sense. Walking and cycling have always been my exercise of choice purely through necessity. Before becoming a mother I always worked physically strenuous jobs, on my feet for 12 hours a day with plenty of heavy lifting and carrying. Even the pushchair years kept me fit and living in the city meant cycling to get around. Several years ago, location and circumstance made it unnecessary to walk or cycle and various failed attempts at making exercise part of my schedule left me pretty much sedentary for the first time in my life.

I have had chronic knee and neck pain for years and have strong prescription medication to keep this under control. I therefore knew that incorporating exercise was going to be tricky for me. However, I decided to try both Tabata and Yoga as they were recommended to accompany the 12 week programme. I had decided at the start that I would go into this with an open mind and would be willing to try anything in order to transform my health and wellbeing.

Due to my knee pain I knew that Tabata may cause an issue for me. I therefore started off slowly and spent time discovering which exercises I could do without causing myself any pain. I found that I really enjoyed the structure of the work outs; the fact you only have to be active for 20 seconds before you rest is great – although exhausting! I still have to be cautious about what exercises I can do, and I cannot do everything to the same ability as others, but I really enjoy what I am able to do and I love the feeling of energy that it gives me.

I found that Yoga was perfect for me; the combination of stretching and breathing techniques was incredibly relaxing and also very therapeutic. I found that it really helped to control my aches and pains. Being able to keep this under control meant I felt comfortable to reduce the medication that I was taking as I no longer needed such large amounts to numb the pain.

I believe that following a Paleo lifestyle helped significantly with being able to reduce the medication, and incorporating an exercise regime was an important part of that. As I progressed through the weeks, I found that my neck pain had disappeared completely. I was shocked. My knees are still painful as I have small kneecaps that don't track properly in the joint but the pain is much more bearable and manageable.

I feel so much better as a result of incorporating exercise into my routine. I have more energy, I feel awake and full of life and it makes me feel better about myself. I have also found that it is a good stress reliever! It has really assisted with my weight loss and I can visibly see that I am more toned and have a better posture than I did to start with. I would recommend it to everyone – even if you think you can't do it, or have been inactive for a while, please give it a try!"

SECTION 5

Enjoy Real Food

Depending on what currently graces your dinner table, your reaction to the thought of preparing food from scratch every day could range from excitement to sheer terror. Many people under the age of forty, and even quite a few people over, were simply not taught to cook or how to manage a household. Once upon a time home economics was a vital part of learning and those that missed it at school learnt about food at the family kitchen table.

Cooking should not be difficult or done under duress. Real food is born of good simple ingredients and is as much a matter of intuition as technical skill. A little understanding and an interested mind go a long way; learn about how each ingredient works, approach the task with calm confidence, and you will never go far wrong.

Cooking is about taking great raw ingredients and bringing out the best in them. Find a good greengrocer, a butcher with integrity, a decent fishmonger and a sharp knife. From there begins great food. Paleo food is no different.

Paleo food has to be one of the most misunderstood ways of eating. How many of these questions can you identify with?

- Isn't Paleo food really restrictive? I want to enjoy my food
- Won't all that meat and fresh produce be really expensive?
- How can cutting out several major food groups be healthy?
- Why would I want to eat like a caveman?
- Won't cooking take up all my time? I have very little time as it is?
- What about feeding the rest of the family?

You most likely have other questions such as "how can I eat fat and lose weight?" and these will be addressed further down the line. For now we will focus on looking in more detail at the issues raised above.

Isn't Paleo food really restrictive? I want to enjoy my food

Paleo offers a vibrant and varied blend of 'clean' ingredients free of the toxins known to damage human health. Visually stunning and full of fresh vital flavours, a Paleo meal of meat or fish and plenty of fresh vegetables will neither weigh you down nor send you to sleep. If by variety you mean an endless parade of starches and sugars in the form of grains, breakfast cereals, bread products, and cakes or biscuits, then yes we can see why you may feel that way. Once you make the switch to a Paleo diet you will really understand how these starchy sugary foods actually offer little variety at all when really all they are variations on a theme.

Won't all that meat and fresh produce be really expensive?

Shopping for food is all about choosing the best ingredients that you can find within the budget available. There are certainly ethical considerations and matters of health to address that we shall look at more closely in Section 6. The important thing to remember is that swapping your processed food for fresh produce, whatever its pedigree or provenance, is the single best thing you can do for your health.

How can cutting out several major food groups be healthy?

The concept of food groups is an outdated one; foods, in relation to the human body, translate into macronutrients and micronutrients. All foods are made up of a variety of these components and some are richer sources than others. *Introduction to Paleo* looked at how nutrients work to fuel the human body and we will revisit the subject in Section 8 where we look at choosing nutrient dense foods.

Why would I want to eat like a caveman?

That is actually a perfectly valid question that really underlines some of the confusion that surrounds the subject of the Paleo diet. The Paleo movement was founded upon the basis of evolutionary science and medicine; research that now underpins much of the current thinking in modern nutritional science and other health related disciplines.

The entire Paleo principle is to choose foods that are genetically right for you as an individual; not to subscribe to some rigid dogma. Yes, many Paleo followers strictly adhere to a framework that questions what our Palaeolithic ancestors would do in certain situations and there are those at the other extreme that miss the point entirely and continue to eat a vastly unhealthy diet composed of over processed foods made with Paleo friendly ingredients. But what Paleo is really telling you is this...

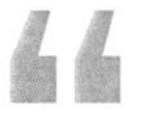

Paleo is not really about living like a caveman. It is about eating natural foods that are not irritable to the human form and realising that the blame for most modern diseases can be laid at the door of industrial agriculture and food processing.

Won't cooking take up all my time? I have very little time as it is?

Cooking need not be an "either or" scenario; if we are to regain our health and that of our planet then we need to loosen the grip of the food industry, and the only way to do that is with a return to cooking. Preparing food, especially when well-planned and provided for, can be an enjoyable event at the end of the day or provide pleasant respite from the monotony of the working week.

Paleo recipes include lots of vegetables, which are some of the quickest and easiest foods to cook that you will find. Meat is equally quick and simple to prepare; even when it needs longer it is often just a case of closing the oven door. Without the ravenous hunger and light headed impatience of a starch fuelled diet, you can enjoy taking a little time in the kitchen rather than rushing about trying to get food on the table as quick as possible. Home should be your haven and the kitchen at the heart of it; pottering about over a warm stove whilst rain lashes against the window can hardly be called hardship now can it? Leave your stress and troubles at the kitchen door and sink into something creative and nurturing instead; it is a valuable lesson that we all could learn.

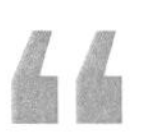

Make your kitchen your haven; somewhere to escape the stresses of the world and find the calm nurturing space within. Food is healing in more ways than one.

What about feeding the rest of the family?

If you are responsible for feeding others, your transition to Paleo can only do them good. Even if they do not join you, as the provider of food in the household your habits will have an impact. Money is more likely to be spent on fresh ingredients rather than junk and you may realise just how much your unhealthy habits have affected everyone else. It is most likely that everybody's health will improve as a result of your efforts.

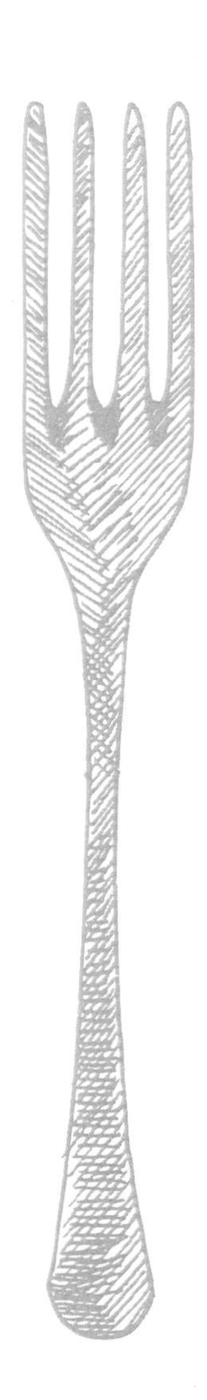

Case Study

"I didn't find the transition to cooking Paleo meals too difficult as I have always been a capable cook. I did find cooking for myself a problem though. For years I had spent money on the foods that the family preferred and not really thought about myself. I always made sure that there were plenty of chocolates and biscuits for everyone to enjoy as they felt the urge. Only now do I realise how true the phrase "killing with kindness" actually is; killing with cupboard love might be more apt.

Once I realised just how unhealthy abdominal fat actually is and stopped denying the poor health of myself and my family, I was utterly horrified; knocked down by guilt. My husband can be tricky to feed; as a colon cancer survivor with severe intestinal damage he has trouble with fibrous foods. But by increasing the vegetables that he can tolerate and removing most sugar and starches from his diet he has lost a lot of weight and has more colour in his cheeks; not to mention a rare feeling of energy. My son's diet has improved in small ways too; he has lost most of his big belly and tries harder with his food.

I would urge anyone to make these changes; it often isn't until you look at things from a new vantage point that you really see things clearly. Once you have a family it is really hard to prioritise your own needs but realising that everyone is better for it can be a huge revelation.

Cost was a big issue for me as we live on a pretty low income. Some weeks are better than others, but even on the really tight weeks I would never stray back to cheap carbs or pulses. My appetite has decreased and I am now satisfied with just enough. I have found that eliminating toxins has made me much more in tune with my body and its needs. Therefore, if my nutrient levels start to drop I can feel it and know that on my next shop I will need a really big boost of fruit and vegetables. I have found that this does not have to be expensive and a small amount goes a long way and I can make several meals out of one dish which is perfect.

Processed food is not cheap. I found that by cutting out all the packets of chocolate, cereal, and bread that ends up in the bin, there was more than enough to buy fresh produce. I looked into sourcing seasonal produce and found that this was a great way to try new things at a really good price. Contrary to popular belief about the Paleo diet, I was not eating loads of meat and in fact I was eating far more vegetables. This was reflected in the glow of my skin and the massively increased energy levels I was experiencing.

Once I past the early days where my hunger was at its peak, I started to buy smaller amounts of high quality meat rather than vast amounts of the industrially farmed stuff; I found that the cost really does level itself out. My entire outlook on food has changed; even treats have become something like an addition of cheese to a meal. I honestly wouldn't thank you for a custard slice; at one time I would have wrestled you to the ground for it."

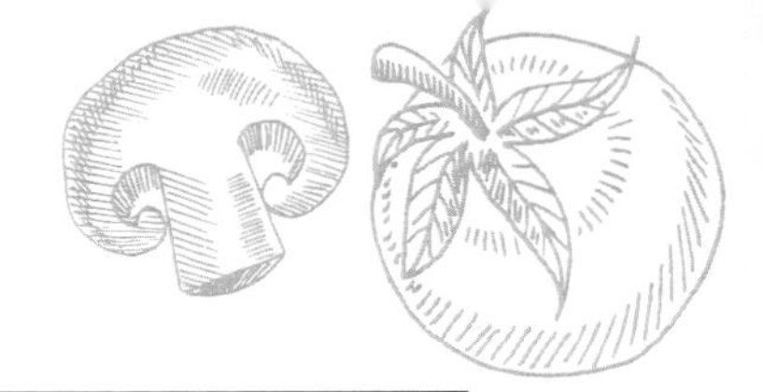

SECTION 6

Build a Better Future

The drive towards local and organic foods gains momentum every day. What once used to be the province of rich folk and hippies has finally become a concern that is felt at virtually every level of society. The connections between food and health are becoming blatantly clear but they cannot truly be separated from issues of sustainability and the environment. The subject of food is a vast and complex one and when studied closely it becomes blindingly obvious that each of its parts interconnect.

Organic food was once considered to be at the top of tree in terms of sustainability and nutritional content, but the diluting of the principles by the major supermarkets led to a new food hero; local food. The very concept of organic, taking at its truest meaning, indicates food which is grown without toxic additions but that also embraces the very ethos of local food too. Distorted out of all recognition from its essential meaning, the term organic could encompass all manner of things. One thing you are guaranteed of course is that the food is pesticide free; which certainly isn't without merit.

So how do you untangle the facts and know which foods will bring the greatest benefit in terms of nutrition, value for money and environmental load?

Local food may be better than organic

Local food is fresh and seasonal. Many farmers, especially in the UK, will farm with integrity using traditional methods and generations of expertise. These farmers may not be able to afford costly organic certification but grow crops that are only one degree off the mark. With local food, especially when you buy at a farmers market, farm shop, or box scheme, the produce will be relatively freshly picked and therefore nutrient value and flavour will be at its peak. Local seasonal food will not be that expensive, especially if you shop around for a trusted source.

Organic food may have flown halfway across the world

Although guaranteed to have organic certification and therefore a higher degree of certainty that you won't encounter unwanted chemicals in your food, a lot of organic produce will be off season and flown thousands of miles to reach your plate. Not only does produce such as this lose much of its nutrient value with its long storage time after harvest, but it clocks up a fair few food miles too.

Organic is not necessarily more nutrient dense

Studies cannot agree on whether a nutrient-rich soil grows nutrient-rich produce; regardless of nutrient loss after harvest. It does offer a guarantee against pesticides, additives and antibiotics which is more valuable in some produce than others, but nutrient content is variable. Organic standards have slipped somewhat since their conception and Big Food got hold of it as a marketing strategy and empty goodwill gesture; produce need only meet minimal standards to pass legislation.

Just how far away is local?

In the UK practically anything grown in this country can be considered local due to the fact that we are a relatively small country. We are lucky enough therefore to be able to count locality in food metres and fresh local produce from a reputable source means exactly that.

How do I know what is in season?

If you buy local produce, then whatever is available is going to be seasonal. Off-season food will have been flown across the world and often (but not always) quite obviously something that won't grow in our climate. In Summer, foods from warmer climes come from Europe and are shipped by rail or sea; this makes them a fairly viable choice to add a bit of sunny variety. Seasonal food is good value and often actually cheap; it also adds variety throughout the year.

Buying meat

Meat is an important subject to the Paleo cook and most likely will be the portion of your food bill that you pay particular attention to. Look to local food as your first port of call. Buying at the farm gate, shop or market pretty much means that your local meat has been grass fed; at least for a good proportion of the animal's life. This meat will have a better flavour and a greater density of beneficial nutrients; a grain fed animal will be flabbier and far more likely to have been intensively farmed and be full of antibiotics and hormones. Once you have spent some time reviewing the options you will be able to determine what is best for you.

Some tips for buying meat

Buy grass fed local meat if you can find it and can afford it.

Choose organic supermarket meat above non-organic.

Do not be afraid to buy conventional meat if it is all you can afford; trim off surplus fat though as it can be toxic.

Lamb is a good choice, whatever the source; it is virtually impossible to intensively farm lamb.

Buy meat in bulk. freezing half a lamb is economical; or share a side of beef between a few of you.

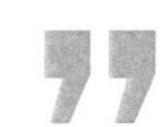

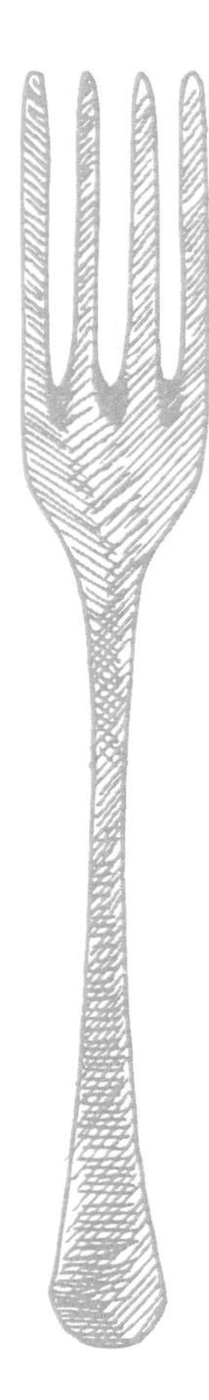

Case Study

"I was really intrigued about sourcing local products and started to take a keen interest in the food that was around me. I became much more aware of adverts for farmers markets and delivery box schemes and looked into all of them to see what they had to offer. I was impressed by how much choice there was and how good the products were, plus I really liked the idea that the food had been grown or reared locally and I therefore knew where it had come from.

I had started to really feel the benefits of cooking good food from scratch and it made me much more aware that what you put into your body will affect how you feel, look and behave. I found this concept really fascinating.

I found a local farmer who had just opened up part of their farm as a tea room and farm shop and thought I would give it a go. I found that the meat was of a fantastic quality and was cheaper than I was paying in the supermarket. Getting to know the owners meant that they would recommend new things to me and also provided me with lots of cheaper cuts when my budget needed this. It is amazing how good a cheap cut of meat can taste when slow cooked in a casserole with a few vegetables.

My recommendation is to simply be aware of what there is around you. We are all programmed to go to the supermarket as this is the easier option. I am not saying it is a bad option, I do the same all the time, I just think it is a shame if you do not get the chance to explore what else is on offer in your local community."

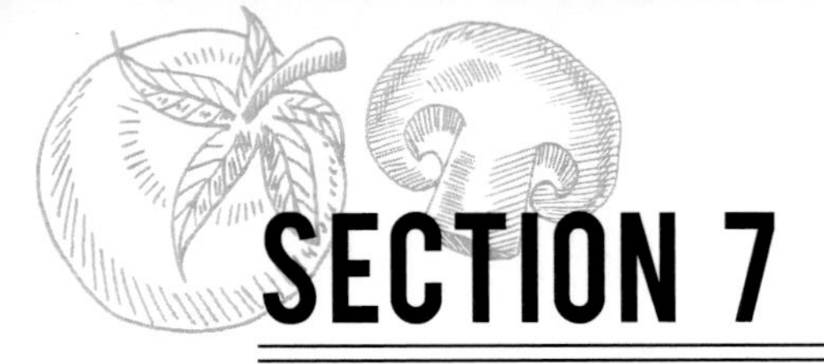

SECTION 7

Avoid Toxins

A fundamental principle of the Paleo diet and the reason why it works so well for weight loss and improved health is that it aims to eliminate all sources of toxins from the diet. There are various sources of potential toxins in our diet; some from an imbalance of macronutrients, some from additives in processed food, and even those in foods considered by many to be perfectly healthy.

Toxins in food cause havoc within the body but many people will not even realise that their health is under attack. Being overweight is not particularly pleasant, and most of us understand that it causes us to be unfit and at risk of certain diseases, but how many of us really understand the extent of the actual and potential damage caused by active fat tissue.

Introduction to Paleo looked in detail at the various metabolic processes behind our food regulation and at the chemical changes that occur in the metabolically challenged system. As we found out, if you are overweight, obese, or simply carrying a little excess abdominal fat, then it is likely that you ARE suffering from a biochemical imbalance.

The foods of the Paleo diet are designed to keep the toxic load as light as possible by eliminating those foods that are shown to be harmful. We set out in this section information about the foods which are toxic and show the effects that consumption of these can have on the body.

Wheat

Out of all the foods that create havoc within the body, wheat is one of the worst. Modern wheat is a long way genetically from ancient wheat (for ancient read before 50 years ago – that's how quickly our food supply has deteriorated) and contains many different proteins which have to be processed into our system. Once broken down within our system particles of these proteins have been shown to cause serious damage to the body. Modern wheat also has far fewer nutrients than its forefathers. Avoid it; always.

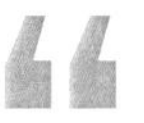

Modern wheat contains highly inflammatory proteins that cross the gut membrane.

Modern wheat contains highly addictive substances that increase appetite.

Modern wheat plays havoc with insulin levels and is at the root of hormonal imbalances.

Sugar

Another key toxin, right up there with wheat and even part of the same story, sugar comes in many forms. Dietary sugar and starch are classified together as carbohydrates and to the human body they are more or less ALL THE SAME. We will deal with the acceptable face of dietary carbohydrate in Section 8, but for now we will concentrate on the downside. *Introduction to Paleo* looked at insulin and its role within metabolism, and also at the repercussions of insulin resistance.

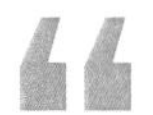

Some facts about sugar

Most forms of sugar come with very little nutrient value.

Sugar causes the insulin surges that create insulin resistance and hormonal imbalance.

Excess sugar is stored as fat.

Sugar activates reward systems that lead to overeating in search of a pleasure response; in other words, feeding an addiction.

Minimising sugar intake to reverse insulin resistance will ensure that your hunger signals are functioning efficiently.

Sugar does not activate the fullness signal to the brain.

Sugar is a source of excess calories that provide little nutrient value and takes the place of other nutrient dense foods.

Regaining control of your biochemical impulses is the key to sustainable weight loss. The only way to do this is to restrict carbohydrate intake to paleo approved sources.

Sugar and starch are one and the same.

Grains

This includes all grains other than wheat. Not all grains are gluten free, so treat those with the same caution as you would wheat. All grains (including wheat) contain certain irritants and anti-nutrients; as well as a predominantly carbohydrate nutrient profile and all of its associated issues. This can cause damage and inflammation to the lining of the gut.

A damaged gut does not always present obvious symptoms and is a major contributor to ill health. Damage to the gut lining means unwanted particles can pass through into the bloodstream and also tampers with nutrient intake. The balance of good bacteria to bad will fall in favour of bad.

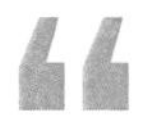

Some facts about grains

Lectins found in grains are damaging to the gut lining and cause inflammatory issues as well as bacterial imbalances.

Phytic acid is also present in grains and humans lack the ability to digest it. Phytic acid binds to certain essential minerals and carries them out of the body.

Legumes

As well as a source of dietary carbohydrate, legumes also contain lectins and phytic acid (as above) and are also a cause of irritation to the gut. Legumes also contain saponins (yes, just like soap) that are found in all plant foods but are abundant and harmful in some more than others. Such as legumes.

Saponins in legumes create holes in the cells of the gut lining and increase permeability. They also cross the gut barrier and initiate an inflammatory response.

Soy and Peanuts

These are the assassins of the legume world, despite soya now being one of the most commonplace dairy substitutions of the world. Both soy and peanuts (which is not actually a nut but a legume) make common appearances on the ingredients lists of manufactured foods and peanut oil is widely used as cheap processed oil.

Peanuts can be harbouring growth of aflatoxins. A group of mycotoxins, aflatoxins are a known carcinogenic. As well as a possible contamination of peanuts, they are also known to be present on corn, especially tortillas and other masa products.

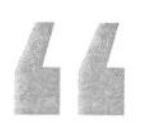

Some facts about soy

Modern soy is one of the main crops of monoculture, pesticides and the gm debate. Traditional soy was a locally grown part of a traditional diet that was always fermented for consumption.

Soy contains phytoestrogens; a group of substances of which some are thought beneficial yet others considered harmful.

Phytoestrogens in soy are known hormone disrupters; as there can be no agreement about the longterm effects they are best just avoided.

Dairy

We find it only prudent to mention the potential issues with dairy produce, although the jury is out even within the Paleo community. The recommended approach is to eliminate to begin with and reintroduce it gradually to identify any intolerance; a subject we return to in Section 15.

Raw dairy is different from processed conventional dairy products. It comes from grass fed animals, not those on grain, so is higher in nutrients and beneficial substances. Raw dairy contains lactase, the enzyme needed to process the sugars in milk, whilst pasteurisation kills it off.

An alternative to milk that is Paleo friendly is almond milk. This can be used as a substitute for milk. We have used almond milk as an ingredient in our Paleo friendly smoothie recipes which can be found in the recipe section.

Some facts about milk

Milk contains potentially allergenic substances, the most well known of which is casein. If you react to gluten then it is also likely that you will react to casein.

Lactose is the sugar in milk. Intolerance to lactose comes in two forms and you can react to one or the other; or both.

The body needs lactase to digest milk sugars but most of us do not produce this enzyme. Raw milk contains lactase.

If gut health is out of balance and you have bacterial overgrowth, then these unwanted bacteria ferment lactose; A major cause of wind and bloating.

What's the problem with processed food?

You would be far closer to the mark if you asked the question "what isn't the problem with processed food?" The reach of the industrial food industry is far and wide, with implications for agriculture, environmental health, human health, and food policy, to name but a few. In short, there is barely a part of our world that is not affected by the power of Big Food.

One of the major issues with processed food, whatever part of the market sector it comes from, is that it requires a growing list of additives to make it shelf stable. All of the toxins mentioned previously find their way into food in the form as fillers, enhancers, flavourings and the like; they may not even come by names you recognise. Barely a factory in the world does not process wheat, so many foods are gluten contaminated by default.

Then there are the other additives; all of the other forms of chemical enhancements that comes with food from a packet. Many are benign, with processing and labelling far stricter than before, but they certainly could not be viewed as necessary. These foods have no place in the real food kitchen, although the odd safe shortcut here and there is just part of surviving the modern world; most of these foods are not food at all but simply poor imitations of the real thing.

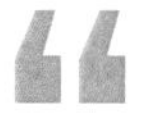

If it needs a label you are already a step removed from real food.

Read labels with care; the longer the list of ingredients, especially those that you cant pronounce, the less wise a purchase it becomes.

Don't be fooled by seemingly unprocessed products. Conventional meat, for instance, comes from intensively farmed animals that are fed highly processed feed that affects content and quality.

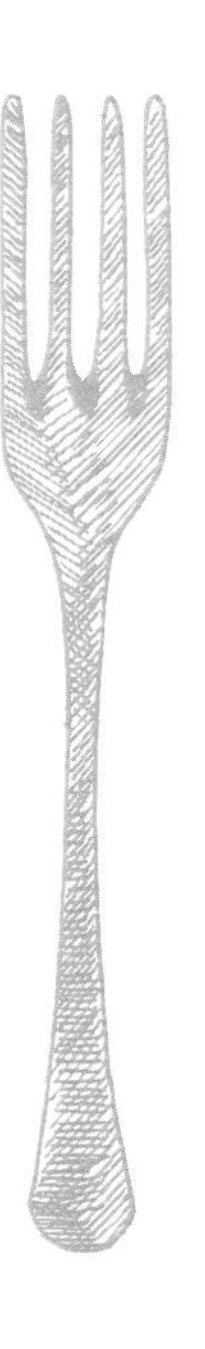

Case Study

"Never before have I given up certain foods when trying to lose weight. Even when trying with mainstream slimming groups there has always been the option, encouragement even, to have those few slices of bread or a low-calorie chocolate bar.

In my first case study entry I went through the side effects that I experienced when I gave up wheat, sugar and dairy. It was not pleasant but once it is done, then it is done and you feel so much better for it. I then found that I had no more cravings because I had cut them out completely. That has been a revelation to me and something which took me a while to get my head around! As a lifelong carb lover I would never have thought that my cravings would disappear completely – I just didn't think it was possible. But then I had never truly looked into why my body was craving those foods to begin with. Until you have gone through the process of re-setting your system you cannot image how good you will feel on the other side."

SECTION 8

Choose Nutrient Dense Foods

Although a balanced Paleo diet will provide you with the nutrients that you need, and counting calories or nutrient content is not necessary, an understanding of human nutrition is essential to get the most from your diet and to be able to fine tune your personal requirements.

The components of food that nourish your body can be broken down into two categories; macronutrients and micronutrients. The macronutrients are fat, protein and carbohydrate. Micronutrients are everything else; vitamins, minerals, phytochemicals and supporting nutrients. Macronutrients tend to be thought of as essential building blocks, although they also provide fuel for energy. Micronutrients provide the fine tuning that prevents eventual breakdown. A diet can contain enough macronutrients to keep you from passing out but that doesn't necessarily mean you are getting the nutrition that you need. An optimal balance that suits you alone is required for a healthy body and mind.

It is ingrained upon us that the balance of our diet needs to be composed of food groups and that to be healthy this means eating certain amounts of particular groups. But foods are rarely a pure form of one macronutrient and ratios vary from group to group and food to food; it is these ratios that are important. We have set out below details of the macronutrients along with the common vitamins and minerals that make up the micronutrients that you need for a healthy diet. The list of micronutrients is complex so we have tried to keep it focused on the main players that you may want to consider and learn more about.

Macronutrients

Carbohydrates

Wheat and grains, although containing a little protein, are predominantly carbohydrate. Legumes, in the form of beans and pulses, are considered a protein food but are also predominantly carbohydrate. When you fill your plate with these foods you are basically taking up the space that could be used far more efficiently by fats, proteins and micronutrients. It is micronutrients, of which vegetables are the richest source, that make the difference between vital health and just getting by. Fats and proteins provide essential nutrients but if you omit rich micronutrient sources from your diet you will feel the consequences.

Contrary to popular opinion, Paleo is not a low-carb diet although some people do thrive on such. Sources of carbohydrate such as grains and legumes come with irritant toxins and little else but sugar that goes straight to your abdominal fat stores. Vegetables, on the other hand, contain much of the carbohydrate that your body needs but with a good balance of fibre and micronutrients too; they are what is known as nutrient dense. Certain vegetables, and most fruit, are rich sources of carbohydrate that provide more sugars than others but can be eaten without the irritating effects of grains and legumes. Known as safe starches, many find that they do better with more in their diet and some with less; sweet potatoes, squashes and root vegetables are all rich sources of safe carbohydrate.

There are two sides to the carbohydrate story and optimal intake differs widely between individuals.

Carbohydrate intake should be kept within the realm of safe starches and vegetable/fruit sources. Fruit should be kept to a minimum for weight loss and lower sugar sources such as berries are optimal.

Too low a carbohydrate intake may lead to fatigue and trouble sleeping. Conversely, too high an intake may result in cravings and excess fat storage.

Fibre

Part of the carbohydrate question is that of fibre. Conventional dietary wisdom ties whole-grains in with fibre so along with the belief that we should get the bulk of our calories from carbohydrates comes the idea we need plenty of bran type fibre too.

Fibre comes from plant foods and is essentially indigestible carbohydrate. There are two varieties of dietary fibre; soluble and insoluble. Soluble fibre reacts with water and forms a gel that coats the intestines and slows down the passage of food. Insoluble fibre swells when it comes into contact with water and speeds up the passage of food.

Soluble fibre is also beneficial to the gut flora by acting as a source of food for the bacteria. It increases production of butyrate in the colon. Also found in butter, butyrate is a short chain fatty acid that aids appetite control and metabolism. An important mechanism in gut healing and digestive health, butyrate provides an energy source for the cells of the colon and is also shown to aid muscular function of the bowel.

Both types of fibre are important to digestive health. Fruits and vegetables are excellent sources of dietary fibre and apples in particular are a prime source of soluble fibre. Although it cannot be denied that grains are a good source of fibre, the Paleo diet does not recommend them for reasons already outlined in previous debate.

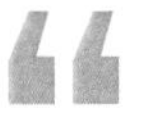

Sufficient dietary fibre can be obtained from a diet rich in fruits and vegetables

Protein

Protein is absolutely vital to the human body and a function is rarely performed without it. A massive subject, protein metabolism is behind something as simple as the cells of your skin right up to the complexities of gene expression; by which your genetic code instructs your body how to function.

All protein is composed of smaller units called amino acids. Joined together by simple chemical bonds, the amino acids form structures that range from simple chains to large complex folding structures; all of which are proteins. There are 20 known amino acids; nine are essential, five can be manufactured within the body, and six become essential under certain conditions such as growth and illness. The nine that are essential must be part of the diet and they are required for manufacture of the others within the body.

The protein molecules in food are broken down by digestion into their component amino acids. Once metabolised within the body they are then built back up again in to the proteins required by the human body. Without all of the amino acids present, the body cannot make the correct proteins.

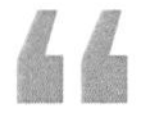

All nine essential amino acids must be available to the body in order to function optimally.

Animal sources of protein are complete and provide all nine of the essential amino acids. To intake all nine from plant sources you would need to eat an array of legumes and grains. The proteins in animal foods are not only complete but are more readily available for use in the human body; meaning that they are more easily and effectively absorbed.

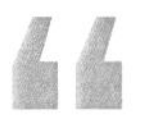

Animal sources of protein provide all of your essential amino acids in a readily available state.

Introduction to Paleo looked at the role of protein in appetite control; a process largely controlled by hormonal and biochemical function. All of these regulatory molecules are made from amino acids (as well as fat) so an adequate supply of complete protein is essential.

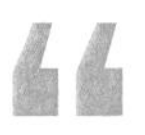

Adequate protein in the diet ensures a plentiful supply of glucagon that results in decreased appetite and effective fat burning.

Protein consumption also triggers cck - a hormone that makes you feel fuller for longer.

As we have seen, adequate protein is essential for optimal function but care must be taken not to overdo it. The recommended Paleo intake of protein is between 10 to 20 percent of your overall food intake; a figure that differs for every individual. In the face of fat-phobia there can be a tendency to consume large amounts of lean protein but this can inadvertently bulk up percentage protein intake. Fat helps the body to process protein so eating fat with protein is essential.

Fat

We have learnt that it is important to keep carbohydrate intake to your optimal minimum and also to regulate protein intake. That leaves us with one thing; fat. Minimal consumption of fat is one of the most ingrained dietary assumptions on the planet and we have already considered the huge failure of the conventional high-carb/low-fat diet in *Introduction to Paleo*. When you consider that protein intake needs to remain at a constant level then the balance has to swing the other way. Before you finish reading this section, you need to have banished your fat-phobia forever as fat will now make up over 50 percent of your diet. Can you really eat fat and lose weight? Yes you can and it is good for you.

What follows is an overview of dietary fats and how they function within the body. Fats may be one of the most misunderstood components of our diet so gaining a deeper understanding can help you to appreciate how important they are in your diet and that dietary fat does not have to equal body fat. Even since the original Paleo framework the thinking on saturated fats has changed and current views now suggest that they are not the bad guy.

What is fat?

Generally speaking, at room temperature, fats are solid and oils are liquid. Trans-fats are oils that have been chemically altered to behave like fats; a good enough reason to stay well away. Grouped together under the term lipids, all of these structures are made up of fatty acids; single units composed of hydrogen, oxygen and carbon. Fatty acids have short, medium or long 'tails' composed of carbon and hydrogen and it is the hydrogen component that determines the type of fat.

Types of fats

When you hear about particular fats and oils, you will come across terms such as mono-unsaturated (MUFA), poly-unsaturated (PUFA), and saturated (SFA). In actual fact what these terms describe are the fatty acids, not the fats themselves.

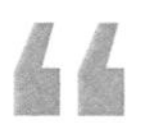 *All fats and oils are made up of a range of fatty acids.* 

Saturated fats (SFA) are usually animal fats, but there are exceptions such as palm oil and coconut oil. Solid at room temperature, saturated fats are composed largely of saturated fatty acids but also contain varying amounts of MUFA and PUFA. Saturated fatty acids have tails that are completely saturated with hydrogen (hence the name); a fact that makes them rigid and also the most stable. We will look at what this stability means for your health shortly.

Mono-unsaturated fatty acids (MUFA) have tails that lack one hydrogen atom and contain a carbon-carbon double bond instead. This effectively creates a space in the tail, making it more fluid than a rigid SFA, and more easily oxidised or degraded. Fats and oils with a large concentration of MUFA are considered healthy oils but are best served as cold dressings or used only in low temperature cooking. Hazelnut and extra virgin olive oil are examples of fats with a large proportion of MUFA. In contrast, fats and oils with a higher ratio of PUFA, such as avocado oil should only be used cold as a dressing or for dipping.

Poly-unsaturated fatty acids (PUFA) can have any number of missing hydrogen atoms, making them the most fluid and the least stable of all. Omega 6 (O6) and Omega 3 (O3) are both PUFA and are essential for optimal heath in a ratio of roughly (O6:O3)1:1 but no more than 4:1. Omega 6 is inflammatory whilst Omega 3 is anti-inflammatory; when you consider that the average ratio in the modern diet is as much as 40:1, it makes sense that most modern diseases are inflammatory conditions. Cheap oils such as sunflower, vegetable and corn oil are not only all highly processed but contain massive ratios of Omega 6; sunflower oil in particular has 130 times more Omega 6 than Omega 3 and is in practically all processed foods as well as the modern cooking oil of choice.

What does cooking temperature have to do with it?

Fats without a full complement of hydrogen bonds are far more susceptible to damage and oxidisation; the processes that make them rancid. Oxidisation in molecules occurs when they are exposed to heat, light and air so incorrect storage or cooking at high temperatures of unstable oils with a large concentration of PUFA essentially means that you are ingesting harmful substances as well as a high concentration of inflammatory Omega 6.

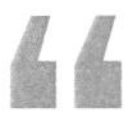

To minimise the harmful effects of inflammation choose solid saturated fats (such as cocunut oil or animal fats) for cooking and use healthy oils high in mono-unsaturated fats (such as extra virgin olive oil) for eating cold, such as on salads.

Your body needs poly-unsaturated fats but choose Omega 3 rich sources (such as walnut oil or flaxseed oil or from sources such as oily fish) and keep Omega 6 to a minimum.

But won't saturated fats give me heart disease?

The links between saturated fat intake and heart disease are gradually being refuted one by one and there is no evidence that shows a link between the two. Studies that informed the past fifty years of nutritional thinking have been exposed as inaccurate and even flawed, and the mainstream media can now often be found reporting on the non-existent link between saturated fat and heart disease.

And what about cholesterol?

Cholesterol is another complex subject and if there is one thing to grasp when it comes to biological processes, and hence that of nutrition, it is that nothing works in isolation and is part of a huge complex system of interactive processes. That said, when you hear about cholesterol, you are hearing about two different things. The first is dietary cholesterol and the second is serum cholesterol (a measure of lipoproteins in the blood).

Recent reports show that dietary cholesterol is not responsible for measures of cholesterol in the blood. The categories of lipoproteins in the blood are LDL (low-density lipoprotein) and HDL (high-density lipoproteins). HDL are commonly known as good cholesterol whist LDL are known as bad; it is however small particle LDL that causes problems, not all LDL. What this essentially means is that dietary cholesterol such as that found in eggs is not connected to the levels measured in the blood.

Why fats are essential for health

As well as being the preferred energy source for the body, fats are essential components of cell membranes and vital molecules. Without healthy membranes cells simply cannot support the functions necessary to life, including communication of regulating hormones; which as we have seen are vital to weight control and optimal health.

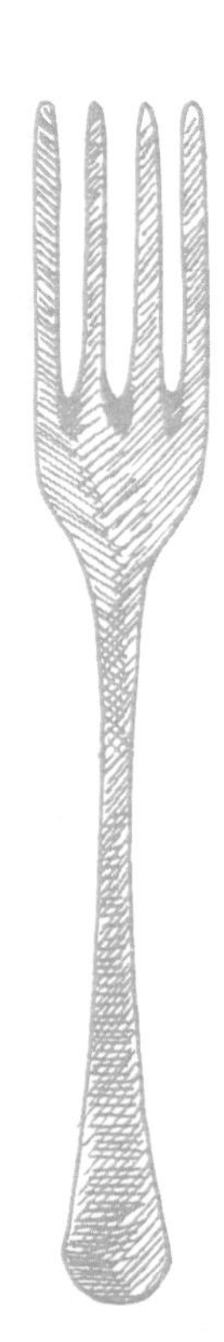

Case Study

"Like many I had to readdress my mind set on fat and the role it had to play in my diet. I had always been indoctrinated to believe that a low fat diet was the only way to lose weight and that a high fat diet ultimately had to equal being fat and unhealthy.

I actually found, on the whole, I welcomed this concept with open arms. I had always found it really restrictive and unrealistic to cook with the 1 tbsp of oil that most diets allow you to have for the day so this actually made more sense to me from a cooking perspective.

I soon realised that all the fats I was eating were incredibly good for me and vital to the functioning of my body. The image portrayed of a high fat diet is that of eating chocolate bars and crisps and processed fatty meats. This was a world away from the fats that I was consuming such as avocado, nuts and coconut milk. These ingredients were not harming me but helping me to address the nutrient deficiencies I had gained over the years. If you take one thing from Paleo it needs to be that fats are good for you. My advice? Embrace it and get cooking!"

Micronutrients

What are vitamins?

Vitamins are nutrient molecules that occur naturally in the living organisms that we eat as food. They are required for chemical processes within the body to function. If the vitamins are lacking then the system cannot function effectively; it is likely that you may not even notice a slight deficiency but there is a broad chasm between disease and wellness. The ultimate goal may be to be disease free but it also makes sense to strive for optimal wellness; dragging around the middle ground is the default for setting for so many of us.

The benefits of optimal vitamin intake, in balance with the other micronutrients we look at later, are felt immediately; skin starts to glow, unknown vitality asserts itself, and quite simply you will feel alive.

Which vitamins are essential?

There are 13 vitamins, divided into two groups; fat soluble and water soluble. The fat soluble vitamins (A, D, E, and K) are stored in fat cells within the body and are therefore readily available. The water soluble vitamins (C, B, biotin and folic acid) are not stored as such and excess amounts are excreted via the urine; these vitamins, need topping up regularly to avoid deficiency.

Vitamin A

Vitamin A plays a vital role in visual function, growth and development (including healthy skin), hormonal function, nervous function and cellular growth.

Vitamin A that can be used by the body is present in liver but vegetable sources contain carotenes that can be converted.

Paleo sources of vitamin A and carotenes are liver, dark green leafy vegetables, squash, carrots and sweet potatoes.

Vitamin D

The body can produce vitamin D by the action of sunlight on the skin. It stimulates the absorption of calcium and therefore plays a vital role in bone health.

Paleo sources of vitamin D are cod liver oil, oily fish and egg yolks. There are vegetable sources but animal sources are preferable.

Vitamin E

An anti-oxidant, vitamin E protects against cell membrane damage and is much lauded by conventional thinking as a must have supplement. The interesting thing here is that the need for vitamin E increases with consumption of PUFA; essentially to protect against the inflammatory damage of Omega 6. So whilst vitamin E provides excellent anti-oxidant protection, you can lower the need for that protection by getting the Omega 6 and Omega 3 ratios in balance.
Paleo sources of vitamin E are avocado, asparagus, spinach and tomato.

Vitamin K

The often forgotten nutrient, vitamin K comes in three forms. K1 comes from plant sources, K2 is produced by our gut bacteria, and K3 is synthetic. All three play a role in blood clotting, but K1 is also important for bone health and osteoporosis prevention.

Paleo sources of vitamin K1 are kale, broccoli, spinach and green tea.

Vitamin B1

Essential for energy production, carbohydrate metabolism and nerve cell function, a deficiency of vitamin B1 manifests as fatigue, depression, constipation and numbness in the extremities.

Paleo sources of vitamin B1 are nuts and seeds, pine nuts, brazil nuts and sunflower seeds in particular.

Vitamin B2

Important in the production of energy, a deficiency of vitamin B2 shows as cracked lips and a swollen tongue. Visual disturbances such as light sensitivity are also common.

Paleo sources of vitamin B2 are offal, mushrooms, almonds, green leafy vegetables and herbs.

Vitamin B3

Essential for energy production and manufacture of hormones, vitamin B3 can be made in the body by the amino acid tryptophan.

Paleo sources of vitamin B3 are offal, eggs, fish, nuts and seeds.

Vitamin B5

Vitamin B5 plays a vital role in energy production and metabolism as well as the manufacture of hormones and red blood cells. Also crucial to optimal adrenal function, vitamin B5 plays a role in the stress response.

Paleo sources of vitamin B5 are offal, meat, fish and poultry. Also present in nuts as well as broccoli and cauliflower.

Vitamin B6

Vital in the formation of proteins, hormonal balance, immune and nervous function and many conditions such as asthma can respond well to supplementation. Modern living plays host to many vitamin B6 antagonists that block the uptake or function of vitamin B6; amongst these are certain food additives and prescription medication.

Paleo sources of vitamin B6 are seeds, nuts, bananas, avocados, green leafy vegetables, peppers, sweet potato and cauliflower.

Folic acid

In conjunction with vitamin B12, folic acid provides critical support for cell division. The most common vitamin deficiency in the world, inadequate amounts of folic acid lead to poor growth, diarrhoea and anaemia.

Paleo sources of folic acids are offal, asparagus, walnuts, spinach, kale and broccoli.

Vitamin B12

Only small amounts of vitamin B12 are required but deficiency can leads to depression and mental confusion.

Paleo sources of vitamin B12 are liver, kidney, fish, eggs and meat.

Biotin

An essential nutrient for optimal metabolism of fat and protein, biotin is manufactured in the intestines from the bacteria of the gut.

Paleo sources of biotin are offal, mushrooms, cauliflower and walnuts.

Choline

Manufactured in the body from certain amino acids, choline is an essential nutrient for efficient metabolism of fats.

Paleo sources of choline are offal, beef and egg yolks. Good vegetable sources are oranges and cauliflower.

Vitamin C

Vitamin C is essential for the manufacture of collagen (a vital structural protein) in the body. Necessary for wound repair, gum health and prevention of bruising, vitamin C is also important for function of the immune system, neurotransmitters and hormones. An important vitamin, it is also responsible for regulation and function of many other nutrients within the body and is a powerful antioxidant. Vitamin C is destroyed by air, so pre-cut fruit and vegetables have already lost most of their content.

Paleo sources of vitamin c are chillies, guava, red pepper, kale, parsley and broccoli. Orange, spinach, strawberries and cauliflower also contain smaller amounts.

Minerals

There are many different minerals, not all of which are essential to human nutrition and many others that can actually be harmful. Found largely in plant food, which in turn derive them from the soil, mineral content in foods is variable and dependant on several factors. Minerals that occur in plants are often found bound with organic molecules that make the minerals more readily available to humans.

Minerals are essential to human health as part of a balanced intake of nutrients; vitamins and minerals work in tandem and often one can be rendered useless without the other.

Calcium

The most abundant mineral in the body, existing largely in the bones, calcium also plays a crucial function in most of the chemical reactions of the body. Low calcium intake is known to contribute to high blood pressure and osteoporosis.

Paleo sources of calcium are leafy greens, nuts and seeds.

Phosphorus

Also found largely in the bones and teeth, phosphorus is essential for absorption of calcium and vital for energy metabolism. The ratio of calcium to phosphorus is key and should be twice as much calcium to phosphorus.

Paleo sources of phosphorus are fish and meat long with nuts and seeds.

Magnesium

One of the most important minerals for cell function, magnesium works closely with calcium and phosphorus. Predominant in muscle and bone, magnesium is important for electrical balance within the body and is involved in many cellular functions including enzyme activation. Magnesium deficiency includes mental confusion, irritability, painful periods, muscle cramps, headaches and insomnia. Deficiency is common as magnesium is only present in whole foods and destroyed by modern processing.

Sea vegetables and nuts are the only reliable sources of magnesium in the diet so supplementation is recommended.

Potassium, sodium and chloride

Grouped together as electrolytes, these minerals play many vital roles within the body; heart, muscle, nerve, and kidney function all rely on these minerals that are also essential for fluid balance; they work in pairs so finely tuned balance is important. The modern diet results in twice as much sodium as potassium yet for optimal healthy function potassium should outweigh sodium by five to one.

Paleo sources rich in potassium but low in sodium are avocados, tomatoes, bananas, apricots and spinach.

Sulphur

The last in this overview of major minerals is sulphur, a mineral found in certain amino acids. Essential for protein formation, sulphur-containing amino acids are found in the body within structural proteins such as skin, hair and nails. They also contribute to hormones and several other biological molecules.

Paleo sources of sulphur are eggs, garlic, onions and cabbage.

Chromium

The first of the trace minerals, chromium is major determinant of insulin sensitivity that can help to lower body weight and improve glucose tolerance. Most individuals are deficient in chromium and levels are further depleted by refined sugars and flours.

Paleo sources of chromium are liver, green peppers, apple, parsnips, banana, spinach and carrots. Fruit and vegetable sources contain only low levels so supplementation may be needed.

Iron

Iron plays an essential role within red blood cells and in enzyme activity. Deficiency is common, either through increased need or insufficient intake. Signs of deficiency are anaemia, impaired immune function and decreased energy. Even a slight deficiency can lead to a reduction in productivity. Heme iron, found in animal foods is absorbed efficiently by the body whilst non-heme iron from vegetable sources is poorly absorbed.

Paleo sources of iron are liver, steak and prawns with leafy greens such as swiss chard and spinach providing non-heme iron.

Manganese

With a key role in many enzymes, including those that regulate blood sugar, energy metabolism and thyroid hormone, manganese is also a vital anti-oxidant. The body's need for manganese increases with inflammatory conditions.

Paleo sources of manganese include tea, pecans, brazil nuts and almonds.

Zinc

Much of the body's enzyme activity relies on adequate levels of zinc. Necessary for immune function, protein synthesis and cell growth as well as maintenance of vision, taste and smell. Often thought of as the male mineral, zinc is indeed essential for male sex hormone and prostate function. Zinc also plays a role in skin health and can help in acne prevention.

Paleo sources of zinc are seafood, beef, lamb, pork, chicken, spinach, cashews and mushrooms.

There are many more minerals, phytochemicals and supporting nutrients that make up the category of micronutrients. It is beyond the scope of this book to review them all in detail so we have covered the main micronutrients that you need for a healthy diet and this can be used a starting block if you wish to venture into this subject further.

A word on supplements

It is best to get nutrients from whole foods wherever possible and choosing from a wide range of natural ingredients should provide you with everything that you need. Isolated nutrients do not provide the same benefits as whole foods and there are many complex components in whole foods that we have not begun to understand. The concept of synergy is one that is popular in aromatherapy and it basically means 'more than the sum of its parts'; two or three compounds taken separately and without their supporting cast of other biological secrets will be far less effective than a range of whole foods known to contain these compounds.

After three, or even six months, when you have reset your health you may wish to explore the benefits of supplementing individual nutrients but for now we recommend that you consider the following nutritional support in the form of supplements. The range of supplements from a good health food store will be far superior and in more bio-available forms than the cheaper alternatives from the supermarket.

We recommend that you consider the following supplements to see you through your transition to Paleo and optimal health: A good probiotic with several different strains of bacteria; magnesium and cod liver oil (for Omega 3 and Vitamin D). These will be available from your local health food store.

Making nutrient dense choices

The nutrient information that you have just read shows how vital it is to include a wide range of whole foods in the diet. Whilst concentrating on so-called superfoods is not a good idea, it cannot be denied that certain foods provide a denser nutrient quota than others.

Taking non-Paleo foods out of the equation, starting with the highly processed packaged meals and refined carbohydrates, is the best starting point to illustrate nutrient density. Devoid of vitamins, minerals and supporting nutrients these foods are nutritionally empty as well as potentially harmful.

Moving on to grains and legumes, the point here is to avoid potentially irritant substances, but also that other foods such as meat and vegetables provide the nutrients found in these foods but with a whole lot more besides.

When choosing meat, a grass-fed animal will have better nutritional quality than an industrially farmed equivalent, but any meat at all will provide higher quality protein than a portion of chickpeas. Eating from a range of meats, including offal, will ensure that you get the full benefit from their varying nutrient content, but if you know that you need iron then head straight for the red meat on that particular day and remember to include it on a regular basis.

When choosing produce such as fruit and vegetables don't stick to the same old choices; a basket of carrots, bananas, broccoli, onions and apples each week is a great start but will be limiting in terms of nutrients. Where is the parsley, the avocado, and the garlic? Make sure to include varieties that provide a wide range of nutrients as described above.

Don't forget to add in a range of nuts and seeds. They may seem extraneous but they contain essential minerals that you may not find in such rich sources elsewhere.

Paleo, and any healthy diet, is not just about omitting the empty calories and the additives, it is about increasing nutrient intake to optimal levels. Sticking to a narrow range of foods, however Paleo friendly they may be, will not support your health and vitality as much as you need.

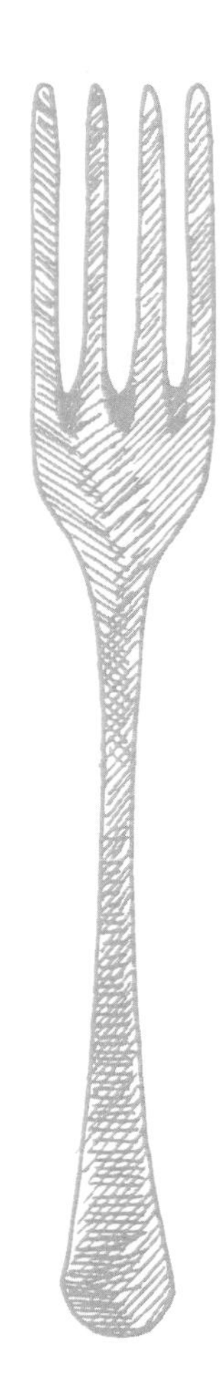

Case Study

"I have always been aware of how quickly I feel energised after eating lots of fruit and vegetables but after giving up work to be a stay at home mum and losing my husband's income too it always seemed that I couldn't prioritise fresh produce. My husband was unable to tolerate any fresh produce for years and my son would turn his nose up so I really felt that I couldn't afford to buy fruit and vegetables for myself.

I realise now of course that if it wasn't for the crisps, ice cream, soft drinks etc that I was buying then I would have been able to afford those things and supported the health of my family too. It isn't always easy to see what is staring you in the face, especially when you think you are doing the right thing.

Since starting the Paleo diet I have become much more aware of the difference between a body that is just "getting by" and a body that is fully functioning and full of life. Since I re-introduced all the lost vitamins and minerals into my diet I have felt what it is like to experience an energised body and mind. I find it difficult to put into words just how much difference that in itself has made to my life. I have been able to come off prescription pain medication and feel awake and alert every day. I am in tune with my body and know when something is wrong. I feel I am much more equipped to deal with everyday life and it takes a lot to stress me out nowadays. I feel so much more in control of my life. Once you add this to the weight loss and glowing skin it really couldn't get any better."

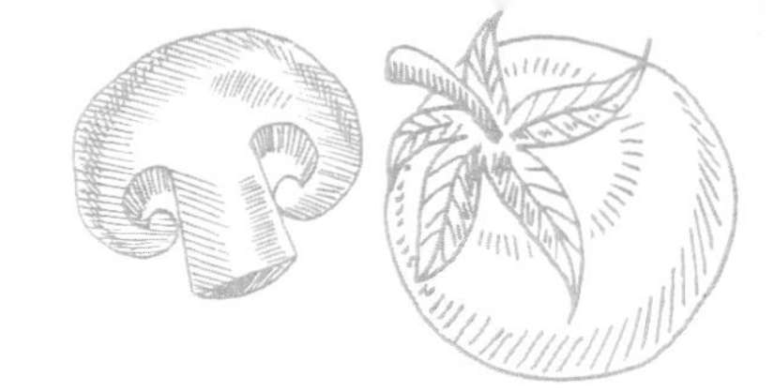

SECTION 9

Understand your Actions

The Paleo lifestyle stands upon a base of academic research and knowledge that explains the motives behind everything it does. So far, we have tried to present as much of that knowledge as possible to give you a broad understanding of the nutritional theory upon which the Paleo ethos rests, but science and ideas are constantly evolving just as you will constantly evolve through your changing needs and desires.

The approach that we take to both our teaching of the Paleo diet and the way that we follow it ourselves, rests on far more than nutritional evidence, food issues and kitchen skills. As the key to lifelong change, we view this Paleo transition as an all-embracing way of life that encompasses self-management and self-awareness techniques on a path to a healthier, more vital, life.

With that approach in mind, the message here is *to question and aim to understand all that you do*. The modern workplace has begun to take an increasingly holistic approach to professional life, with continued professional development, coaching techniques and lifelong learning becoming very much the norm. In the field of healthcare in particular, trainee practitioners are expected to practice ongoing reflection and planning as part of their remit, whilst there is not a higher education course in the land that does not consider personal development a part of the curriculum. *So why do we not put in as much effort with the other areas of our lives?* We try, try, and try some more to be the best that we can be in our working lives but when it comes to our health and our mental wellbeing we just muddle along regardless.

Learning to make personal development a part of your everyday life is not as rigid as it may sound; in fact the very opposite. Being self-aware and self-managed is about flexibility and fluidity not rigid attention to an unwavering schedule. The first step to taking responsibility for your own health and wellbeing is knowledge; the key to making informed choices.

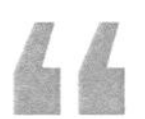

Understanding the processes behind your actions is an important part of learning and growing; ultimately it improves your chance of success.

What we would advise is that you understand the foods that you eat and choose them accordingly. Of course there is a basic Paleo framework of foods that we have covered in some detail already, but if you come across an ingredient or a food that you have to question, then at least explore its nutritional value and potential effects rather than looking for a black and white answer.

Make it your mission to explore the theory behind nutrition, health and wellbeing. Use this knowledge to inform your own decisions about what is right or wrong for you as an individual. Conversely use your own experiences to fuel further questions and exploration. The world has evolved on questions and answers; progress made by those who dare to challenge.

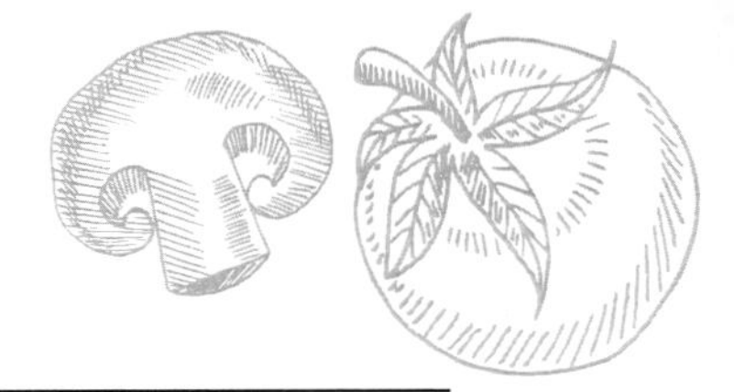

SECTION 10

Prioritise Quality Sleep

Introduction to Paleo explored some of the ways in which you can improve the quality of your sleep and we also touched briefly on the hormonal impact of lack of sleep or poor quality sleep.

We have all been there; tired and grumpy, or completely washed out, it is the fast track to hot buttered toast followed by half a packet of digestives. Oh, and perhaps a spoonful of sugar in the all-important mug of tea; just this once.

Being permanently tired through not prioritising sleep, patches of extreme exhaustion due to sleep issues or overwork, or not even realising that you need more or better quality sleep can all be vital clues as to why you overeat or make poor food choices. It is literally impossible to make any kind of positive choice when you are over tired; especially when it is chronic, ongoing disruption. Not only will you make poor food choices but all of your self-development and stress management strategies are likely to fly out the window too. Your entire world view becomes distorted.

So, instead of constantly battling against yourself in a vicious circle of overeating and guilt, take steps to improve the quality of your sleep. Make it a priority.

What can I do to improve my sleep quality?

The first step is to examine your current sleep patterns and environment. See how many of the following statements apply to you and read through the explanations, with possible solutions, below.

- I do not have a regular bedtime
- I try to catch up on sleep at the weekends

Your circadian rhythm is responsible for your sleep/wake cycle. Revolving around natural cycles of light and dark, and regulated by biochemical processes such as hormones and neurotransmitters, this sophisticated system is responsible for making sure you feel awake in the morning and sleepy at night. Cortisol (the stress hormone) is responsible for wakefulness, whilst the opposite action is performed by melatonin.

The main themes here are rhythm and balance. By constantly varying your sleep/wake times you are upsetting a sensitive and cyclical rhythm and disrupting hormonal balance. The simple answer is to go to bed at the same time each night and get up at the same time each morning. This may seem utterly impractical, even impossible, but sleep is as important as food, heat and light and needs to be afforded the same priority. Try your best to work within the boundaries that you have and see what a difference it makes. Working shifts may need a longer term solution but watching box sets at midnight can easily be resolved.

> *Going to bed at the same time each night and waking at the same time each morning is one of the kindest things you can do for yourself.*

- I do not have a bedtime routine

Introducing, or changing, your bedtime routine can make all the difference to a good night's sleep. Make the last few hours before bed about relaxing your body and mind to better induce sleep. Have a bath, read a book, dim the lights. Give your body every chance to do what it is designed to do; lower your cortisol levels and increase melatonin.

- I work on my computer late at night
- I watch TV before bed

The light from a computer screen and the fact that the brain is still working overtime is not conducive to sleep. If you must occasionally work at night then use a program to change the spectrum of light coming from the screen. TV may seem like a relaxing to do before bed but the noise and visuals are stimulating your body and stopping production of sleep inducing melatonin. To be in a restful state for sleep your body needs as little stimulation as possible.

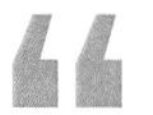

> *Try to turn off the screen at least two hours before bed. Preparing for sleep is vital for hormonal balance.*

- Light comes in through my bedroom curtains
- The street is noisy at night

Light and noise are both disruptive to sleep, even if you are not consciously aware of the fact. You could be tossing and turning all night but think you have had your eight hours and wonder why you feel so tired. For deep motionless sleep to occur, the conditions must be conducive to sleep; dark and quiet. Try black out blinds or heavy curtains, even an eye mask if necessary. If noise is bothering you then invest in a pair of earplugs; the foam types used by swimmers are excellent.

> *Block out noise and light at night as they effect quality of sleep.*

- I am under a lot of stress at the moment

The links between stress and sleep are well documented and the resulting constant flow of cortisol is not conducive to sleep. Follow all of the measures that we cover in this section and embark on a stress management program too. Unfortunately, there are no instant answers and is something that must be worked through; with a health professional if necessary.

- I sleep fitfully

A fitful night isn't pleasant for anyone and there are even times when you don't realise that you had a night of poor quality sleep. This is where quantity over quality comes into play. There could be many reasons for a fitful night and covering all of the steps in this section should resolve the problem. There are many apps on the market now that monitor sleep patterns using motion technology and can prove useful to pinpointing where your problems lie.

As we fall asleep, we move through several phases of the sleep cycle. REM sleep (or rapid eye movement) is the dreaming phase where we are closer to consciousness. This is light sleep, easily disrupted and not particularly restful. Non REM sleep is deep sleep, some of which is deeper than others as we move through the cycle; the time for really deep sleep is in the hours before midnight so an early night really does make a difference to sleep quality.

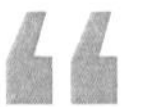

> *It is quality of sleep, not quantity, that counts. Getting an early night can make all the difference.*

- I can't seem to settle down at night
- My bedroom is chaos

Is your bedroom a sanctuary or a repository for unwanted furniture and unsorted junk? Making your bedroom into a relaxing calming place is essential to a good night's sleep and you should take every step possible to make your bedroom conducive to a good night's rest.

If you have problems settling down then you could be uncomfortable. Perhaps the room is too cold or too warm? Or the room temperature is fine but the blankets are stifling. When did you last replace the mattress or check that it is suitable for your needs? How old are your pillows, and do they provide the right support for you?

> *Sometimes the only clue to poor quality sleep is that you feel tired during the day. Consider your sleeping environment and ways in which it could be improved.*

As well as considering the efficacy of your bed and bedding, take a look at your surroundings. Is the room full of clutter or things that do not really belong there? Consider ways in which you could make your bedroom into more of a restful haven. It doesn't have to be expensive; a clear out and a lick of paint can work wonders. A soothing colour scheme, clean lines and an uncluttered space are all helpful in the quest for a good night's sleep.

- There is a TV/computer in my bedroom
- I have an LED alarm clock

However unnoticeable you think they may be, the standby light on electronic devices or the neon glow of a clock radio can be as disruptive to sleep as light streaming in through the windows. Use a different style of clock and, if you must have electronics in the bedroom, switch them off at the wall. You will find the bedroom a far more restful place if you remove them altogether.

- I eat dinner late
- I wake up hungry in the night
- I snack in the evening

Hunger levels, and blood sugar levels, can be linked to restless nights. If your body is struggling to digest a heavy meal late at night then you may have difficulty getting to sleep. Disrupted insulin balance can effect sleep, waking you in the night with a dip in blood sugar causing a craving for sugar or keeping you up late on a sugar high.

Most sleep disruption at night due to hunger can be controlled with a Paleo diet that gets your hormone levels back into balance; no more blood sugar issues. A diet too low in carbohydrates can cause sleepless nights so introducing safe starches such as sweet potato is a good idea if you suffer from this particular problem. A magnesium supplement at night can also aid a good night's sleep. Eating dinner too early may mean you actually feel hungry late at night, or eating too late could make you too full; finding the perfect balance for you is a matter of trial and error.

- I smoke
- I like an alcoholic drink in the evening
- I take prescription/non-prescription medication

Cigarettes, alcohol, caffeine, and some medications, are all stimulants that will prevent you from relaxing at night. Alcohol may appear to relax you and send you into a welcome coma but once the body begins to metabolise the alcohol it has a stimulating effect. A cup of coffee at midday can be enough to prevent you sleeping at bedtime; most advice regarding caffeine recommends stopping caffeine intake after 2pm, or eliminating it entirely.

We have learnt that rather than struggling against your environment and getting stuck in a cycle of weight gain and despair, it is often far more effective to deal with external issues first. It is easier to stay on track with positive choices when you can cope with the curveballs that life throws you. We all know how easy it is to attend to our health when life runs smoothly but when the pressure starts piling on it is a whole new story; and pressure is there more often than not. Managing your environment and your responses is a vital part of weight management that make it easy for you keep making those healthy choices.

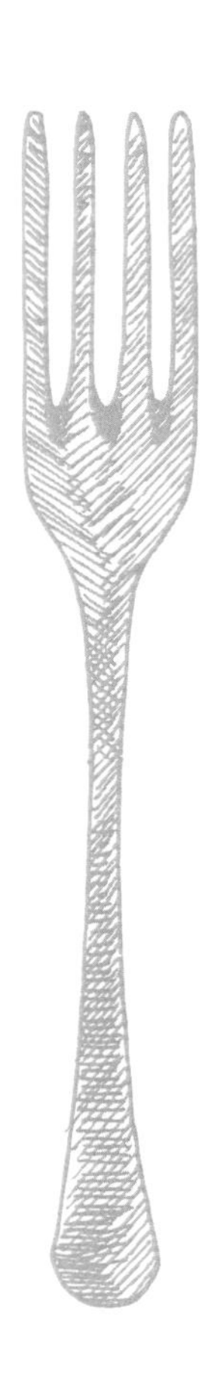

Case Study

"Sleep has always been important to me and I know that if I don't get my eight or nine hours then I can't function well. Everyone always asks me how I cope with some of the stuff life throws at me and I always say it is because I always make sure I get enough sleep. I'm never afraid to say 'right, I'm off to bed now' even if it is 9pm and the party is just getting started.

I notice that once my workload builds up that I start to experience restless nights and I know that this can then lead to the possibility of weight gain. I have now learnt that when I feel this process happening that I need to give myself a proper day off and focus on getting a few goods night sleep. I find that once my attentions are re-directed onto prioritising sleep and time to rest that I will inevitably notice a difference in my skin and even my weight almost immediately.

My bedroom was a tip for many years; full of old wardrobes and clutter. I tidied it up and painted during the 12 week programme and I found that it makes a big difference to the atmosphere and I now love my tranquil space. My favourite sleep tip? Audiobooks; take time to find a narrator with a soothing voice and have an hour each night before sleep. It has now become a cue for me and my body knows that is bedtime. I find it better than reading because you can turn the lights out."

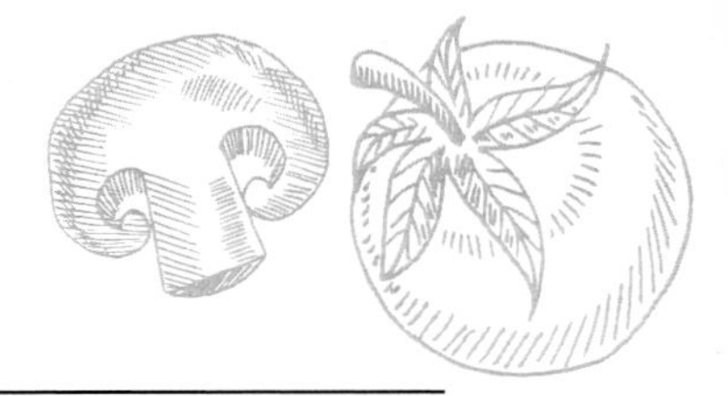

SECTION 11

Manage Stress

Learning to manage stress is a vital part of any health improvement plan and could be the key to implementing sustainable lifelong change. If you have not done so already, we would recommend that you read *Introduction to Yoga* alongside this section as this will provide you with a detailed insight into the control and management of stress that you encounter as a result of everyday life.

Our mechanisms that deal with stress are designed to cope with acute immediate situations of danger. They are not designed to cope with the chronic relentless attack of modern life. Stress hormones are stuck in the on position and this over exposure leads to an imbalance that wreaks havoc in every part of the body.

As we noted earlier, direct health implications of stress aside, it becomes virtually impossible to stick to healthy goals when stress is making a mockery of all your good intentions. Stress hormones not only increase heart rate and blood pressure but have severe implications for weight management too. Blood sugar levels and storage of visceral fat (the worst kind of fat stored around your waist) are increased, the mechanisms that increase hunger, cravings and food intake kick in, and your body becomes less efficient at burning fat. Even with the best will in the world you just don't stand a chance.

What is the answer to dealing with stress effectively?

Unlikely as it is to go away any time soon, and considering its negative role in human health as well as the part it has most likely played in the global obesity epidemic, it is unbelievable that so many of us are ill equipped with the skills required to manage it.

Introduction to Yoga provides an insight as to how to use relaxation and breathing techniques alongside Yoga poses to combat stress that we cannot eliminate from our lives. Throughout the remainder of this section we will be showing you how to incorporate stress management techniques into your routine. You will be able to explore the possibility as to whether you are able to eliminate or reduce some stress triggers and will learn about how to cope with those elements which cannot be avoided.

What is stress management?

Stress management involves working through a series of logical steps and taking the time to explore the sources of stress in your life and how you deal with them. Just like stress management has implications in how well you sleep, which in turn has links to how well you eat, it also segues seamlessly into self-development and the tools that help with one can shed light on the other.

Introduction to Paleo provided an insight to the idea of reflection and its vital role in development; essentially by making a habit of noting things down we have a record that can be used for exploration and further planning. What worked? What didn't work? How could I have done that differently? Could the outcome have been more positive for all involved? All of this comes through the practice of reflection; our memory is not as accurate as we like to think and without a record, vital information can be lost. The point here of course is that reflection is a valuable tool in stress management.

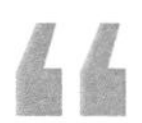

Stress management is all about taking control of how you react to situations.

An ongoing plan for stress management

Consider keeping a stress journal. Use it to record all of your thoughts about how you handle stressful situations and any exercises that you do within your stress management program.

Identify all of your current sources of stress. Anything that elicits a stress response, however seemingly trivial, should go down here. *Introduction to Yoga* contains advice and help on how to identify areas of stress if you are not able to identify the stress trigger. It is not uncommon for symptoms of stress to appear but without there being a single notable trigger. You will then need to take steps to identify the specific trigger by paying close attention to your symptoms and your daily activities.

Once you have identified sources of your stress, think about how you cope with each in turn. Do you have different reactions to different sources? Are they healthy reactions or could you find healthier ways of coping.

Stress management strategies

Now that you have explored the stressors in your life and identified the ways in which you tend to react the next step is to work out if there is a better way of coping with the problem.

We have set out below some strategies that you can apply to try and deal with the stress triggers that you have identified. Start at the beginning and work through sequentially until you have reached a potential solution; each stressor will require its own process.

Once you have come up with a plan for dealing with these sources of stress now is the time to put them into action, feedback the information into your stress journal and explore the efficacy of your revised strategies.

Strategy 1 – AVOID the stressor

The first thing to consider is how many sources of stress you can actually eliminate from your life. Could you…

- ➥ avoid unnecessary stress?
- ➥ stop taking on more than you can handle? Learn to say no.
- ➥ avoid people that bring you negativity and stress?
- ➥ prioritise your tasks?

Strategy 2 – ALTER the situation

Obviously not all sources of stress can be eliminated but there are techniques that can be employed to help you assess and alter the situation. Could you…

- ➥ express your concerns?
- ➥ reach a compromise?
- ➥ be more assertive?
- ➥ employ time management techniques?

If you struggle in any of these areas then you could consider taking a short course or finding the information to help you teach yourself. Ask at your workplace about self-development training; skills such as these are often under one umbrella and many are provided free by your local authority; look up adult or lifelong learning. Learning to communicate effectively is a worthwhile skill that could open many doors.

Strategy 3 – ADAPT to the situation

If your attempts at improving communication or time management do not relieve you from the stressors then it is time to think about altering the way that you look at a given situation. Most of these techniques come under the subject of REFRAMING. A vital skill that can get you through the most relentless of times, reframing becomes second nature once you have had enough practice. It may sound obvious, but once your vision is skewed by stress it can be difficult to remember to stand back and take a different view.

Look at the big picture. Where does this situation rank in the grand scheme of things? For that matter what is the grand scheme of things.

Adjust your standards. Are your expectations realistic? Don't worry if you come to the conclusion that yes they are; no one is asking you to compromise your integrity but simply consider all the angles and judge each situation in context.

Focus on the positive. If you look hard enough you can always find a positive angle even if it is only to chalk this down to experience. If you never faced problems then you would never change; and without change there can be no growth.

The last part of adapting to stressors is to pay careful attention to your internal dialogue. If you must have a conversation with yourself, and trust me we all do it, then make it a positive one. Instead of plotting your office manager's downfall and unleashing the sulky teenager within, use your inner dialogue to work through the situation and give yourself a pep talk. Learn to make your inner self someone you can trust.

Strategy 4 – ACCEPT the things you cannot change

These steps are all part of learning to accept that there are bits of life that you just cannot change. You have to deal with it and move on. If you can't do that, then you need to keep digging until you find resolution. Stress management is an ongoing process; something that once learned becomes a natural part of the way you live your life.

Remember that you can't control everything. The universe is a huge, weird and wonderful place that you are just one tiny part of; enjoy it.

Try to see challenges as an opportunity for personal growth. Let go of negative energy. Harbouring resentment or storing up old ills will prevent you from moving forward; forgive, forget and move on. Be aware of your own energy; by viewing the world through a positive lens and letting go of some of the weight on your shoulders you will have a positive effect on everything around you.

Don't forget that these steps form part of a process and as such are cyclical in nature. After working through and reaching the final strategy you may come to realise that you cannot reframe or accept a certain situation. You may have learned that in order to get through this you will have to consider enormous change such as new career or the breakdown of a relationship. That's hard; but taking control often is. But now you are armed with the self-knowledge to inform your decision and guide you through your choices. Before we move on to look at self- awareness, there's just one more thing.

Make time for leisure

Nurturing yourself is a necessity; not a luxury or something that you have to earn. Make sure that you spend time amongst positive people, embrace every opportunity that comes your way, and do something that you enjoy every single day.

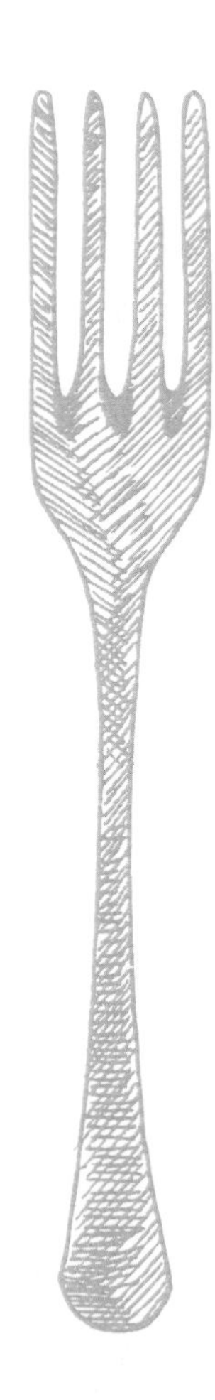

Case Study

"Like many other women who look after families whilst also holding down a demanding job I was used to having a high level of stress in my life. I always thought that it was inevitable and just something that happened as part of everyday life. It was not until I took some action to try and relieve some of the stress that I realised what a physical toll stress can take on you.

Once I started the Yoga work outs I found that this was really helpful to block out the stresses of the day and just focus on myself for a while. It would leave me with a calm sense of wellbeing and would put me back on track after a stressful day. I would really recommend Yoga to anyone. It doesn't take long and you don't even need to leave your house.

I have been working on using the strategies for coping with stress and I am getting better at being able to eliminate some sources of stress from my life. I have learnt that I really can't let myself get upset about everything and am focusing on the fact that I can only be responsible for my own actions and that I cannot possibly control the actions of others. This is useful for me to remember and I am feeling the benefits of this. As with everything it is difficult to suddenly try and change your mind set especially when we are all stuck in our ways. I would just recommend that you keep an open mind about the possibilities of stress reduction and to explore the benefits it may have for you as it is really working for me."

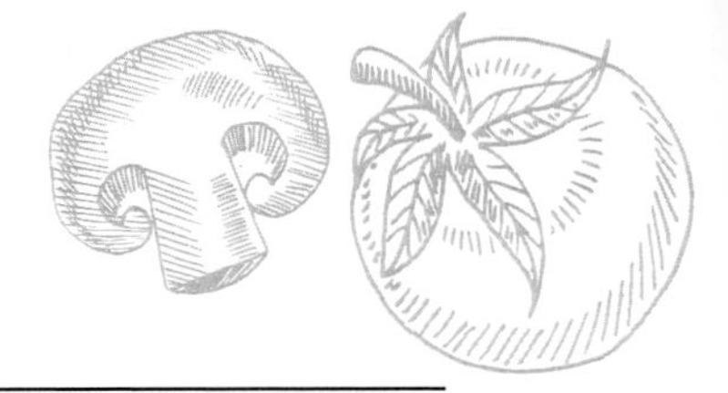

SECTION 12

Practise Self Awareness

If you want to get the best from life, make the most of opportunities, and feel good in your own skin, then you need to practice self-awareness. Those people that seem to know who they are and have the courage to just be themselves? Chances are it didn't come handed to them on a plate and they have spent a good portion of time working it all out. Experience and age bring with them plenty of opportunities for learning about yourself and how you fit best into the world but there are plenty of useful tools around to aid the process.

Rather than a set of problem solving tools that render you instantly self-savvy, the process of self-development is something that stays with you for life. It becomes part of who you are; someone who takes a pro-active role in their own life as opposed to just letting it pass by. It isn't about being self-absorbed or obsessive, it is simply about making the most of the opportunities available and being the best version of you that you can be.

We realise that to many people this seems like something that "other people do". This is a normal reaction to have when we are faced with something new that we have not tried before. Having feelings of hesitation and doubts as to its efficacy are completely normal. All we ask is that you keep reading with an open mind. You may be surprised at what you learn about yourself if you accept this method into your lifestyle and embrace wholeheartedly. What have you go to lose?

A questioning mind

We made a point earlier on that without change there could be no growth but there is one vital component missing from that statement; questions. In counselling and coaching circles there is a term for the dialogue between client and practitioner; it is called "the therapeutic dialogue". It basically means that the setting required for change to take place is one built upon questions; it is an ongoing conversation between two people in which finding the answers to questions moves the dialogue forward. It is also very much about finding the right questions.

Without a professional prompting you with questions, it is up to you to act as both sides of the conversation and all it needs is an enquiring mind. There are plenty of resources out there to help you frame revealing questions and you can learn a lot about yourself just by working through some simple exercises.

What does all of this have to do with my Paleo diet?

We have already ascertained that the links between body and mind are unbreakable so any process of change and development must address the system as a whole. This holistic approach is at the forefront of the Paleo movement and is one which the Paleo Diet and Fitness Plan embraces wholeheartedly. Our ethos throughout is that your transformation to a sustainable and healthy lifestyle rests upon finding the right path to health for you as an individual.

When we look at the biochemical patterns beneath the surface, we have seen that changes in our environment or our physical health can all effect our control over what we eat and how our body stores food. Learning to manage stress is just one branch of self-awareness; finding ways to ensure better quality sleep is another. Taking the time out to follow a new way of eating such as this one also comes under the heading of self-development. Call it life coaching, lifelong learning, or self-development, it all encompasses the same tools and boils down to one thing; working towards a deeper understanding of yourself to enhance your life.

Some useful tools for self-development

The coaching wheel

Used as it is in so many development arenas as a starting point for personal exploration, the wheel of life seems a bit of a hoary old chestnut. It is however a very useful old chestnut and its very popularity and longevity stand testimony to its relevance. Starting with the bigger picture and working your way down to the specifics is a good way to hone in on the areas that need attention. You may think that you already know, and there is every chance that you do, but taking the time to map out a broad view can often throw out some interesting revelations.

Using the coaching wheel serves to underline the fact that everything is linked and encourages the view of life as a whole. You could search the internet for a wheel of life diagram and print it off but we think that the drawing of the wheel marks an investment of time into the process. You will need nothing more than a piece of paper and a pen. Begin by drawing a circle with enough space around it to comfortably label your diagram and then split the wheel equally into eight sections by drawing lines to form quarters and then halfway across each quarter to equal eight. Now split the wheel again by drawing two concentric circles of equal distance apart thus segmenting each wedge into three compartments. You should now have a circular diagram that looks like a simplified dartboard.

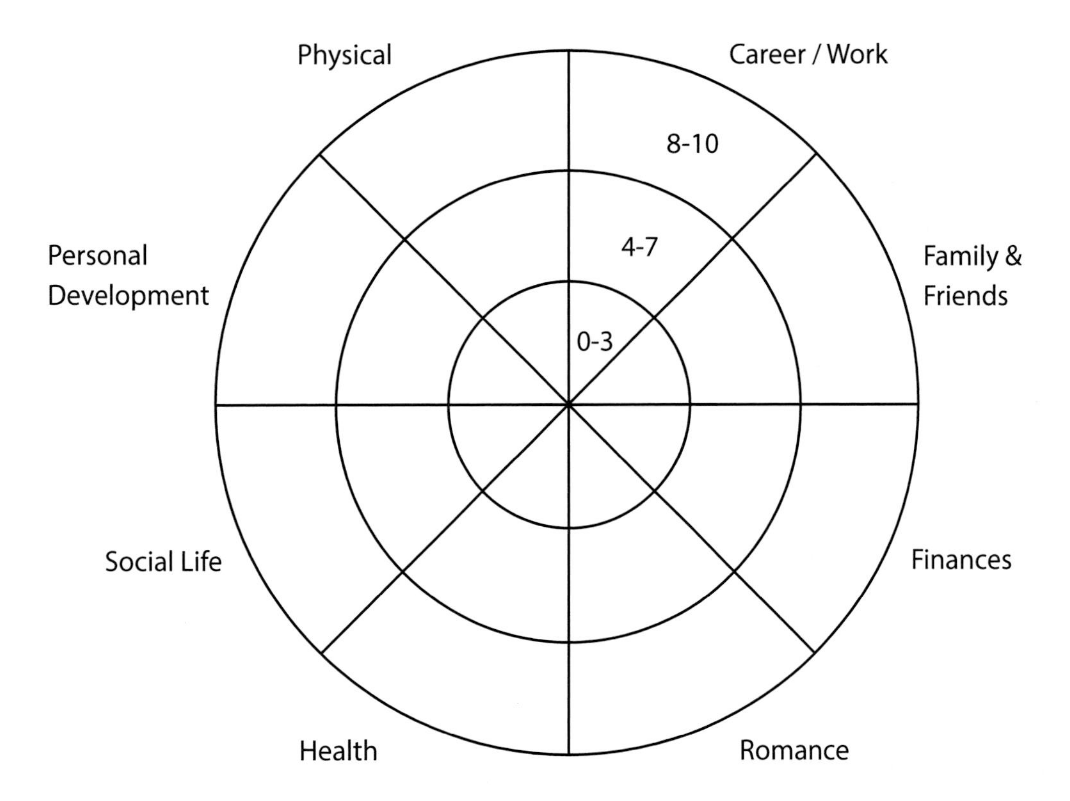

In one of the wedges, working outwards from the centre, label the sections 0-3, 4-7, 8-10, respectively. Now, around the edge, label the wedges as shown in the diagram. Interpret each as you wish; this is your life, nobody else's.

Spending time to consider your answers, rather than following ingrained knee-jerk responses, give each area a satisfaction score. A useful way to represent this is to colour up to the relevant section of the respective wedge. What you end up with is something like a bar chart, but curving around a circle. It serves as a graphical representation of how happy you are with your life and which areas need the most work.

The diagram also shows connections between areas, in that satisfaction in one area can lead to satisfaction in another; you may love your job that causes your finances to thrive but the result could be less than satisfactory personal relationships. This is not a test, or a quest for the perfect life; it is just a tool to be used in discovering a deeper understanding of your life. Not something that you do only once, the coaching wheel can be completed at various intervals as part of your overall reflection practise.

Focus on specifics

The next stage of using the coaching wheel is to further explore the areas of life and the reasons behind your scores. Can you break each category down further and examine each part? Perhaps there are bits that you feel satisfied with whilst others are lacking. Looking at life in this way not only helps identify specific areas for change but can make you realise that there are certain areas that make you really happy; without conscious positive thought, the good is almost always overshadowed by the bad. Try to develop several statements, negative or positive, for each area. Take another look and see if the results in the original wheel have changed in terms of areas scoring the least in satisfaction.

Goal planning

Following on from the work with the coaching wheel and part of identifying what you want from life and how you intend to get there, goal planning is a crucial part of any self-development program. Using the thoughts that you generated in the work on specifics, ask yourself what steps you could take to increase satisfaction in these areas. To be successful, goals should be specific and measurable and you should write them down.

Research has shown that those who write their goals down are more likely to achieve them. Even better success has been shown by those who shared those goals with a friend and provided a weekly update on their progress. They were 33% more likely to achieve their goals. This is an astonishing figure and shows how much power is associated with putting something into writing and making a commitment to making it happen. *Tabata Transformation* provides in depth advice on how to set specific and measurable goals and we would recommend that it is reviewed in conjunction with this section.

The first step is to decide on a goal for each area and a time frame in which they can reasonably be achieved. From there you can break the goals down into specific tasks that must be accomplished in order to reach your target. Reflection, as outlined below, is the ideal tool for evaluating your progress.

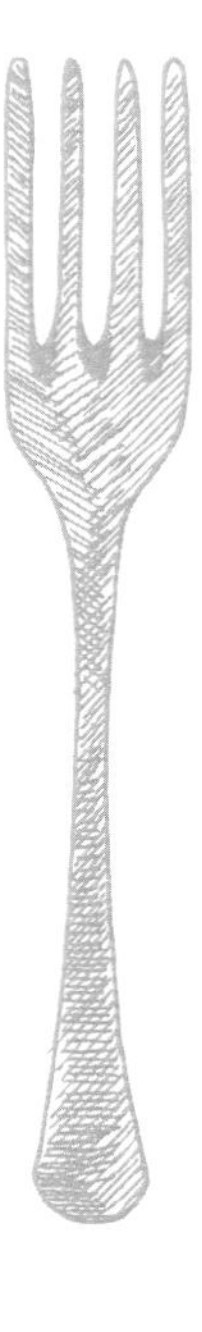

Case Study

"I was intrigued about the concept of setting goals by writing them down. I was amazed at the statistics that showed the success of people who did this. So I went ahead and wrote out my goals nice and neatly and for a while I just kept them in my note book and would come across them every now and again. One day I realised this was more than likely not the intention of the exercise and so I took the piece of paper and put it into one of the photo frames on the wall in my kitchen. This meant I would see it every day and most importantly when I was cooking. I did find it more motivational than I thought I would, especially as the weight started to drop off and I was getting nearer to my goal. It was almost like having a calendar where you cross off the dates to your holiday – it created the same anticipation and excitement. I don't know if writing the goals down were the reason for my success but I know it certainly boosted me along the way."

Reflection

Nothing mystical or deep, although it can be if you like, reflection is simply the action of keeping a diary or journal and using it to ask questions of yourself with a view to learning and making possible improvements. Writing it down means an investment of time on your part but it also gives you a valuable record of a certain point in time that may or may not stick in your mind.

There are several ways to use this method of recording and questioning but regularity is the key. You can write about events as they happen, and then question them later or you can do it all at once; you will probably end up doing a mixture of both. Reflection isn't just for recording situations that went wrong, examining the things that you felt happy with is just as important. Why did you feel such a sense of achievement on that particular instance? What can you learn from the event that will give you confidence in the future? If a situation went less than well, consider what could have been done differently and how the outcome could have better for everyone involved.

Reframing thoughts

We looked at the technique of reframing in Section 11 in the context of stress management, but it is such a powerful technique in so many ways that we thought to include it here. This version is about changing your mental perspective so that you can learn from your experiences, however seemingly mundane, and take a broader view. It also ties in nicely with the subject of inner voice too. So, for example, instead of asking "which one is better" you would ask "what are the merits of each". Rather than seeking blame you could consider what each person may learn from the situation. It is about bearing in mind that things are not simply black or white and that being judgemental prevents learning and growth.

We all have a lot to learn about ourselves and how our body and minds interact. How you view yourself is often much distorted to how others will describe you. We often hold ourselves up to a much high standard than we would expect from anyone else and put immense pressure on ourselves. It is inevitable that we cannot always live up to our own high expectations and this can lead to feelings of disappointment and failure which are unnecessary and unjust and the hardest to dismiss. By taking steps to understand and alter our approach we can learn to deal with situations more effectively and improve our health and happiness along the way.

Learning how to explore who we are and the "how's and whys" of what makes us function is a long but interesting road that we all should walk once in a while.

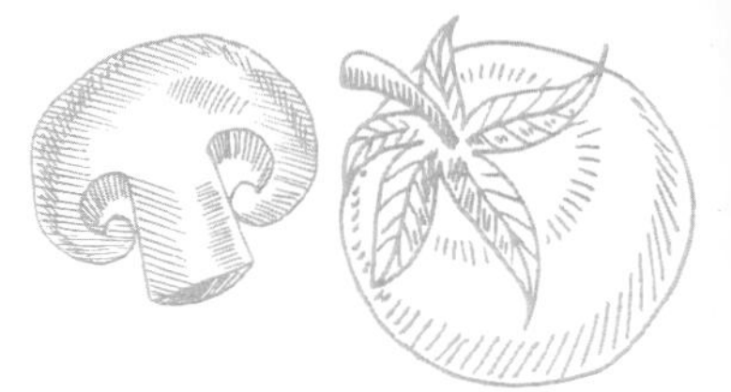

SECTION 13

FAQ

We have set out below some of the questions that we frequently get asked in relation to the Paleo programme. Hopefully these will answer any questions that you may have which have not already been covered elsewhere.

Can I still have tea or coffee?

When following a Paleo lifestyle, caffeine falls into a category of consume in moderation. Therefore, you do not have to cut it out of your routine completely but you should try to limit it to one cup a day. If you take milk then try using almond milk or coconut milk as an alternative to the traditional dairy version.

You are able to drink as many herbal or decaffeinated hot drinks as you like throughout the day. Why not try experimenting with a few herbal teas – they can be quite addictive once you have given them a chance.

What if I am hungry between meals?

In these first few weeks of your transition you will probably find that you eat a lot more than you will once your body has adjusted. Eat when you feel hungry but take on board what you have already learned about biochemical behaviour and learn to question if it is hunger you are feeling or merely cravings.

If you have had very little in the way of nutrients over the past few months (or even years) then your body will continue to crave food until its reserves have been topped up. Choose nutrient dense snacks such as cooked meats, hard boiled eggs, nuts or fruits or check out our tasty snack and smoothie recipes for something a bit different.

Will I feel any side effects?

The answer is possibly. This is known as the low-carb flu and the symptoms are aching muscles, headache and low energy levels. Not everyone feels this way, but some do. It is a result of a combination of detox and physical withdrawal from substances that you may have become addicted to such as wheat and sugar. Not much comfort at the time, but be assured if this is happening to you then you really need to be making these dietary changes; severe withdrawals are a sure sign that if you carry on with these toxic foods then you are heading for serious ill health in later life. Keep yourself well hydrated and listen to your body, rest if you need to and the symptoms should pass within a few days. You will get through it!

Do I have to follow the meal plans?

The meal plans are there to give you a helping hand in the transition to a Paleo lifestyle. We have set out everything that you will need to complete your 12 week programme down to meal plans and even shopping lists. We have done this to make the process as easy as possible for you. We know that many people are not overly confident in the kitchen or are just short on time so by providing recipes for every meal it takes away the excuses.

All of our recipes have been created to provide a balance of nutrition and a variety of Paleo friendly foods. However, if you want to adapt the recipes to suit your needs or even come up with your own recipes, this is fine. You will need to make sure that you understand the Paleo principles and that these are applied to your recipes. Try to keep a varied diet, this will mean that you are getting a wide variety of nutrients and trying new things is always good for you.

What if I don't like all of the foods used in the recipes?

The chances are that you will come across a few ingredients in the recipes that you are not overly keen on. There will also be a few that you have probably never tried and then some more that you have never even heard of. In the first instance we would urge you to try the recipe with all of the ingredients. It may be the case that you discover that you actually do like the ingredient you were dreading. The foods that we have included are all full of vitamins and goodness and we would love everyone to eat and enjoy them wholeheartedly. You should bear in mind that it only takes a couple of weeks for our tastes to become adapted to a new way of eating so the avocado you can't stand in week one could be a new favourite by week three.

Give it a try but if you really can't eat something then you are able to substitute it for any Paleo friendly ingredient that you wish.

What if I have a bad few days and eat non Paleo foods?

Now let's get one thing straight from the start. You are only human. We all have good and bad days and we all have situations whereby we are tempted to eat and drink things which we know are bad for us. The Paleo Diet and Fitness Plan is not about depriving yourself and sticking to a rigid regime for the rest of your life. We provide you with the information that you need in order to make sensible decisions about the food that you want to eat.

If you do find that you fall off the Paleo wagon for a day, or even a few days, then first of all stop beating yourself up about it. It has happened and there is nothing you can do about it. The chances are that you will be feeling the effects of the non-Paleo foods for a few days and will remember just way you eliminated them in the first place. There is nothing like a few days of being bloated and sluggish to get you back on track.

What you should not do is revert back to old ways and go eat everything in sight on the basis that you will "start again tomorrow". You need to re-educate yourself about your attitude towards food. The Paleo Diet and Fitness Plan will help with that but it can take time. You need to consider what made you slip up and try to put systems in place to eliminate or reduce your exposure to the same trigger event. Remember that mistakes are there to learn from. You need to pick yourself up and just start again. Do not think it is pointless and give in. Taking control is the only way to make a positive change.

SECTION 14

Troubleshooting

We have included this section as a troubleshooting "checklist" so that you can revert to this if you feel that your Paleo transition is stalling and you cannot work out why. We cannot emphasise enough the fact that every single person is individual and therefore everyone (and we mean everyone) will respond differently, in varying time frames, to a change in lifestyle.

If you are starting your Paleo journey with a friend you will most likely see that there are differences in how your bodies respond to the change in diet and lifestyle and that one of you may take to the transition quicker than the other. If this happens please be reassured that this is completely normal. You will get there in the end so please do not be disheartened. You should always try to avoid comparisons with others but we know that this can be difficult. Just be safe in the knowledge that you are doing something incredibly positive for your body and you will see the benefits of your hard work.

If you are unsure as to whether you need to be doing something different then why not have a look through the "checklist" that we have set out below which can help to identify some areas that you may need to focus more attention on.

Are you drinking enough water?

In the early stages of the Paleo transition it is easy to make sure that you are drinking enough water; you feel thirsty as your cells eliminate toxins and you shed excess water too. Once you are on an even keel though it can be simple to forget to keep your water intake topped up and therefore you will start to retain water which will show on the scales.

Do you take any medications?

If you take medication, especially prescription ones for specific conditions, it is important that you continue to take them whilst you adapt to this new way of eating. Even if you feel an easing of symptoms it is important to discuss medication with your doctor. Some medications can be responsible for increased appetite or water retention so if you do take any then make sure to drink plenty of water, cut down on salt and be aware of any persistent issues with cravings and hunger. If you have any concerns about your medication then please see your doctor or health care professional.

Do you need to consider a probiotic supplement?

The ability to shed toxins and eliminate food waste efficiently can have a direct impact upon your weight loss. If you find that weight loss stalls then a probiotic supplement may help. Choose a quality supplement with several strains of bacteria rather than just one; most good ones contain various enzymes too.

Do you need to consider your overall food intake?

Although our plan covers a broad range of ingredients and an optimal range of nutrients, it cannot take into account individual needs. If you are not losing weight or your weight loss has stalled you may wish to consider your overall food intake; perhaps you are eating too much or too little? Maybe you are snacking too much? Are you including enough fat in your diet?

Do you need to consider your nutrient intake?

You may notice that as your nutrient intake tops up and levels out that you are better able to control your cravings. This is because if any micronutrients are lacking in your diet your body will simply request more food. You may wish to consider various nutrients that may still be deficient in your diet: a high strength cod liver oil will cover your Omega 3 needs as well as vitamin D; magnesium is often lacking in the healthiest of diets due to poor soil content or depleted nutrients in produce. Iodine is also essential; if you don't intake sea vegetables or plenty of seafood then consider reintroducing table salt.

Have you lost inches rather than pounds?

The scales may tell a completely different story to the tape measure or the fit of your clothes. This can become especially relevant when you are incorporating exercise such as Tabata into your routine. It may well be that you are turning fat into lean muscle and are therefore seeing a reduction in measurements but not a corresponding reduction in the scales. This is completely normal and happens to the majority of people.

It is actually a really good position to be in as it shows that your body is responding well to the exercise and you are developing lean muscle mass. We discuss how to measure weight loss accurately in *Tabata Transformation* and we would recommend that you review this. It may be that you should invest in some body composition scales to assist with making an accurate record of your progress.

Are you weighing yourself too often?

Whilst the scales are a relevant overall marker, do not become too reliant on them as weight fluctuates on a daily and even hourly basis for all sorts of reasons and being a martyr to the scales is not particular healthy. Use your clothes to gauge your progress and leave the scales for once a month; every two weeks if you must. Remember that women are subject to weight fluctuations before, during and after a menstrual cycle which is caused by hormonal changes in your body. If you weigh yourself too often you are likely to get caught up in the tiniest of fluctuations that are completely normal and unavoidable.

Are you exercising?

Have you managed to incorporate exercise into your weekly routine? Did you start out with good intentions and then let this slide? Or have you found that you are not putting as much effort into the work outs as you should be? If this is the case then you need to make a commitment to ensure that you incorporate enough exercise into your weekly routine. We know it can be difficult but it really will not take long for you to complete a Tabata or Yoga work out. We do not know of a single person who has not felt better after doing a work out – you just need to get up and do it. Make sure that you follow the exercise programme to the letter for the next couple of weeks and see if that makes a difference.

Are you sleeping?

Do you have trouble sleeping? We have looked in some detail at how lack of quality sleep can sabotage your weight loss efforts but it can be easy to focus on food. If you have followed our tips on restful sleep but are still not sleeping well then that may explain why your weight loss has stalled. Try a magnesium supplement at night or introducing more starchy vegetables.

Are you under stress?

We have also looked in detail at the ways that stress can derail your weight loss or even cause weight gain. Stress management is a continuous process and issues in this area could explain why you are not losing any weight. Try consulting a professional for a stress management plan if your own efforts are overwhelming you.

Could you further reduce your toxic load?

Are you sure that you have eliminated all sources of potential toxins in your diet? Have you unwittingly retained sources of processed vegetable oil or missed certain ingredients on labels? It can be easy to think that a little mayonnaise from a jar or tuna in sunflower oil may not make a difference but if you aren't seeing the results you expected then it may be time to take another look.

Is your carbohydrate intake right for you?

Getting the carbohydrate balance just right for you can be tricky. It may take a little more or a little less to kick start your weight loss. There are only moderate carbohydrates on our plan so you may want to try going up rather than down. Add in extra sweet potatoes here and there or a few extra bananas. If that doesn't work then try eliminating all starchy vegetables and fruit.

Are you getting enough fat?

If you are using less fats and oils than stated in recipes or choosing lean sources of meat from habit then you may not be taking in enough fat to support your metabolic processes. Or you may simply need a little more than the standard level in the plan; remember everybody is different so it is important to find what is right for you.

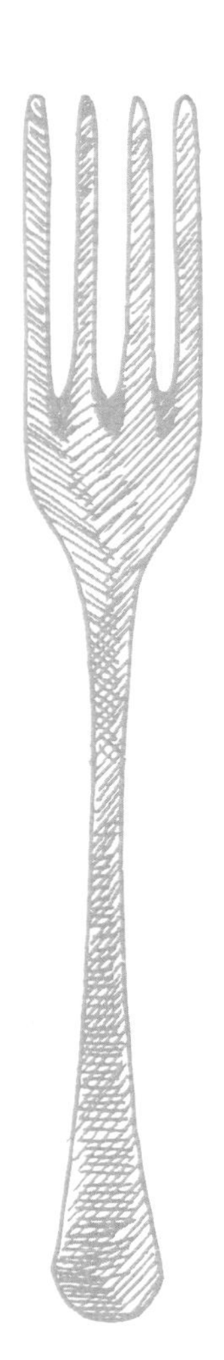

Case Study

"I won't lie and say that the 12 weeks were issue free and plain sailing. I had a few stumbling blocks along the way and needed to consider and evaluate what the issue may be to get me back on track. After looking at my situation carefully I decided to try taking a probiotic when my weight loss began to stall. I found that this really helped and once I started taking it my weight loss ramped up again.

I find that I tend to lose more weight with a lower carb diet although I feel physically better when I increase the starchy vegetables. It was important to me to take the time to find the balance that worked best for me. I realised that as long as the weight was going in a downwards trajectory then it didn't matter how long it took me to reach my final goal as I knew I would get there by eating what was right for me.

Having done many previous diets where the weight comes off quickly but you feel terrible I found for the first time ever that feeling good was just as important as the weight loss. It was also comforting to know that I had the tools and knowledge to make sure that I saw the weight loss through. I had always just felt a feeling of impending doom on previous diets knowing that it could never last as it simply wouldn't stand up to my cravings for chocolate cake!

I also found that increasing the fat content of my diet helped to kick-start my weight loss again which is something I never thought I would get to say! It is true that when you don't crave foods it can be easy to under-eat. I started to incorporate a few snacks to help increase my fat intake, again this is not simply a case of eating chocolate! I would have things such as a handful of nuts or some crudités and guacamole and I was shocked (but pleasantly surprised!) when this actually boosted my weight loss."

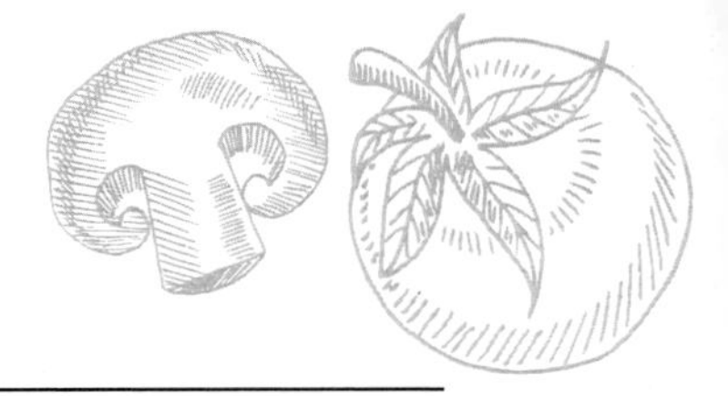

SECTION 15

Make It Individual to You

This is where knowing yourself is of vital importance and is when you become "self-managed" which is the ultimate goal of any self-development initiative. Over the 12 week programme your body will have had time to heal and repair, giving you the opportunity to really understand and connect with the links between body and mind as well as discover the benefits that optimal nutrition can bring.

The main goal of *Paleo: 12 Weeks to Change Your* Life is to help you make that transition to a truly sustainable and healthy lifestyle that can be maintained forever. This is the holy grail of the diet world and something which we truly hope you will be able to achieve.

The reason that we chose to implement a 12 week plan is that your body takes time to adjust and changes do not always occur as quickly as we would like. It takes time for new behaviours to become established and to become habit forming and reintroducing certain foods too early could result in cravings that you cannot cope with or inadvertently lead you back to where you started. Everything that you do during the 12 week programme is designed to lead you to a point where you are able to take control of your health and make sensible choices to fit you and your lifestyle. You will need to take everything that you have learnt and put it into practice. You will be surprised at how easy it has become and how much you want to keep going with the Paleo lifestyle. It is addictive and truly life changing.

Reintroducing foods

You may wish to consider reintroducing some of the foods that have so far been completely eliminated from your diet such as dairy. There are some toxic foods that you really don't want to be reintroducing such as highly processed packaged foods, refined sugars or processed oils; even if you do have the occasional dabble some of you may be affected more than others so be prepared! But there are certain foods that you may find suit you as part of a moderate diet. You may find that you tolerate cheese, butter and yoghurt perfectly well or that the occasional side dish of rice or cous-cous is something that you want to enjoy. Bread may have been one of the hardest foods to eliminate but when you try to reintroduce it you may discover you are completely intolerant to wheat or gluten; if that is the case you may find you have less of a reaction to pumpernickel or sourdough bread.

Introducing foods is a slow, very specific process. You need to be sure that a particular food (perhaps even right down to the producer) is responsible for certain symptoms or, conversely, utterly benign. The only way to do this is one food at a time.

Reactions can happen anywhere between a few minutes and a whole day. Mixing up foods to reintroduce gives you no way of knowing which food caused what reaction. We would suggest that you initially try to reintroduce one new food each week; this will then give you plenty of time to listen to your body and to determine whether the food is causing any reaction. This will differ for each person so just listen to your body carefully and do what feels right for you. Just please don't try re-introducing all the eliminated foods in one blow out meal. This will not end well!

Keep a note of the foods that you reintroduce and write down symptoms as they occur. It may be that a food causes no initial symptoms but as you progress it turns out that it doesn't suit you too well after all. It is all about continual assessment and getting to know when something is out of kilter with your body. You will most likely find that your body becomes very highly tuned and you will begin to notice even the smallest of "off days" which to most would just be considered as being normal. You should embrace the fact that you can be so in tune with your body. It is a rare thing and you have worked really hard to achieve it.

Only reintroduce foods when you are on an even keel; eating bread for the first time as a reaction to the stress of a new job is neither a healthy mindset or a good indication of how it may affect you. Be aware of why you make the choices that you do, especially if you have had an unhealthy relationship with food in the past.

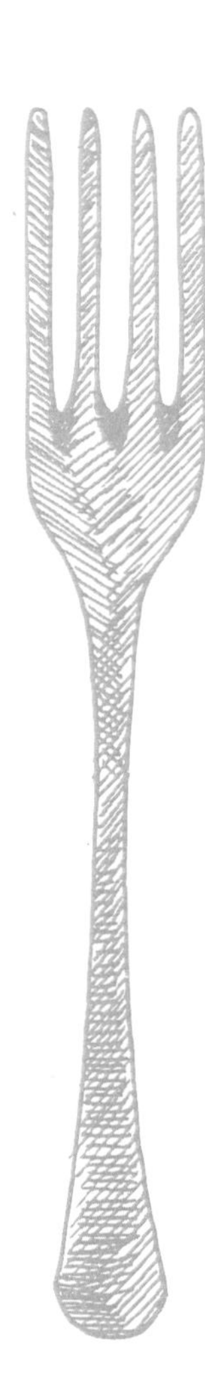

Case Study

"Once you get to the end of your 12 week programme it can be exciting at the thought of introducing some foods back into your diet. If you are anything like me and have struggled with eating issues all your life you will need to exercise some caution and restraint! If you decide to reintroduce food such as bread it can be easy for the balance to tip from moderation to becoming a daily habit. I found myself falling into this trap and had to take stock and realise how the change was affecting my body and making me feel bloated and lethargic. A feeling I had long since banished. Even knowing I felt better without it – it still takes time to readjust your mind set to get back on track.

I found that after completing the 12 week programme that I was much better equipped to deal with this situation but I can see that it would still be easy for me to slip back to old habits given the right circumstances. So just be careful of this.

I have found that caffeine is an easy habit to slip back into. After giving it up completely I now go through periods of drinking tea or coffee instead of herbal or decaffeinated and it definitely shows in my face and my skin. The decision for me is therefore what effects I find acceptable and to create a system of balance that works for me.

I think the one piece of advice I can really pass on is to just think carefully about what you want to introduce and why. Think about how good you feel without having that food in your diet and make a sensible and reasoned decision and when you do start reintroducing foods – do it slowly and remember moderation!"

A question of balance

It is not entirely realistic for most mere mortals to maintain a complete Paleo diet 100% of the time; this isn't about rigidity and unwavering self-control but rather about living a healthy life that comes naturally and with ease. We are after all only human and life is for enjoying. You will probably find that your craving for 'treats' will change; where once only ice cream would do, the ultimate comfort food becomes a piece of cheese or a bowl of porridge. Follow your Paleo plan 80% of the time and let the other 20% take care of itself.

The greatest quest in this life for most people, and often the hardest to achieve, is that of balance. If you can lose the weight, improve your health and energy levels, live your life and still make room for the things (including food) that really bring you pleasure then we have done what we set out to do. And so have you.

Clean detox reset

The final word, after congratulating you on taking part in this journey, concerns what to do if it all falls apart. Many people take on this challenge effortlessly, discover newly found vibrant health, and never look back. There is however a strong possibility that what brought you to the Paleo lifestyle was a life-long struggle with food issues and weight; you are after all the very person it was written for, and we have been there too.

If you find that you have gone way beyond the 80/20 balance and after reintroducing dairy and a few grains you suddenly realise that you have also reintroduced chocolate, crisps, soft drinks and the odd entire packet of biscuits, all you have to do is hit reset and start again. You know it works, you know how it works, and you also know how it fails. Get back on the horse, be kind to yourself, and start again…

Because there is no such thing as failure; just chances to learn and grow

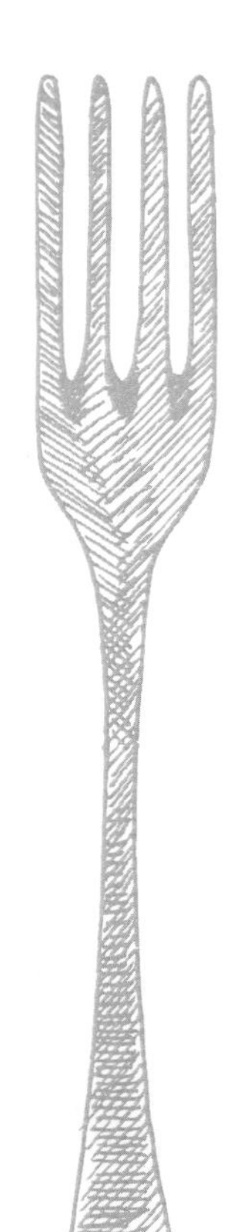

Case Study

"So here we are at my final case study entry. Well I am guessing that what you want to know is whether I achieved my goals? The answer is yes. At the end of my 12 week programme I had lost lost nearly two stone which equated to a loss of several inches in terms of body measurements. Throughout the 12 weeks I had managed to reduce my pain medication, eliminated my neck pain altogether and got my knee pain to a manageable state. I had learnt the importance of good food decisions and had rekindled my love for cooking. My skin was glowing and I had a new found confidence that made me smile so much more than I used to. I could not have been happier with my results.

I love the fact that Paleo is such an individualised approach. It makes it so different to every other diet I have previously tried. The flexibility of Paleo and the concept of making it individual to you makes it easier to move forward with Paleo as a life choice. I do not think of myself as being on a constant "diet", what I am doing is not dieting – it is simply eating what is good for my body.

I still allow myself treats and allow myself to enjoy the foods I love. If it is not a Paleo food I eat in moderation, this is something you will learn to do, it can be difficult but you will have the necessary tools to make these decisions. If your balance becomes skewed beyond moderation then you know what you have to do to change the situation and it can be rectified. No-one is perfect and we will all be there at times!

It is really not the rigid lifestyle that many would have you believe and I never feel deprived. I have learnt much more about food and nutrients and making sensible choices than I ever thought I would and feel empowered with this knowledge.

For me, three things really stick out about the Paleo diet. First, the biochemical information was a turning point for me making it much easier to make the right choices. Secondly, the feeling of being truly nourished and having your body fully functioning is a fantastic feeling. Being able to live your life with the energy and clarity of mind that it creates is something everyone should experience, but so few get to. Thirdly, it's not a diet. It is a lifestyle and a very flexible and satisfying one that I thoroughly enjoy.

All that remains is for me to wish you luck on your own Paleo journey. I know it can be tough, especially at the beginning, but you just need to stick with it. I am so pleased I made the transition and I know you will feel the same. Good luck".

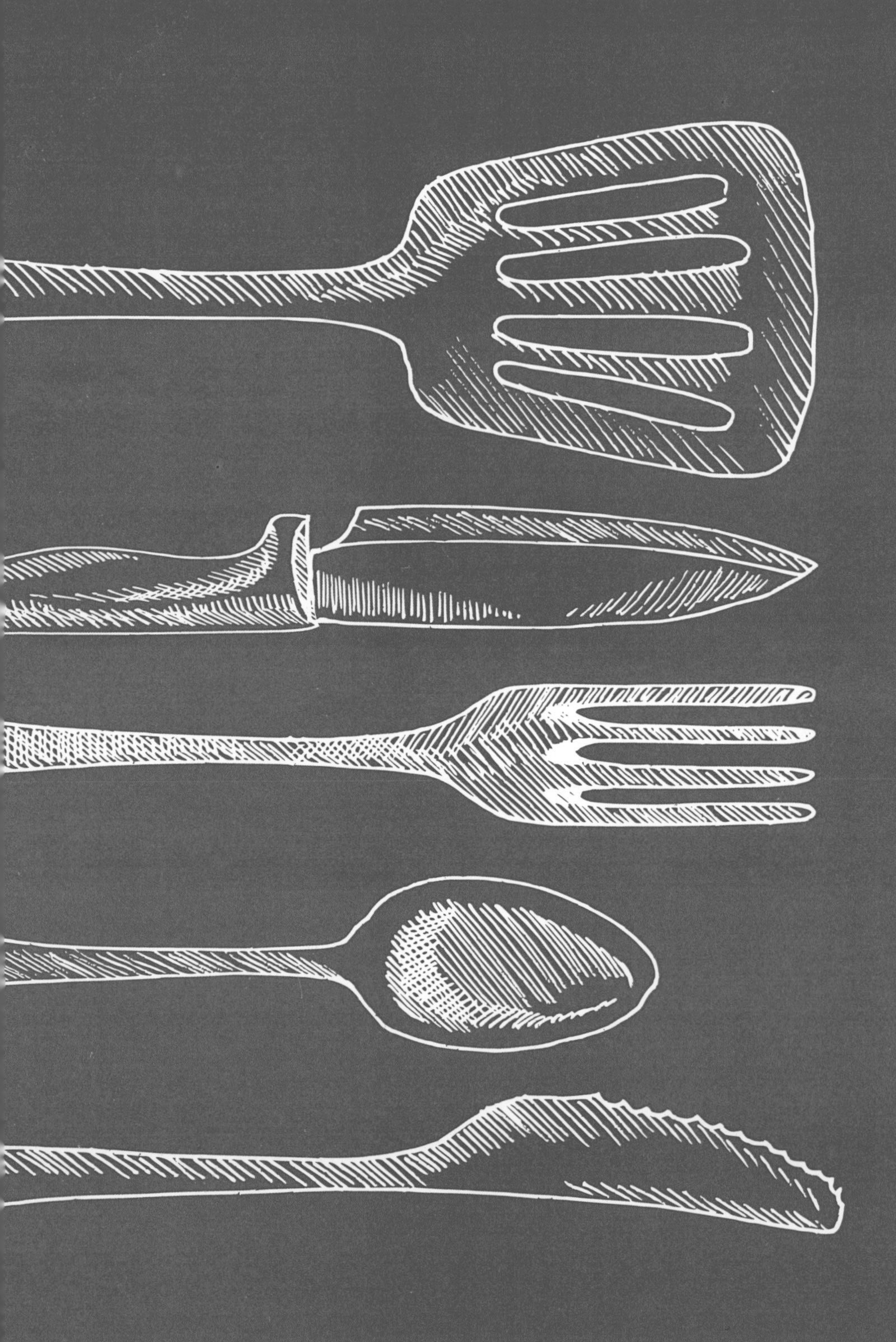

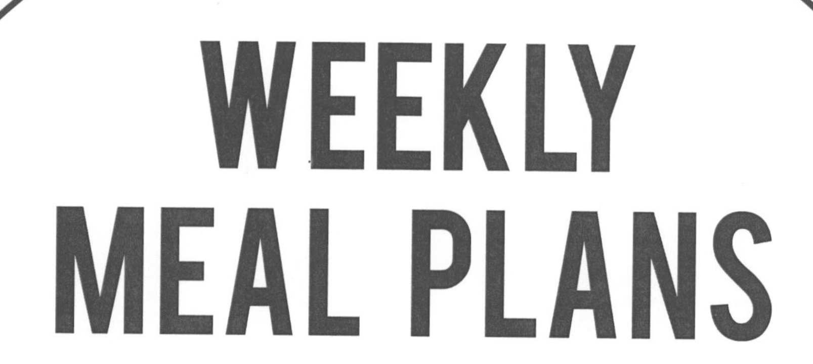

WEEKLY MEAL PLANS

We have provided a convenient weekly meal planner for you so that you can see what meals you will be having week by week.

If you want to swap any recipes around then please do so, there are plenty for you to choose from and you will soon discover your favourites. We would recommend that you try to keep your food choices varied as this will make sure that you are obtaining all the essential nutrients that you need. Plus it is always good to try something new.

We have included two dessert recipes for each week. You do not have to have them but there are there if you are having a sweet craving. Remember that you can always have a simple fruit salad or a small piece of dark chocolate for dessert if you prefer.

As snacks are down to individual need, we have not made provision for them on the weekly meal plans but they are of course there if you need them.

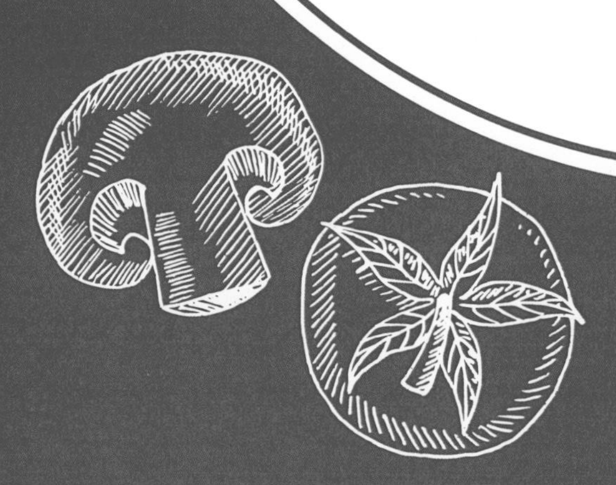

ONE

	BREAKFAST	LUNCH	DINNER	DESSERT
MONDAY	ushroom melette	Beef, Horseradish and Tomato Salad	Roast Chicken Roasted Roots Balsamic Green Beans	
TUESDAY	Scrambled Eggs with Spinach and Tomato	BLT Wrap	Lemon and Garlic Scallops Green Beans with Lemon	Lychee, Pineapple and Coconut Cream
WEDNESDAY	Breakfast Smoothie	Mustard Chicken Salad	Indian Lamb Burgers Tomato and Spring Onion Salad	
THURSDAY	Grain-Free Granola	Avocado, Tomato and Basil Salad	Fragrant Herb Chicken Curry Cauliflower Rice	
FRIDAY	Chopped Eggs with Olive Oil and Herbs	Chicken, Bacon and Mango Salad	Persian Chicken Kebabs Roasted Cauliflower with Mint Baba Ganoush	
SATURDAY	Baked Eggs Peperonata	Chilli Chicken Stir Fried Greens	Smoky Baked Chicken Basic Side Salad	Grilled Peaches with Cinnamon
SUNDAY	Full English	Squash and Bacon Soup	Cajun Cod Pan Steamed Carrots Pan Steamed Broccoli	

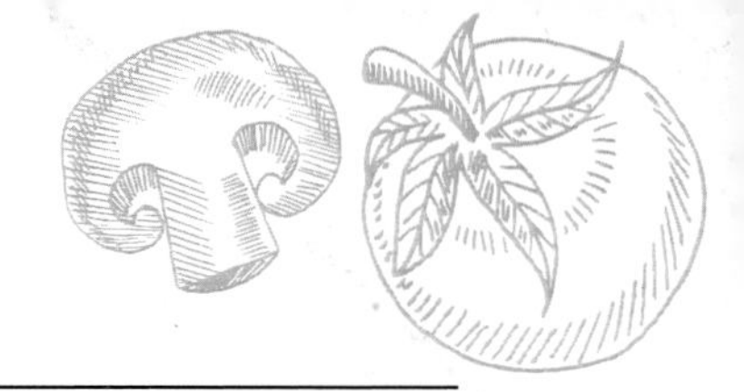

WEEK TWO

DAY	BREAKFAST	LUNCH	DINNER	DESSERT
MONDAY	*Ham and Tomato Omelette*	*Smoky Baked Chicken (leftover from Saturday)* *Avocado and Apple Salad*	*Sausages with Caraway Cabbage*	
TUESDAY	*Breakfast Salad*	*Lamb Meatballs* *Greek-Style Salad*	*Salmon with Tomato and Caper Dressing* *Spinach with Garlic and Raisins*	*Pan Fried Apples*
WEDNESDAY	*Scrambled Eggs with Mushrooms and Peppers*	*Leek and Celeriac Soup*	*Easy Lamb Curry* *Cauliflower Rice* *Tomato and Spring Onion Salad*	
THURSDAY	*Sausage Egg and Tomato–on-the-Run*	*Prawn and Avocado Salad*	*Turkey Burgers* *Sweet Potato Fries*	
FRIDAY	*Warm Spiced Apricot Compote with Granola (left over from Week One)*	*Mackerel and Watercress Salad with Horseradish*	*Garlic and Herb Chicken Breasts* *Simple Leaf Salad*	
SATURDAY	*Bacon and Eggs*	*Sesame Chicken Cakes* *Asian Dressing* *Simple Raw Slaw*	*Grilled Fresh Trout with Lemon and Parsley* *Peas with Onions and Bacon*	*Grilled Papaya with Lime*
SUNDAY	*Smoked Salmon Florentine*	*Scallops with Frisee and Bacon*	*Cocoa Steak* *Root Mash* *Pan Steamed Broccoli*	

WEEK THREE

DAY	BREAKFAST	LUNCH	DINNER	DESSERT
MONDAY	*Breakfast Smoothie*	*Herb Omelette Tuna Wrap*	*Fragrant Asian Steaks* *Sharp Asian Slaw*	
TUESDAY	*Chopped Eggs with Olive Oil and Herbs*	*Crab, Grilled Grapefruit and Rocket Salad*	*Gammon Steaks* *Roast Cinnamon Apples and Squash*	*Coconut Hot Chocolate*
WEDNESDAY	*Grain-Free Granola*	*Carrot and Ginger Soup*	*Baked Italian Chicken* *Simple Leaf Salad*	
THURSDAY	*Mushroom Omelette*	*Apple, Ham and Parsley Salad* *Mustard Vinaigrette*	*Aromatic Fish Parcels* *Broccoli with Mustard Seeds*	
FRIDAY	*Scrambled Eggs with Spinach and Tomato*	*Baked Italian Chicken (leftover from Wednesday)* *Simple Raw Slaw*	*Mushroom and Pepper Burger* *Simple Leaf Salad*	
SATURDAY	*Baked Eggs Peperonata*	*Roasted Root Salad with Orange and Thyme*	*Slow Baked Shoulder of Lamb* *Middle Eastern Herb Salad*	*Baked Banana Split*
SUNDAY	*Full English*	*Roast Chicken* *Roast Parsnips with Thyme and Bacon* *Pan Steamed Carrots* *Simple Kale*	*Bubble and Squeak*	

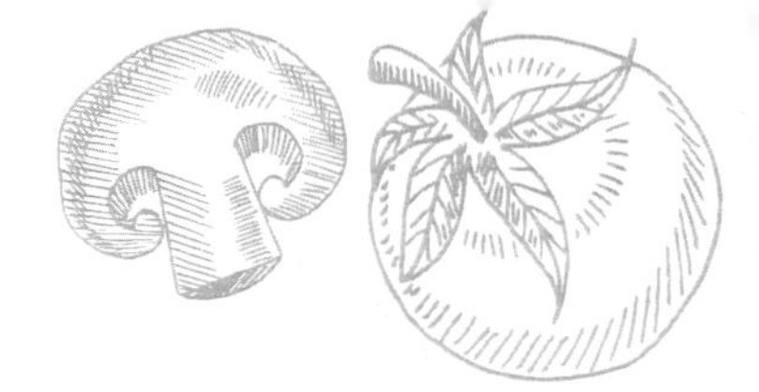

WEEK FOUR

DAY	BREAKFAST	LUNCH	DINNER	DESSERT
MONDAY	*Sausage Egg and Tomato-on-the-Run*	*Slow Baked Shoulder of Lamb (left from Saturday)* *Carrot and Coriander Salad* *Simple Leaf Salad*	*Pork Tenderloin with Sage and Tomato* *Beetroot and Peach Salad*	
TUESDAY	*Ham and Tomato Omelette*	*Chopped Italian Style Salad*	*Lemon and Parsley Baked Salmon* *Pan Steamed Carrots* *Pan Steamed Broccoli*	*Coconut Mango Sorbet*
WEDNESDAY	*Warm Spiced Apricot Compote with Granola (left over from Week Three)*	*Spinach Soup*	*Cinnamon and Black Pepper Chicken* *Roasted Mediterranean Vegetables*	
THURSDAY	*Breakfast Salad*	*Mediterranean Vegetable Salad*	*Middle Eastern Lamb Meatballs* *Cauliflower Rice*	
FRIDAY	*Scrambled Eggs with Mushroom and Peppers*	*Cinnamon and Black Pepper Chicken (leftover from Wednesday)* *Simple Leaf Salad*	*Beanless Beef Chilli* *Baked Sweet Potato* *Tomato and Spring Onion Salad*	
SATURDAY	*Bacon and Eggs*	*Prawn and Avocado Salad*	*Mexican Spice Burgers* *Guacamole* *Simple Raw Slaw*	*Warm Berries and Orange Compote*
SUNDAY	*Smoked Salmon Florentine*	*Italian Wrap*	*Beef Bourguignon* *Pan Steamed Broccoli*	

WEEK FIVE

DAY	BREAKFAST	LUNCH	DINNER	DESSERT
MONDAY	*Chopped Eggs with Olive Oil and Herbs*	*Papaya Prawn and Red Pepper Salad*	*Peri-Peri Chicken Skewers* *Coleslaw*	
TUESDAY	*Grain-Free Granola*	*Egg Salad*	*Sausage and Squash Lasagne* *Pear and Walnut Waldorf Salad* *Simple Leaf Salad*	*Roast Plums with Star Anise and Cashew Nut Cream*
WEDNESDAY	*Mushroom Omelette*	*Peri-Peri Chicken Skewers (leftovers from Monday)* *Roasted Pepper, Onion and Tomato Salad*	*Carne Asada* *Fennel, Almond and Pomegranate Salad*	
THURSDAY	*Breakfast Smoothie*	*Avocado and Bacon Wrap*	*Grilled Pork Chops with Peaches* *Roast Cauliflower with Turmeric* *Green Beans with Lemon*	
FRIDAY	*Scrambled Eggs with Spinach and Tomato*	*Carne Asada (leftovers from Wednesday)* *Greek-Style Salad* *Roast Pepper, Onion and Tomato Salad*	*Prawn Curry* *Cauliflower Rice*	
SATURDAY	*Baked Eggs Peperonata*	*Mexican Chicken Soup*	*Steak with Mixed Peppercorns* *Avocado and Apple Salad*	*Raspberry Ice Cream*
SUNDAY	*Full English*	*Ham, Mango and Red Cabbage Salad*	*Lamb Skewers with Herb Dressing* Sautéed Courgettes with Lemon	

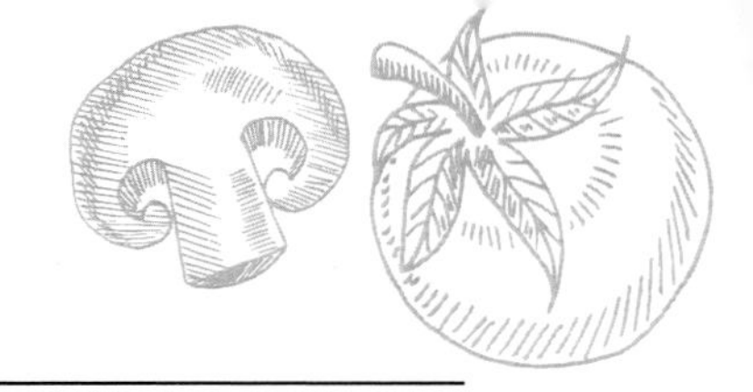

WEEK SIX

DAY	BREAKFAST	LUNCH	DINNER	DESSERT
MONDAY	*Breakfast Salad*	*Italian Wrap*	*Gammon Steaks* *Roast Cinnamon Apples and Squash*	
TUESDAY	*Scrambled Eggs with Mushroom and Peppers*	*Avocado and Bacon Wrap*	*Roast Chicken* *Root Mash*	*Vanilla Pears*
WEDNESDAY	*Ham and Tomato Omelette*	*Apple, Ham and Parsley Salad*	*Baked Italian Chicken* *Balsamic Green Beans*	
THURSDAY	*Warm Spiced Apricot Compote with Granola (left over from Week Five)*	*Chicken, Sun Dried Tomato, Olive and Herb Salad*	*Burger with Watercress Sauce and Butternut Squash*	
FRIDAY	*Sausage Egg and Tomato-on-the-Run*	*Mackerel and Watercress Salad with Horseradish*	*Steak and Eggs* *Sweet Potato Fries*	
SATURDAY	*Bacon and Eggs*	*White Wine and Garlic Mussels*	*Monkfish in Parma Ham* *Peas with Artichokes*	*Rhubarb, Rose and Raspberry Compote*
SUNDAY	*Smoked Salmon Florentine*	*Clear and Calm Soup*	*Classic Beef Stew* *Roasted Roots* *Simple Kale (half recipe)*	

WEEK SEVEN

DAY	BREAKFAST	LUNCH	DINNER	DESSERT
MONDAY	*Grain-Free Granola*	*Asian Tuna Wrap*	*Pan Fried Rosemary Chicken* *Greens with Lemon, Olive Oil and Garlic*	
TUESDAY	*Breakfast Smoothie*	*Squash and Bacon Soup*	*Horseradish and Parsley Burger* *Simple Leaf Salad* *Sweet Potato Fries*	*Lychee, Pineapple and Coconut Cream*
WEDNESDAY	*Mushroom Omelette*	*Pan Fried Rosemary Chicken (leftovers from Monday)* *Tomato and Avocado Salad*	*Salmon with Avocado Salsa* *Basic Side Salad*	
THURSDAY	*Chopped Eggs with Olive Oil and Herbs*	*Mega Mixed Veggie Salad* *Mustard Vinaigrette*	*Stir Fry Duck Breast with Asian Greens* *Sharp Asian Slaw*	
FRIDAY	*Scrambled Eggs with Spinach and Tomato*	*Avocado and Bacon Wrap*	*Chicken Fajita Bowl*	
SATURDAY	*Baked Eggs Peperonata*	*Bacon and Frisee Salad*	*Beef Goulash* *Simple Kale*	*Pan Fried Apples*
SUNDAY	*Full English*	*Chicken Fajita Bowl (leftovers from Friday)* *Simple Leaf Salad*	*Lamb Chops with Cracked Coriander* *Fiery Aubergine Dip*	

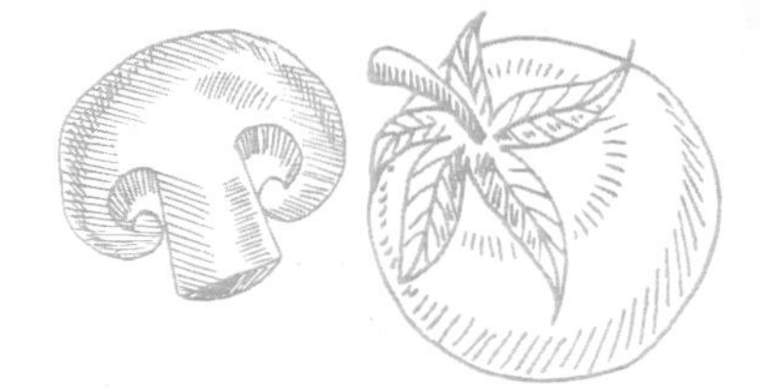

WEEK EIGHT

DAY	BREAKFAST	LUNCH	DINNER	DESSERT
MONDAY	*Sausage Egg and Tomato-on-the-Run*	*Lamb Chops with Cracked Coriander (Leftovers from Sunday)* *Tomato and Avocado Salad*	*BBQ Pork Burger* *Sweet Potato Fries*	
TUESDAY	*Ham and Tomato Omelette*	*Courgette and Mint Soup*	*Garlic Steak* *Red Salad* *Mustard Vinaigrette*	*Warm Berries with Orange Compote*
WEDNESDAY	*Scrambled Eggs with Mushroom and Peppers*	*Fig, Ham and Pistachio Salad*	*Sausage and Pepper Casserole* *Greens with Chilli and Walnut*	
THURSDAY	*Breakfast Salad*	*Chicken, Bacon and Mango Salad*	*Pork with Sage, Apples and Onions* *Wilted Spinach*	
FRIDAY	*Warm Spiced Apricot Compote with Granola (left over from Week Seven)*	*Spinach and Squash Soup*	*Chicken Breast Stuffed with Mushroom, Bacon and Herbs* *Simple Leaf Salad*	
SATURDAY	*Bacon and Eggs*	*Chilli Chicken Stir Fried Greens*	*Easy Lamb Curry* *Cauliflower Rice*	*Baked Banana Split*
SUNDAY	*Smoked Salmon Florentine*	*Peri-Peri Chicken Skewers* *Tomato and Spring Onion Salad*	*Jamaican Jerk Chicken* *Fennel, Almond and Pomegranate Salad*	

WEEK NINE

DAY	BREAKFAST	LUNCH	DINNER	DESSERT
MONDAY	*Chopped Eggs with Olive Oil and Herbs*	*Crab and Avocado Cocktail*	*Fragrant Chicken Kebabs* *Rocket, Cucumber, Pistachio and Pomegranate Salad*	
TUESDAY	*Breakfast Smoothie*	*Salmon, Spring Onion and Cucumber Wrap*	*Olive, Garlic & Lemon Chicken* *Broccoli with Cashew Nuts*	*Coconut Mango Sorbet*
WEDNESDAY	*Scrambled Eggs with Spinach and Tomato*	*Curried Cauliflower Soup*	*King Prawns with Paprika and Fennel Seed* *Simple Raw Slaw*	
THURSDAY	*Grain-Free Granola*	*Leek and Bacon Soup*	*Marinated Tuna Steaks* *Avocado, Red Onion and Green Pepper Salsa*	
FRIDAY	*Mushroom Omelette*	*Fig, Ham and Pistachio Salad*	*Sweet and Sour Pork* *Cauliflower Rice*	
SATURDAY	*Baked Eggs Peperonata*	*Roasted Root Salad with Orange and Thyme*	*Shepherds Pie* *Sautéed Carrots with Fresh Herbs*	*Grilled Peaches with Cinnamon*
SUNDAY	*Full English*	*Scallops with Frisee and Bacon*	*Kleftiko* *Greek-Style Salad* *Fried Sweet Potatoes*	

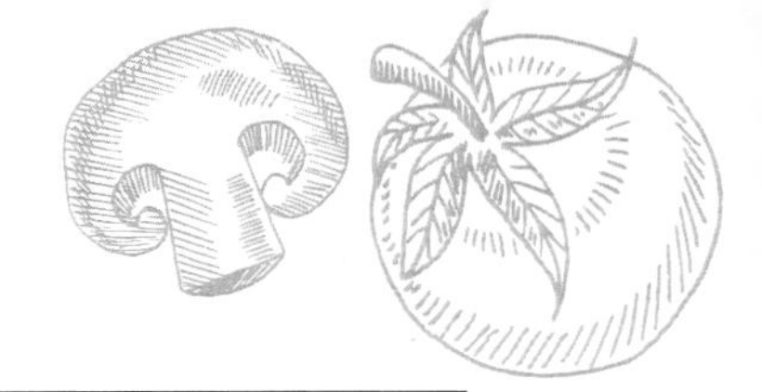

WEEK TEN

DAY	BREAKFAST	LUNCH	DINNER	DESSERT
MONDAY	*Scrambled Eggs with Mushroom and Peppers*	*Kleftiko (leftovers from Sunday)* *Roasted Pepper, Onion and Tomato Salad*	*Roast Chicken* *Coleslaw* *Baked Sweet Potato*	
TUESDAY	*Breakfast Salad*	*Chicken, Tomato and Tarragon* *Simple Leaf Salad*	*Mushroom and Pepper Burger* *Simple Leaf Salad*	*Roast Plums with Star Anise and Cashew Nut Cream*
WEDNESDAY	*Ham and Tomato Omelette*	*Roasted Pepper, Onion and Tomato Salad (leftovers from Monday)* *Greek-Style Salad*	*Sole with Lemon and Thyme* *Pan Steamed Carrots* *Pan Steamed Broccoli*	
THURSDAY	*Sausage Egg and Tomato-on-the-Run*	*Chorizo and Savoy Cabbage Broth*	*Olive, Garlic & Lemon Chicken* Simple Kale	
FRIDAY	*Warm Spiced Apricot Compote with Granola (left over from Week Nine)*	*Prawn and Avocado Salad*	*Sage and Onion Chicken Burger* *Simple Raw Slaw*	
SATURDAY	*Bacon and Eggs*	*Herb Omelette Tuna Wrap*	*Greek Stifado* *Green Beans with Lemon* *Simple Kale (leftovers from Thursday)*	*Vanilla Pears*
SUNDAY	*Smoked Salmon Florentine*	*Sage and Onion Chicken Burger (leftovers from Friday)* *Spinach, Apple and Fennel Salad*	*Awesome Pulled Pork* *Radicchio and Orange Salad*	

WEEK ELEVEN

DAY	BREAKFAST	LUNCH	DINNER	DESSERT
MONDAY	*Mushroom Omelette*	*Awesome Pulled Pork (leftovers from Sunday)* *Coleslaw* *Simple Leaf Salad*	*Roast Chicken* *Roasted Roots* *Balsamic Green Beans*	
TUESDAY	*Chopped Eggs with Olive Oil and Herbs*	*Avocado, Tomato and Basil Salad*	*Lemon and Garlic Scallops* *Green Beans with Lemon*	*Coconut Mango Sorbet*
WEDNESDAY	*Scrambled Eggs with Spinach and Tomato*	*Mustard Chicken Salad*	*Indian Lamb Burgers* *Tomato and Spring Onion Salad*	
THURSDAY	*Grain-Free Granola*	*Beef, Horseradish and Tomato Salad*	*Smoky Baked Chicken* *Basic Side Salad*	
FRIDAY	*Breakfast Smoothie*	*Chicken, Bacon and Mango Salad*	*Fragrant Herb Chicken Curry* *Cauliflower Rice*	
SATURDAY	*Baked Eggs Peperonata*	*Squash and Bacon Soup*	*Persian Chicken Kebabs* *Roasted Cauliflower with Mint* *Baba Ganoush*	*Grilled Papaya with Lime*
SUNDAY	*Full English*	*Chilli Chicken Stir Fried Greens*	*Cajun Cod* *Pan Steamed Carrots* *Pan Steamed Broccoli*	

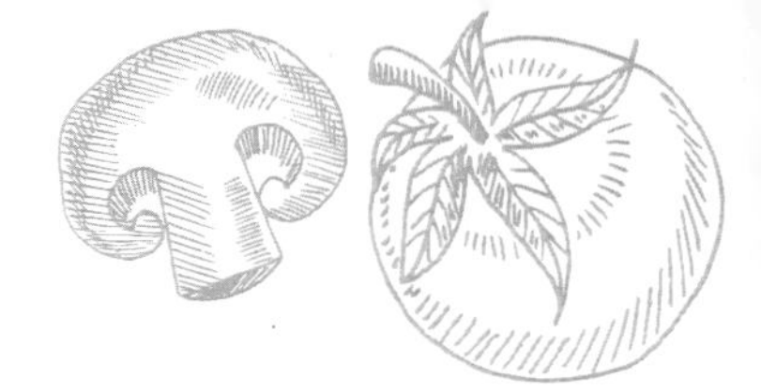

WEEK TWELVE

DAY	BREAKFAST	LUNCH	DINNER	DESSERT
MONDAY	*Breakfast Salad*	*Roast Chicken* *Coleslaw* *Baked Sweet Potato*	*Salmon with Tomato and Caper Dressing* *Green Beans with Lemon*	
TUESDAY	*Scrambled Eggs with Mushroom and Peppers*	*Mustard Chicken Salad*	*Grilled Pork Chops with Peaches* *Greens with Lemon, Olive Oil and Garlic*	*Coconut Hot Chocolate*
WEDNESDAY	*Warm Spiced Apricot Compote with Granola (left over from Week Eleven)*	*Herb Omelette Tuna Wrap*	*Smoky Baked Chicken* *Basic Side Salad*	
THURSDAY	*Ham and Tomato Omelette*	*Smoky Baked Chicken (leftovers from Wednesday)*	*Indian Lamb Burgers* *Simple Leaf Salad* *Tomato and Spring Onion Salad*	
FRIDAY	*Sausage Egg and Tomato on-the-Run*	*Prawn and Avocado Salad*	*Chicken Fajita Bowl*	
SATURDAY	*Bacon and Eggs*	*Sesame Chicken Cakes* *Sharp Asian Slaw* *Asian Dressing*	*Cocoa Steak* *Greek-Style Salad*	*Grilled Peaches with Cinnamon*
SUNDAY	*Smoked Salmon Florentine*	*Scallops with Frisee and Bacon*	*Beef Goulash* *Pan Steamed Broccoli* *Pan Steamed Carrots*	

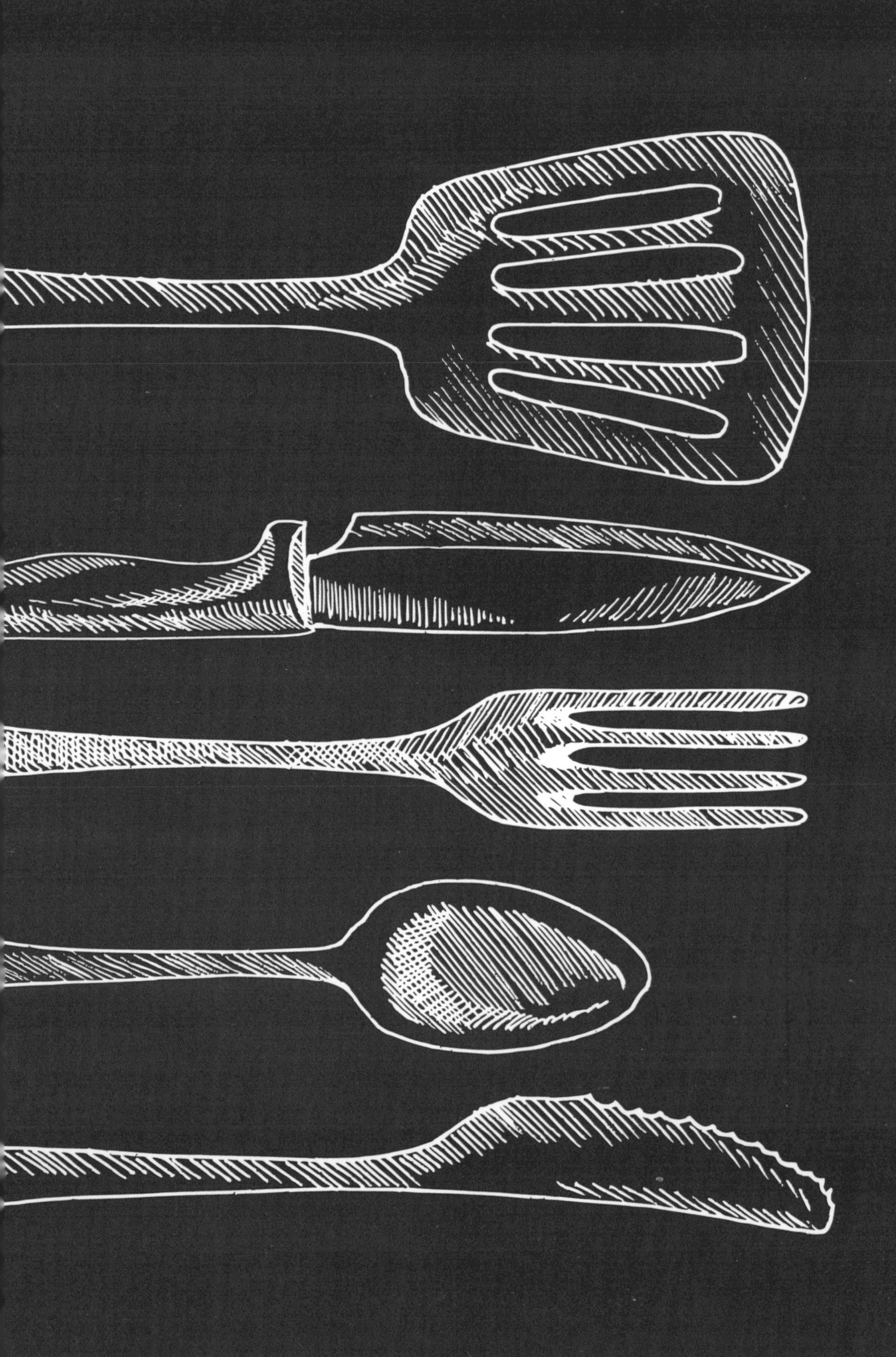

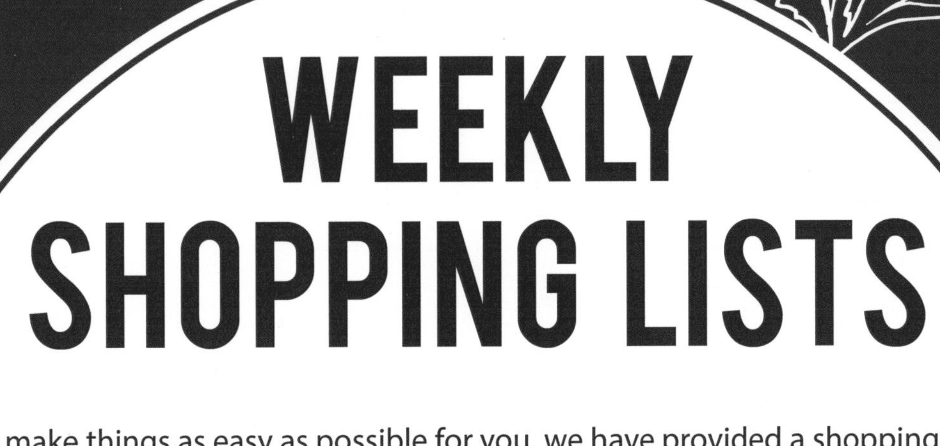

WEEKLY SHOPPING LISTS

To make things as easy as possible for you, we have provided a shopping list to go with each of the weekly meal plans. The shopping list will include everything that you need in order to make the recipes for each week as stated on the relevant meal plan.

We would suggest that you review the weekly meal plan to see if there are any recipes you want to amend or switch around and then remember to adjust your shopping list accordingly.

The shopping list will assume that you have used up all the ingredients from the week before, including store cupboard ingredients, it is therefore a good idea to check what ingredients you have left over and cross those you do not need off the list.

We have not included any ingredients for snacks in the shopping lists as this is a personal choice as to whether you want to incorporate them into your weekly routine. If you would like to include snacks in your weekly shop then please make sure that you add any ingredients you require onto your list.

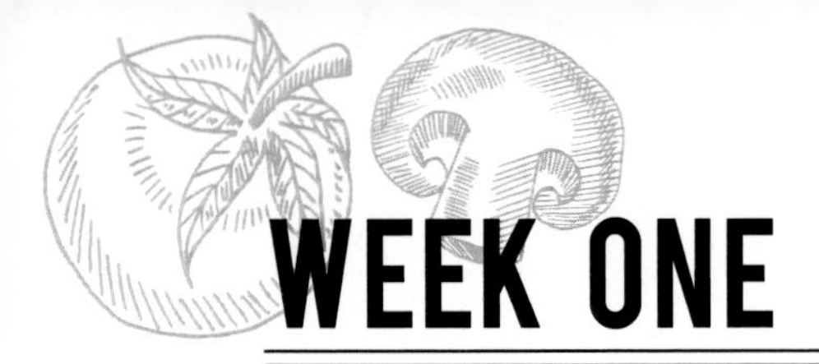

WEEK ONE

Fruit and Vegetables

1 green apple
2 avocados
1 banana
1 orange
2 large peaches
1 pineapple
5 lemons
3 limes
1 mango
1 iceberg lettuce
1 cucumber
2 portabella mushrooms
3 bags mixed salad leaf
1 bag rocket
100g spinach
1 bunch spring onions
4 bok choi
2 punnets cherry tomatoes
20 tomatoes
150g mushrooms
2 red bell peppers
1 bunch coriander
1 bunch basil
3 sprigs fresh thyme
2 bunches mint
1 bunch parsley
2 bulbs garlic
1 small piece fresh ginger
2 green chillies
3 red chillies
1 head broccoli
2 heads cauliflower
1 butternut squash
4 parsnips
1 aubergine
¼ white cabbage
¼ red cabbage
11 carrots
400g green beans
5 white onions
6 red onions
4 shallots

Fresh Seafood

2 cod fillets
400g scallops

Meat and Poultry

20 rashers bacon
8 chicken thighs, boneless with skin on
8 chicken thighs, on the bone with skin on
4 chicken breasts
2 small chickens
400g lamb mince
4 pork sausages

Store Cupboard

400g tin of lychees (or fresh if you can get them)
400g tinned tomatoes
1 tbsp dijon mustard
1 tbsp horseradish
2 tbsp raw honey
400ml coconut milk
1 carton of almond milk
200ml creamed coconut
1 tbsp almond butter
1 tbsp tahini
50g gherkin (pickled in jar)
1 tbsp madras curry powder or paste

Prepared Foods (Homemade if possible, Paleo friendly if not)

500ml chicken stock
Paleo mayonnaise

Cooking Oils

400g lard, beef dripping or goose fat
Coconut oil
Olive oil

Dressings

Extra virgin olive oil
Balsamic vinegar
Walnut oil

Eggs

2 dozen eggs

Deli

300g cooked beef
100g kalamata olives

Dried Fruit

30g dates
50g dried cranberries

Nuts and Seeds

50g flaked almonds
50g ground almonds
50g cashew nuts, unsalted
50g pecans
50g pumpkin seeds
50g sunflower seeds
100g walnuts
50g flax seed
50g coconut flakes

Spices and Seasonings

2 bay leafs
Black pepper
2 tsp cayenne pepper
1 tbsp chilli powder
3 tsp coriander seed, ground
3 tsp garlic powder
2 tsp ground cinnamon
1 tsp ground ginger
1 whole nutmeg
3 tsp ground oregano
3 tsp turmeric
1 tsp paprika
1 tsp ground cumin
2 tbsp smoked paprika
Sea salt

Frozen Fruit

100g frozen berries

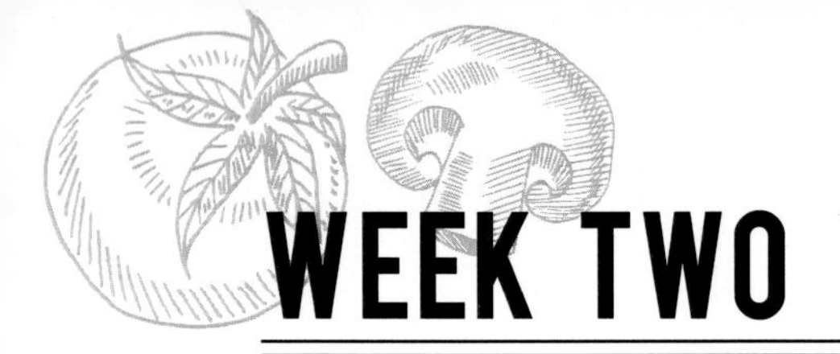

WEEK TWO

Fruit and Vegetables

7 green apples
2 oranges
1 papaya
9 lemons
4 limes
6 avocados
1 cucumber
2 red bell peppers
6 mushrooms
18 tomatoes
2 bunches spring onions
1 bag frisee curly leaf salad

3 bags mixed salad leaves
1 bag watercress
1 bag rocket
250g spinach
1 bunch coriander
1 bunch parsley
1 bunch basil
1 bunch mint
50g bean sprouts
1 bulb garlic
3 red chillies
1 small piece fresh ginger

1 head broccoli
1 cauliflower
¼ white cabbage
½ savoy cabbage
½ red cabbage
5 carrots
½ celeriac
3 parsnips
½ swede
2 large sweet potatoes
2 leeks
5 white onions
4 red onions

Fresh Seafood

200g cooked prawns
2 salmon fillets
10 scallops
2 smoked mackerel fillets
2 trout, whole

Meat and Poultry

20 rashers bacon
2 chicken breasts
400g diced lamb
400g chicken mince
400g lamb mince
100g lardons
12 pork sausages
2 sirloin or rib eye steaks
500g turkey mince

Store Cupboard

1 tin chopped tomatoes
2 tbsp capers
1 tbsp horseradish
1 tbsp raw honey
1 tsp unsweetened cocoa powder
2 tbsp rogan josh spice mix or paste

Prepared Foods (Homemade if possible, Paleo friendly if not)

500ml chicken stock

Cooking Oils

400g lard, dripping or goose fat
Coconut oil
Olive oil
Sesame oil

Dressings

Extra virgin olive oil
Balsamic vinegar
White wine vinegar
Walnut oil

Eggs

2 ½ dozen eggs

Deli

100g smoked salmon
100g sun dried tomatoes
200g baked ham
16 black olives

Dried Fruit

100g dried apricots
2 tbsp raisins

Nuts and Seeds

50g almonds
100g sesame seeds

Spices and Seasonings

Black pepper
1 tsp caraway seed
1 tsp chinese five spices
1 cinnamon stick
1 tsp ground cumin seed
1 tsp ground coriander seed
1 tsp ground allspice
2 tsp ground cinnamon
1 whole nutmeg
1 tsp ground oregano
1 tsp ground thyme
3 tsp paprika
1 tsp garlic powder
Sea salt

Frozen Vegetables

200g frozen peas

WEEK THREE

Fruit and Vegetables

5 green apples
3 bananas
2 oranges
50g raspberries
1 ruby grapefruit
4 lemons
3 limes
100g bean sprouts
20 cherry tomatoes
4 baby beetroot, raw
3 bunches spring onions
150g mushrooms
6 portabella mushrooms
3 red bell peppers
1 ½ cucumbers
14 tomatoes
3 bags mixed salad leaves
150g spinach
200g rocket
1 bunch coriander
2 bunches parsley
1 small bunch basil
1 sprig oregano
1 large bunch mint
3 sprigs fresh rosemary
10 sprigs fresh thyme
3 bulbs garlic
1 large piece of fresh ginger
2 sticks lemongrass
3 red chilli peppers
2 sweet potatoes
1 butternut squash
2 heads broccoli
12 carrots
4 parsnips
150g baby carrots
150g baby parsnips
½ white cabbage
¼ red cabbage
200g kale
1 leek
3 white onions
2 red onions
8 shallots

Fresh Seafood

2 cod fillets
200g white crab meat

Meat and Poultry

6 rashers bacon
500g beef mince
8 chicken drumsticks, with skin on
8 chicken thighs, with skin on
2 small chickens
4 pork sausages
1 small shoulder of lamb
4 gammon steaks (thick cut)
2 sirloin steaks

Store Cupboard

1 tin tuna, in spring water or brine
3 tins chopped tomatoes
100g dark chocolate, 60-70% cacao solids
1 tbsp coconut aminos (available in health food stores or online)
2 tbsp raw honey
1 tbsp almond butter
1 carton almond milk
400ml coconut milk
1 tbsp dijon mustard

Prepared Foods (Homemade if possible, Paleo friendly if not)

500ml chicken stock
500ml vegetable stock

Cooking Oils

400g lard, dripping or goose fat
Coconut oil
Olive oil
Sesame oil

Dressings

Extra virgin olive oil
Walnut oil
Balsamic vinegar

Eggs

3 dozen eggs

Deli

100g kalamata olives

Dried Fruit

30g dates
50g dried cranberries

Nuts and Seeds

100g almonds
30g coconut flakes
75g flaked almonds
50g ground almonds
50g cashew nuts, unsalted
50g pumpkin seeds
1 tsp sesame seeds
50g walnuts
30g flax seed
50g sunflower seeds

Spices and Seasonings

5 bay leaves
Black pepper
1 tsp coriander seed
1 tsp ground allspice
1 tsp ground cinnamon
1 tsp ground oregano
1 tsp paprika
Sea salt
1 tsp black peppercorns
2 star anise
1 tbsp mustard seeds

Frozen Fruit

100g frozen berries

WEEK FOUR

Fruit and Vegetables

3 oranges
7 avocados
1 mango
2 large peaches
6 lemons
1 lime
3 red bell peppers
1 yellow bell pepper
100g beetroot, raw
2 courgettes
50g bean sprouts
2 bunches spring onions
½ cucumber
2 bulbs fennel
1 aubergine
1.1kg mushrooms
16 tomatoes
2 bags rocket
1 romaine lettuce
1 iceberg lettuce
4 bags mixed leaf salad
350g spinach
2 bunches coriander
1 small bunch basil
1 small bunch sage
1 bunch parsley
2 sprigs fresh thyme
2 bulbs garlic
2 jalapeno peppers
1 red chilli
2 heads broccoli
1 head cauliflower
¼ white cabbage
¼ red cabbage
9 carrots
2 large sweet potatoes
7 white onions
6 red onions
20 shallots

Fresh Seafood

200g cooked prawns
2 salmon fillets

Meat and Poultry

20 rashers bacon
1.3kg beef mince
8 chicken drumsticks, with skin on
8 chicken thighs, with skin on
500g lamb mince
4 pork sausages
1 pork tenderloin (500g)
500g stewing beef

Store Cupboard

300ml red wine
2 tins chopped tomatoes
100ml coconut milk
1 tube tomato puree
1 small jar roasted red bell peppers
1 large jar artichoke hearts

Prepared Foods (Homemade if possible, Paleo friendly if not)

500ml chicken stock

Cooking Oils

400g lard, dripping or goose fat

Coconut oil

Olive oil

Dressings

Extra virgin olive oil

White wine vinegar

Balsamic vinegar

Eggs

2 ½ dozen eggs

Deli

300g cooked chicken (should be leftovers from week 3 available – please check)

36 black olives
24 slices salami
100g smoked salmon

100g sun dried tomatoes
200g baked ham

Dried Fruit

100g dried apricots

2 tbsp raisins

Nuts and Seeds

50g almonds

Spices and Seasonings

1 bay leaf
Black pepper
1 tsp chilli powder
2 cinnamon sticks
3 tsp ground cumin seed

1 tsp ground coriander seed
2 tsp ground cinnamon
2 tsp ground oregano

6 tsp paprika
Sea salt
1 whole nutmeg
1 tsp dried thyme

Frozen Fruit

400g frozen mango cubes

200g frozen berries

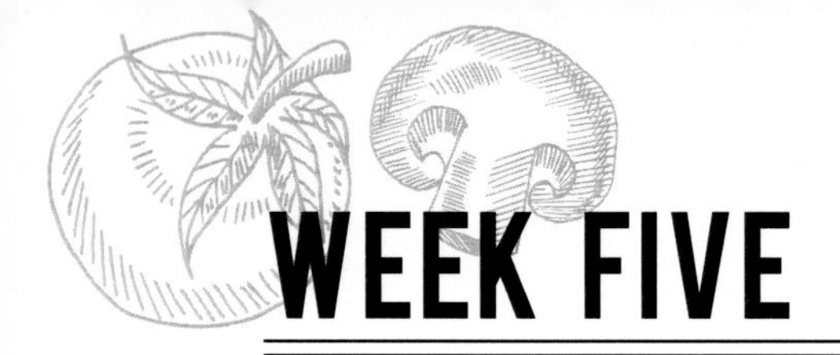

WEEK FIVE

Fruit and Vegetables

2 green apples
2 oranges
1 mango
1 large peach
2 large pears
2 papaya
8 plums
1 pomegranate
2 bananas
5 lemons
6 limes
4 avocados
2 portabella mushrooms
3 red bell peppers
4 courgettes
3 sticks celery
1 ½ cucumbers
1 bulb fennel
150g mushrooms
2 bunches spring onions
17 tomatoes
32 cherry tomatoes
3 bags mixed salad leaves
1 iceberg lettuce
2 bags rocket
100g spinach
2 bunches coriander
2 bunches parsley
1 small bunch dill
2 bunches mint
2 sprigs rosemary
1 small bunch sage
2 sprigs thyme
1 small piece fresh ginger
3 bulbs garlic
10 small red birds eye chillies
3 red chilli peppers
4 green chilli peppers
2 heads cauliflower
½ white cabbage
¼ red cabbage
1 butternut squash
1 carrot
200g green beans
3 white onions
7 red onions

Fresh Seafood

400g king prawns
200g cooked prawns

Meat and Poultry

12 rashers bacon
4 chicken breasts
1 small chicken
400g diced lamb
300g cumberland sausage
2 pork chops (bone in)
4 pork sausages
3 rib eye steaks (200-250g each)
2 sirloin steaks (200-250g each)

Store Cupboard

4 tins chopped tomatoes
2 tbsp raw honey
1 tbsp almond butter
250ml coconut milk
Bamboo skewers
2 tbsp tomato puree
1 carton of almond milk
1 tsp dijon mustard
1 tbsp Madras curry powder or paste

Prepared Foods (Homemade if possible, Paleo friendly if not)

Paleo mayonnaise

Cooking Oils

400g lard, dripping or goose fat

Coconut oil

Olive oil

Dressings

Extra virgin olive oil

Balsamic vinegar

Cider vinegar

White wine vinegar

Walnut oil

Eggs

2 ½ dozen eggs

Deli

400g roasted red bell peppers

300g thick cut ham

28 kalamata olives

Dried Fruit

30g dates

50g dried cranberries

Nuts and Seeds

50g almonds

30g coconut flakes

50g flaked almonds

75g ground almonds

100g cashew nuts, unsalted

50g pumpkin seeds

50g sunflower seeds

100g walnuts

30g flax seed

Spices and Seasonings

1 bay leaf

Black pepper

2 tsp cumin seed

1 tsp garlic powder

4 tbsp curry powder

1 tsp green peppercorns

1 tsp pink peppercorns

1 tsp white peppercorns

1 tsp black peppercorns

1 tsp ground allspice

2 tsp ground cinnamon

2 tsp ground oregano

1 tbsp turmeric

2 tbsp paprika

2 star anise

Sea salt

Frozen Fruit

100g frozen berries

150g frozen raspberries

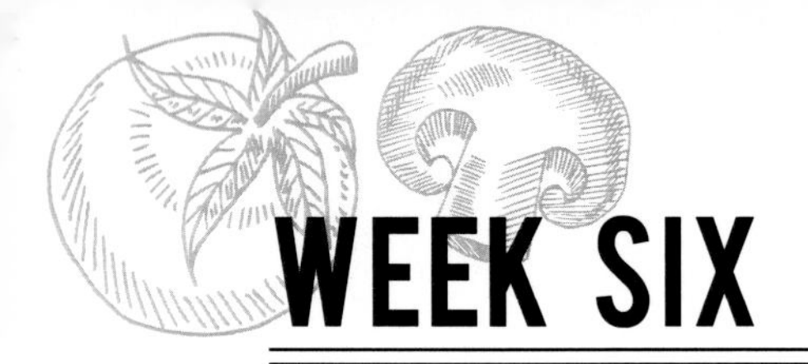

WEEK SIX

Fruit and Vegetables

5 green apples
2 oranges
2 large pears
150g raspberries
500g rhubarb, raw
2 lemons
4 avocados
1 bunch spring onions
6 mushrooms
100g bok choi
1 red bell pepper
14 tomatoes
1 iceberg lettuce
2 bags mixed salad leaves
1 bag rocket
150g spinach
200g watercress
1 small bunch chives
1 small bunch coriander
1 bunch parsley
1 sprig rosemary
2 sprigs oregano
7 sprigs thyme
2 bulbs garlic
2 inch piece fresh ginger
1 stick lemongrass
2 red chilli peppers
2 butternut squash
2 large sweet potatoes
½ swede
11 carrots
11 parsnips
200g green beans
100g kale
2 leeks
6 white onions
4 red onions
4 shallots

Fresh Seafood

2 monkfish fillets
1kg fresh mussels

Meat and Poultry

20 rashers bacon
800g beef brisket
2 small chickens
500g beef mince
4 pork sausages
8 chicken drumsticks, with skin on
8 chicken thighs, with skin on
400g gammon steaks (thick cut)
2 sirloin steaks (200 – 250g each)

Store Cupboard

200ml white wine
1 tsp dijon mustard
1 tbsp horseradish
1 tbsp rose water
1 tbsp raw honey
2 tbsp tomato puree
1 small jar roasted red bell peppers
1 jar artichoke hearts
2 tins chopped tomatoes

Prepared Foods (Homemade if possible, Paleo friendly if not)

1 litre chicken stock
Paleo mayonnaise

Cooking Oils

400g lard, dripping or goose fat
Coconut oil
Olive oil

Dressings

Extra virgin olive oil
Balsamic vinegar
White wine vinegar
Walnut oil

Eggs

3 dozen eggs

Deli

200g kalamata olives
2 slices parma ham
200g baked ham
8 slices salami
300g cooked chicken (if no leftovers available – please check)
100g smoked salmon
100g sun dried tomatoes
2 fillets smoked mackerel

Dried Fruit

100g dried apricots

Nuts and Seeds

100g cashew nuts, unsalted
125g walnuts

Spices and Seasonings

5 bay leaves
Black pepper
1 cinnamon stick
1 tsp ground cinnamon
2 tbsp paprika
Sea salt
1 vanilla pod
1 tsp dried mixed herbs

Frozen Vegetables

300g frozen peas
200g frozen berries

WEEK SEVEN

Fruit and Vegetables

6 green apples
¼ pineapple
1 banana
3 lemons
5 limes
8 avocados
2 portabella mushrooms
6 radishes
7 red bell peppers
200g bean sprouts
4 bok choi
1 aubergine
2 cucumbers
1 bulb fennel
2 bunches spring onions
150g mushrooms
1 yellow bell pepper
13 tomatoes
3 punnets cherry tomatoes
4 bags mixed salad leaves
1 bag frisee curly leaf salad
1 iceberg lettuce
100g spinach
1 small bunch coriander
1 bunch parsley
1 small bunch mint
4 sprigs rosemary
2 bulbs garlic
2 red chilli peppers
2 inch piece fresh ginger
2 large sweet potatoes
1 butternut squash
4 carrots
200g kale
¼ red cabbage
½ savoy cabbage
1 leek
6 white onions
5 red onions

Fresh Seafood

2 wild salmon fillets

Meat and Poultry

20 rashers bacon
4 chicken breasts
8 chicken legs, skin on
2 duck breasts
16 lamb chops
500g minced beef
4 pork sausages
800g braising steak

Store Cupboard

400g tin of lychees (or fresh if you can get them)
1 tin tuna, in spring water or brine
2 tins chopped tomatoes
1 tbsp tomato puree
1 tbsp dijon mustard
1 tbsp horseradish
1 carton of almond milk
2 tbsp raw honey
1 tbsp almond butter
200ml coconut cream
1 tbsp harissa paste

Prepared Foods (Homemade if possible, Paleo friendly if not)

500ml chicken stock

Cooking Oils

400g lard, dripping or goose fat
Coconut oil
Olive oil
Sesame oil

Dressings

Extra virgin olive oil
Balsamic vinegar
Red wine vinegar

Eggs

2 ½ dozen eggs

Deli

12 kalamata olives

Dried Fruit

30g dates
50g dried cranberries

Nuts and Seeds

75g almonds
30g coconut flakes
50g flaked almonds
50g ground almonds
50g cashew nuts, unsalted
50g pecans
50g pumpkin seeds
50g sunflower seeds
50g walnuts
30g flax seed

Spices and Seasonings

2 bay leaves
Black pepper
1 tsp chilli powder
1 tsp chinese five spices
1 tbsp coriander seed
1 tsp cumin seed
2 tsp garlic powder
3 tsp ground cinnamon
2 tsp ground oregano
2 tbsp paprika
1 tbsp smoked paprika
2 whole nutmeg
Sea salt

Frozen Fruit

100g frozen berries

WEEK EIGHT

Fruit and Vegetables

2 green apples
1 red apple
4 oranges
50g raspberries
1 mango
1 pomegranate
2 bananas
4 large figs
3 lemons
5 limes
4 avocados
4 bok choi
6 mushrooms
10 button mushrooms
3 bunches spring onions
3 red bell peppers
1 bulb fennel
2 cooked beetroot (not pickled)
3 courgettes
1 punnet cherry tomatoes
16 tomatoes
4 bags mixed salad leaves
1 bag rocket
400g spinach
2 bunches parsley
1 small bunch coriander
1 small bunch mint
4 sage leaves
4 sprigs fresh thyme
2 bulbs garlic
3 inch piece fresh ginger
10 small red birds eye chillies
5 red chilli peppers
1 head cauliflower
2 large sweet potatoes
½ butternut squash
¼ white cabbage
½ savoy cabbage
¼ red cabbage
2 red onions
5 white onions

Fresh Seafood

200g king prawns

Meat and Poultry

24 rashers bacon
10 chicken breasts
8 chicken drumsticks, with skin on
8 chicken thighs, with skin on
2 pork chops (bone in)
400g pork mince
10 pork sausages
2 sirloin steaks (200-250g each)
400g diced lamb

Store Cupboard

2 tins chopped tomatoes
2 tbsp dijon mustard
1 tbsp raw honey
50g dark chocolate, 60-70% cacao solids
2 tbsp rogan josh spice mix or paste

Prepared Foods (Homemade if possible, Paleo friendly if not)

800ml chicken stock

Cooking Oils

400g lard, dripping or goose fat
Olive oil

Dressings

Extra virgin olive oil
Balsamic vinegar
Apple cider vinegar
White wine vinegar
Walnut oil
Red Wine Vinegar

Eggs

2 ½ dozen eggs

Deli

400g baked ham
100g smoked salmon
300g cooked chicken

Dried Fruit

100g dried apricots

Nuts and Seeds

100g almonds
25g flaked almonds
50g pistachio nuts
100g walnuts

Spices and Seasonings

2 bay leaves
Black pepper
1 tsp celery seed
2 cinnamon sticks
2 tsp garlic powder
2 tbsp ground allspice
2 tsp paprika
Sea salt
1 whole nutmeg
1 tsp sweet paprika
2 tsp habanero powder
1 tsp dried thyme

Frozen Fruit

200g frozen berries

WEEK NINE

Fruit and Vegetables

1 green apple
2 oranges
1 banana
2 large peaches
4 large figs
1 pomegranate
½ mango
¼ pineapple
6 lemons
1 lime
4 avocados
2 portabella mushrooms
4 baby beetroot
50g bean sprouts
1 green bell pepper
3 red bell peppers
150g mushrooms
2 ½ cucumbers
1 bunch spring onions
20 cherry tomatoes
9 tomatoes
1 iceberg lettuce
1 bag mixed lettuce leaves
1 bag frisee curly leaf salad
350g rocket
100g spinach
1 bunch parsley
1 small bunch chives
1 small bunch mint
1 small bunch coriander
2 sprigs rosemary
6 sprigs thyme
4 bulbs garlic
1 small piece fresh ginger
2 red chilli peppers
2 heads broccoli
2 heads cauliflower
¼ red cabbage
¼ white cabbage
150g baby carrots
150g baby parsnips
9 carrots
1 celeriac
2 large sweet potatoes
2 leeks
7 white onions
3 red onions
8 shallots

Fresh Seafood

10 scallops
2 tuna steaks
16 shell on king prawns
200g white crab meat

Meat and Poultry

10 rashers bacon
16 chicken thighs, with skin on
600g lamb mince
8 chicken thighs, no bone
4 lamb shanks
100g lardons
400g pork loin
4 pork sausages

Store Cupboard

1 tsp dijon mustard
1 tube tomato puree
1 carton almond milk
2 tbsp raw honey
1 tbsp almond butter
100ml coconut milk
1 tin salmon
1 tin chopped tomatoes

Prepared Foods (Homemade if possible, Paleo friendly if not)

1 litre chicken stock
Paleo mayonnaise

Cooking Oils

400g lard, dripping or goose fat
Coconut oil
Olive oil

Dressings

Extra virgin olive oil
Apple cider vinegar
White wine vinegar
Balsamic vinegar
Walnut oil

Eggs

2 dozen eggs

Deli

200g sliced ham
100g Kalamata olives
100g green olives

Dried Fruit

30g dates
50g dried cranberries

Nuts and Seeds

30g coconut flakes
50g flaked almonds
75g ground almonds
50g pumpkin seeds
50g sunflower seeds
80g cashew nuts, unsalted
50g walnuts
50g pistachio nuts, unshelled
30g flax seed

Spices and Seasonings

2 bay leaves
Black pepper
1 tsp chinese five spices
2 tsp coriander seed
2 tsp curry powder
1 tsp fennel seed
1 tsp garlic powder
3 tsp ground cinnamon
1 tsp ground ginger
2 tsp ground oregano
1 tsp ground turmeric
2 tbsp paprika
Sea salt

Frozen Fruit

400g frozen mango cubes
100g frozen berries

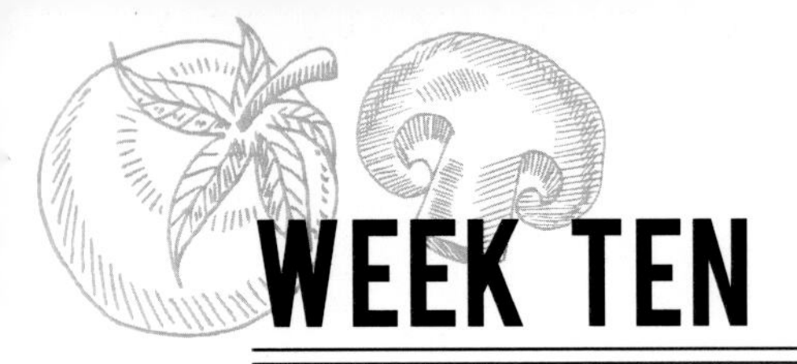

WEEK TEN

Fruit and Vegetables

3 green apples
3 oranges
2 large pears
8 plums
8 lemons
4 avocados
6 mushrooms
4 portabella mushrooms
2 red bell peppers
50g bean sprouts
1 bunch spring onions
1 cucumber
1 bulb fennel
17 tomatoes
4 bags mixed salad leaves
1 radicchio
250g spinach
1 bunch parsley
1 small bunch tarragon
4 sprigs thyme
2 bulbs garlic
2 large sweet potatoes
8 carrots
1 head broccoli
½ red cabbage
½ savoy cabbage
½ white cabbage
200g green beans
200g kale
5 red onions
10 white onions

Fresh Seafood

200g cooked prawns
2 sole fillets

Meat and Poultry

24 rashers bacon
500g beef mince
16 chicken thighs, with skin on
2 small chickens
800g braising steak
2kg pork shoulder
400g chicken breast
400g chicken thighs, no bone
4 pork sausages

Store Cupboard

1 tin tuna, in spring water or brine
2 tbsp tomato puree
1 tbsp dijon mustard
200ml red wine
1 tin chopped tomatoes

Prepared Foods (Homemade if possible, Paleo friendly if not)

500ml chicken stock
Paleo mayonnaise

Cooking Oils

400g lard, dripping or goose fat
Coconut oil
Olive oil

Dressings

Extra virgin olive oil
Balsamic vinegar
White wine vinegar
Walnut oil

Eggs

3 dozen eggs

Deli

150g chorizo
200g roasted red bell peppers
16 black olives
200g baked ham
100g smoked salmon
100g green olives
300g cooked chicken (should have leftovers – please check)

Dried Fruit

100g dried apricots
2 tbsp raisins

Nuts and Seeds

200g cashew nuts, unsalted
50g almonds

Spices and Seasonings

4 bay leaves
Black pepper
1 cinnamon stick
4 tbsp paprika
2 star anise
1 vanilla pod
Sea salt
1 tsp dried sage
1 tbsp ground cinnamon
1 tsp ground coriander
2 tsp ground cumin
1 tsp garlic powder
1 tsp chipotle powder or flakes

WEEK ELEVEN

Fruit and Vegetables

1 green apple
1 orange
1 banana
1 mango
1 large papaya
5 lemons
3 limes
2 avocados
2 bunches spring onions
4 bok choi
1 cucumber
150g mushrooms
2 portabella mushrooms
2 red bell peppers
1 aubergine
30 cherry tomatoes
15 tomatoes
4 bags mixed salad leaves
100g spinach
1 bunch coriander
1 bunch parsley
1 small bunch basil
2 bunches mint
3 sprigs thyme
2 bulbs garlic
2 inch piece fresh ginger
3 red chilli peppers
2 green chillies
1 head broccoli
2 heads cauliflower
4 parsnips
12 carrots
½ butternut squash
½ white cabbage
¼ red cabbage
400g green beans
6 white onions
6 red onions
4 shallots

Fresh Seafood

2 cod fillets
400g scallops

Meat and Poultry

12 rashers bacon
4 chicken breasts
2 small chickens
8 chicken thighs, boneless with skin on
400g lamb mince
8 chicken thighs, with bone and skin on
4 pork sausages

Store Cupboard

1 tbsp dijon mustard
1 tsp horseradish
1 carton almond milk
1 tsp tahini
1 tin chopped tomatoes
3 tbsp raw honey
1 tbsp almond butter
300ml coconut milk
50g gherkin (pickled in jar)

Prepared Foods (Homemade if possible, Paleo friendly if not)

500ml chicken stock
Paleo mayonnaise

Cooking Oils

400g lard, dripping or goose fat
Coconut oil
Olive oil

Dressings

Extra virgin olive oil
Balsamic vinegar
Walnut oil

Eggs

2 dozen eggs

Deli

600g cooked chicken (check for leftovers)
300g cooked beef
12 kalamata olives

Dried Fruit

50g dried cranberries
30g dates

Nuts and Seeds

50g coconut flakes
50g ground almonds
50g flaked almonds
50g pecans
50g cashew nuts, unsalted
50g pumpkin seeds
50g sunflower seeds
75g walnuts
30g almonds
30g flax seed

Spices and Seasonings

2 bay leaves
Black pepper
1 tsp cayenne pepper
1 tsp chilli powder
1 tsp ground ginger
2 tsp coriander seed
1 tbsp madras curry powder
3 tsp garlic powder
3 tsp cinnamon
1 whole nutmeg
3 tsp ground oregano
3 tsp ground turmeric
1 tsp paprika
1 tsp ground cumin
2 tbsp smoked paprika
Sea salt

Frozen Fruit

400g frozen mango cubes
100g frozen berries

WEEK TWELVE

Fruit and Vegetables

2 green apples
2 oranges
3 peaches
5 lemons
6 limes
6 avocados
2 bunches spring onions
6 mushrooms
50g bean sprouts
1 ½ cucumbers
5 red bell peppers
10 cherry tomatoes
15 tomatoes
1 bag frisee curly leaf salad
3 bag mixed salad leaves
175g spinach
1 small bunch mint
1 bunch coriander
1 bunch parsley
1 small bunch sage
1 bulb garlic
2 inch piece fresh ginger
4 red chillies
2 large sweet potatoes
1 head broccoli
10 carrots
½ white cabbage
½ red cabbage
½ savoy cabbage
200g green beans
1 leek
8 white onions
5 red onions

Fresh Seafood

200g cooked prawns
2 salmon fillets
10 scallops

Meat and Poultry

15 rashers bacon
4 chicken breasts
400g lamb mince
8 chicken thighs, bone in, skin on
800g braising steak
400g chicken mince
2 pork chops (bone in)
2 small chickens
4 pork sausages
2 sirloin steaks (200 – 250g each)
100g lardons

Store Cupboard

1 tin chopped tomatoes
2 tbsp capers
1 tbsp horseradish
1 tsp unsweetened cocoa powder
200ml coconut milk
50g dark chocolate, 60-70% cocoa content
1 tbsp tomato puree
1 tbsp dijon mustard
50g gherkins (pickled in jar)
1 tin tuna, in brine or spring water

Prepared foods (Homemade if possible, Paleo friendly if not)

500ml chicken stock
Paleo mayonnaise

Cooking Oils

400g lard, dripping or goose fat
Coconut oil
Olive oil

Dressings

Extra virgin olive oil
Balsamic vinegar
White wine vinegar
Walnut oil
Apple Cider Vinegar
Sesame Oil

Eggs

3 dozen eggs

Deli

300g cooked chicken (check for leftovers)
100g smoked salmon
16 black olives
200g baked ham

Dried Fruit

100g dried apricots

Nuts and Seeds

25g almonds
100g sesame seeds

Spices and Seasonings

Black pepper
1 tsp chinese five spices
1 cinnamon stick
1 tbsp coriander seed
1 tsp cumin seed
1 tsp ground cinnamon
1 tsp ground oregano
4 tbsp paprika
4 bay leaves
2 tsp smoked paprika
1 tsp chilli powder
2 tsp garlic powder
1 tsp Madras curry powder
1 tsp ground cayenne
Sea salt

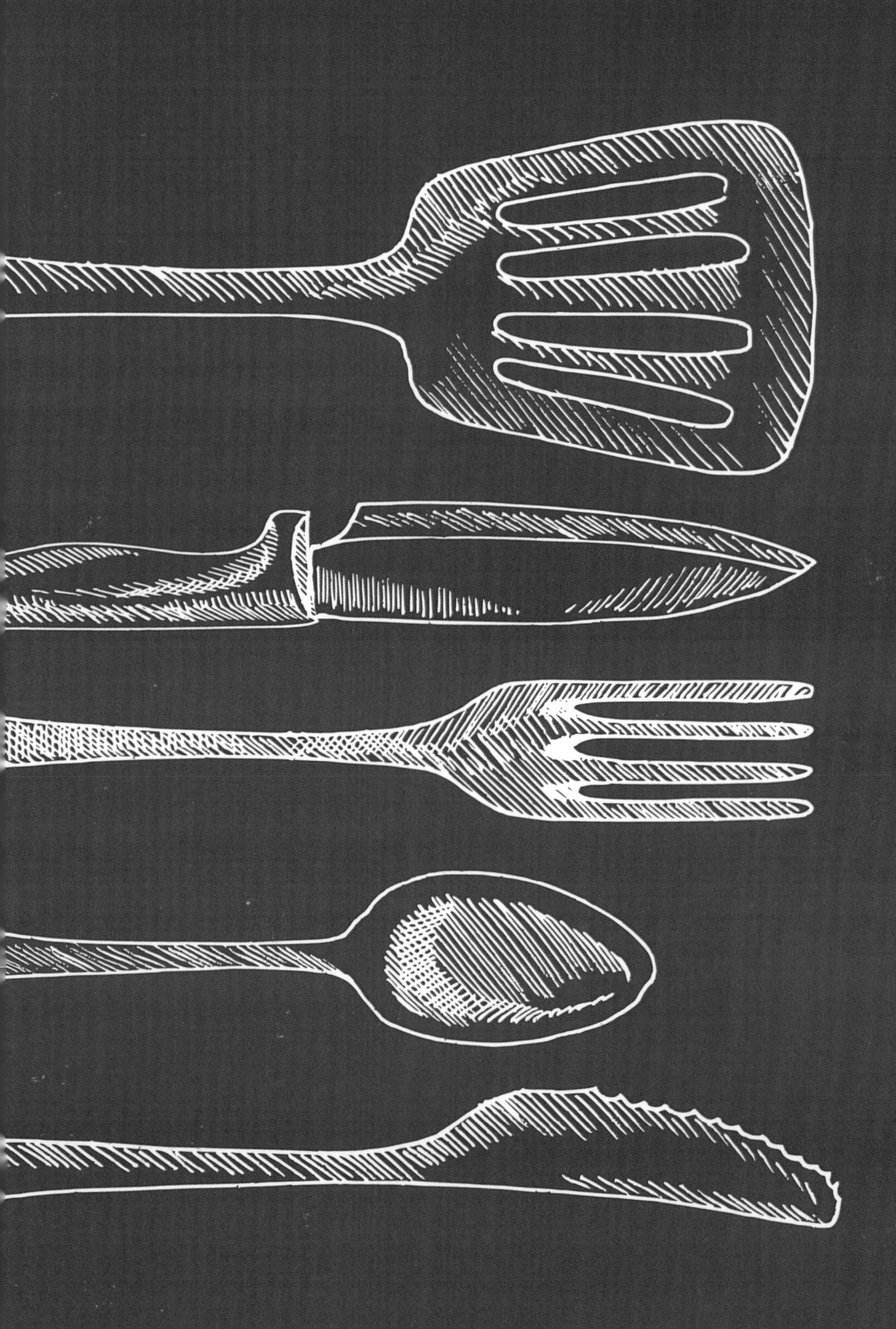

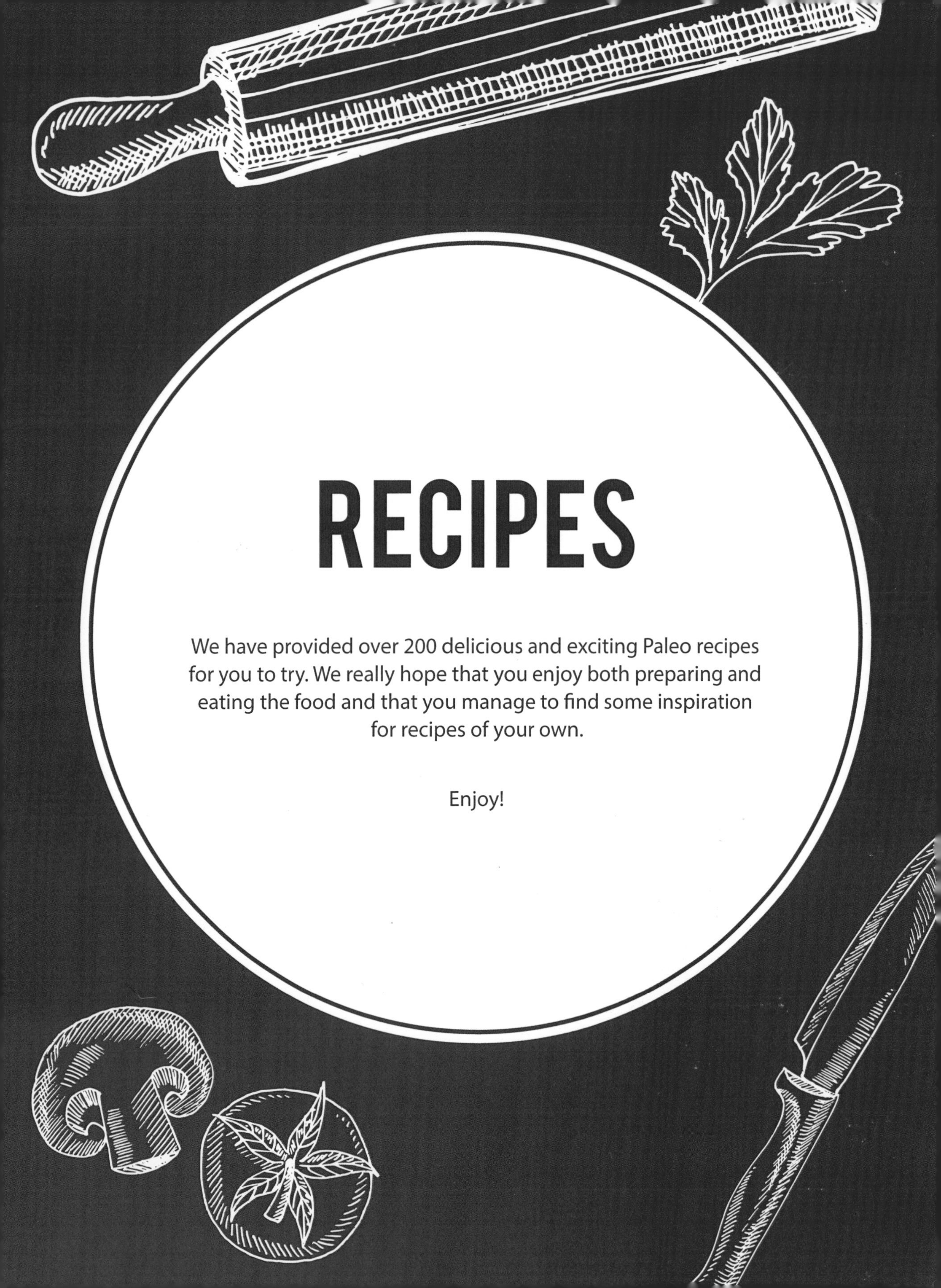

RECIPES

We have provided over 200 delicious and exciting Paleo recipes for you to try. We really hope that you enjoy both preparing and eating the food and that you manage to find some inspiration for recipes of your own.

Enjoy!

BREAKFAST

Breakfast is the most important meal of the day. For some it is a joy whilst others avoid it at all costs. We would suggest that if there is one habit you really have to change for the Paleo lifestyle that is learning to eat breakfast. Yes, it will take a bit more of your time in the morning but once you get used to your routine you will find that you can rustle up something delicious in no time. Even if you do not want to follow all of our recipes every day, creating a simple omelette for breakfast takes just minutes.

Paleo breakfasts are a real treat. You get to indulge in a cooked breakfast of yummy eggs almost every day. You will find that once you get into eating the Paleo breakfasts it will fast become your favourite meal of the day. Nutritionally, our breakfasts have so much to give and you will be full of energy all the way up until lunchtime.

We really hope that you will give breakfast a go – it is a fantastic and scrumptious meal that will set you up for the day whatever you have ahead of you.

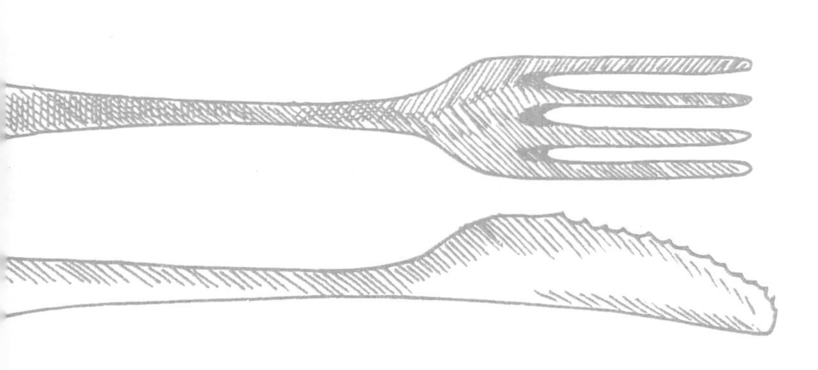

BACON AND EGGS

 *Servings: 2*

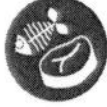 *Preparation Time: 5 minutes*

 *Cooking Time: 15 minutes*

 *Total Time: 20 minutes*

Ingredients

6 rashers of bacon

1 tbsp lard

4 eggs

Preparation

1. Place a large frying pan over a medium heat and melt the fat.
2. Fry the bacon until crisp, remove and keep warm.
3. Cook your eggs to your liking whether scrambled, fried or poached.

BREAKFAST SMOOTHIE

 *Servings: 2*

 *Preparation Time: 10 minutes*

Ingredients

500ml almond milk

1 large banana

1 tbsp coconut oil

100g frozen berries

1 tbsp almond butter

Preparation

1. Blitz all ingredients together in a blender.
2. Pour over ice (if needed as should be cold from the frozen berries) and serve.

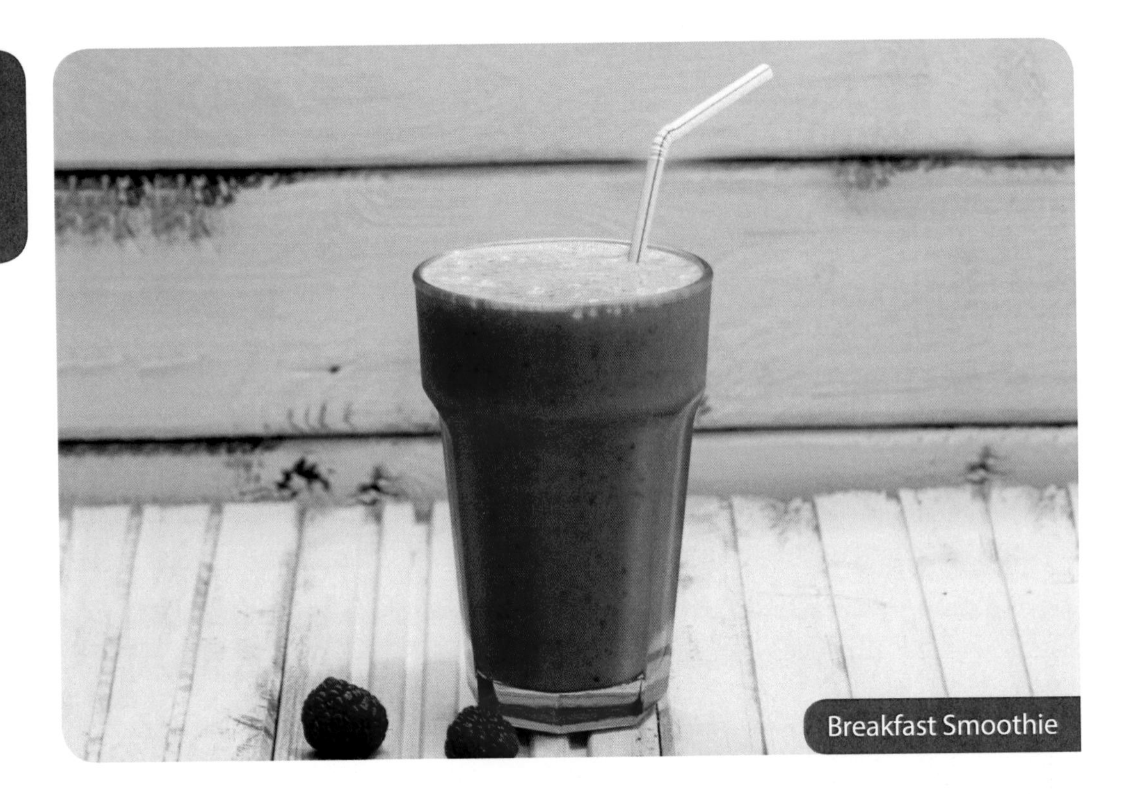

Breakfast Smoothie

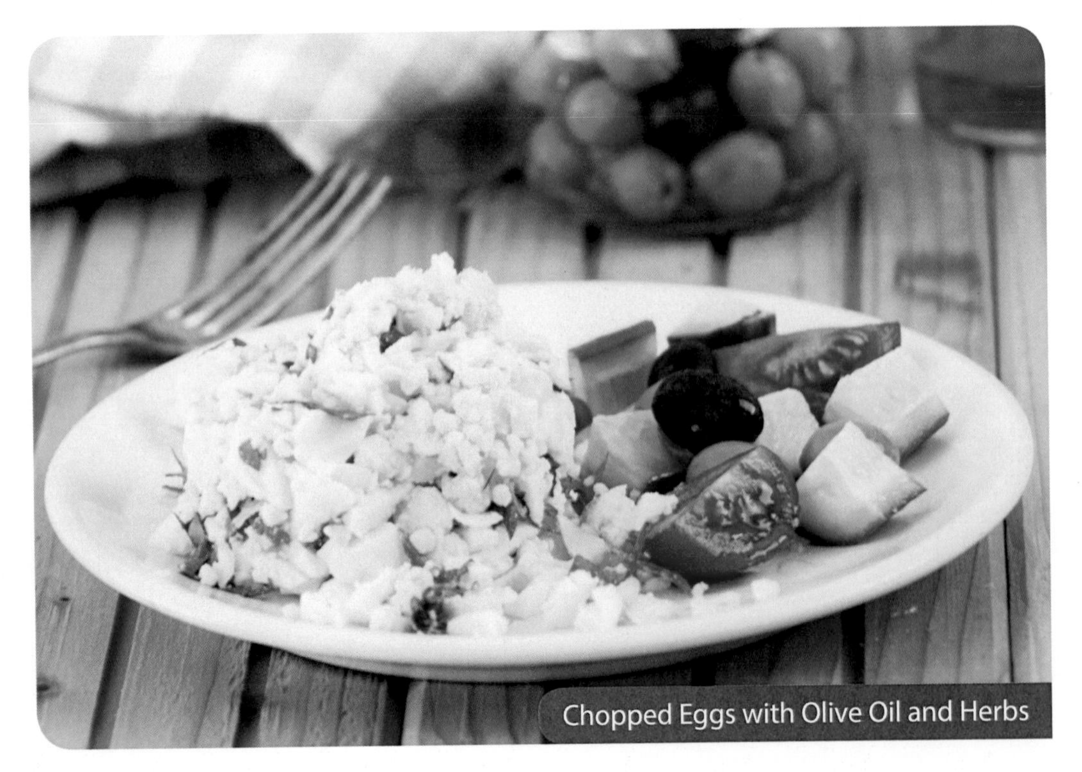

Chopped Eggs with Olive Oil and Herbs

CHOPPED EGGS WITH OLIVE OIL AND HERBS

You can boil the eggs the night before in order to save some time in the morning.

 *Servings: 2*

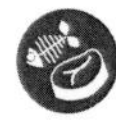 *Preparation Time: 10 minutes*

 *Cooking Time: 10 minutes*

 *Total Time: 20 minutes*

Ingredients

4 eggs, hard boiled and finely chopped

2 tbsp fresh parsley, chopped

1 pinch flaked sea salt

20 cherry tomatoes

12 Kalamata olives

5 spring onions, finely chopped

1 tbsp fresh mint, chopped

2 tbsp extra virgin olive oil

½ cucumber, sliced

Preparation

1. Place the eggs in a saucepan and cover with water. Slowly bring to the boil.
2. Once boiling, the eggs will take 7-10 minutes to cook depending on how hard you like the yolks.
3. Once the eggs are cooked, drain and cool under cold running water.
4. You can leave the eggs in the fridge overnight if preparing in advance.
5. Once the eggs are cooled you can carefully remove the shell and chop into pieces.
6. Arrange the finely chopped egg on a plate and scatter with onions and herbs.
7. Season with a pinch of sea salt to taste and drizzle over the oil.
8. Chop the tomato, olives and cucumber and serve with the egg.

BAKED EGGS PEPERONATA

 *Servings: 2*

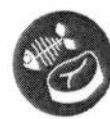 *Preparation Time: 15 minutes*

 *Cooking Time: 45 minutes*

 *Total Time: 1 hour*

Ingredients

4 large eggs
1 red onion, thinly sliced
1 pinch ground oregano
4 tbsp extra virgin olive oil
Fresh parsley, chopped
2 red peppers, thinly sliced
400g tinned, chopped tomatoes
2 garlic cloves, crushed
Sea salt

Preparation

1. Preheat the oven to 200C and prepare the peppers, onion and garlic.
2. Heat the oil in a large pan over a medium heat.
3. Add the peppers, onions and garlic with a pinch of salt and the oregano.
4. Sauté gently for about 10 minutes.
5. Add the tinned tomatoes and cook down slowly until you have a thick glossy sauce.
6. Spread the tomato sauce in the bottom of a heat proof dish.
7. Make 4 indents in the sauce and crack an egg into each.
8. Bake in the oven for about 5 minutes, until the eggs are set.
9. Serve hot with a garnish of fresh parsley.

BREAKFAST SALAD

You can plan ahead and hard boil the eggs the night before to give you more time in the morning. You can also cook the bacon the night before if you want to. To keep the salad ingredients as fresh as possible you should prepare the tomatoes and avocado in the morning.

 *Servings: 2*

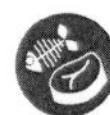 *Preparation Time: 10 minutes*

 *Cooking Time: 15 minutes*

 *Total Time: 25 minutes*

Ingredients

4 hard-boiled eggs, quartered

400g bacon, cooked and chopped

50g baby spinach leaves

2 ripe avocado, chopped

2 large ripe tomatoes, chopped

Preparation

1. Place the eggs in a saucepan covered with water and slowly bring to the boil.
2. Once boiling, the eggs will take 7-10 minutes to cook, depending on how well done you like them.
3. Once the eggs are cooked, drain the water leave the eggs to cool.
4. If you are boiling the eggs the night before you can then place in the fridge.
5. Place the bacon in a frying pan and cook to your desired taste. You should not need to add any fat or oil for cooking.
6. Whilst the bacon is cooking prepare the avocado and the tomatoes.
7. Peel the eggs and cut into slices or chunk, whichever you prefer.
8. Place the avocado, eggs and tomatoes into a bowl and add the spinach.
9. Once the bacon is cooked, chop into pieces and mix together with the salad.

FULL ENGLISH

 *Servings: 2*

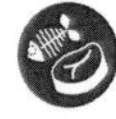 *Preparation Time: 5 minutes*

 *Cooking Time: 30 minutes*

 *Total Time: 35 minutes*

Ingredients

1 tbsp lard

4 pork sausages

2 large Portabello mushrooms, chopped

4 slices bacon

2 large tomatoes, sliced

2 large eggs

Preparation

1. Place a large frying pan over a medium heat and melt the lard.
2. Add the sausages and cook until about half way.
3. Add the bacon and the mushrooms and cook until the bacon is crisp and the mushrooms tender.
4. Remove the cooked sausages, bacon and mushrooms from the pan and keep warm.
5. Add the tomatoes and fry for a few minutes on either side.
6. Remove the tomatoes to keep warm, and then fry the eggs how you like them.
7. Serve hot.

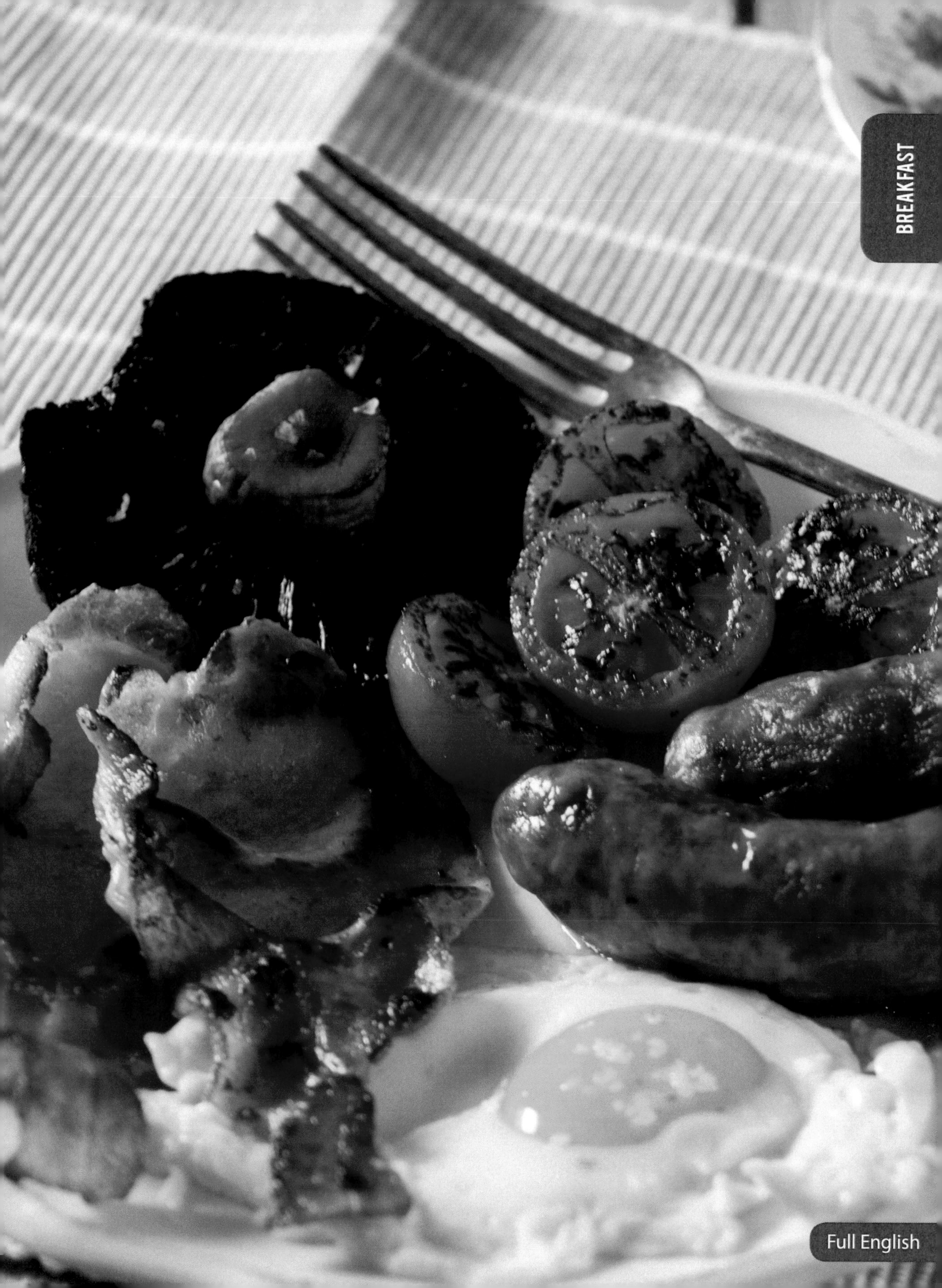

Full English

GRAIN-FREE GRANOLA

This recipe makes about 6 portions of insanely good granola that you can keep in an airtight jar for about 10 days; omit the egg white and it will keep even longer. As it has no grains, just nuts, seeds and fruit, it is seriously nutrient dense and a real sweet treat when your palate has become used to mostly savoury foods. As delicious raw as it is baked, don't be fooled by the sweetness in its raw state; once toasted it does need a little sweetener that also helps it to stick together.

It may take a few goes to get it right should you wish for it to cluster; the egg white helps it along, but the right consistency and bake is also essential. Don't worry if you don't get chunky clusters first time round; it tastes awesome anyway. Use the recipe as a base and tweak it to fit; raw honey or maple is the most effective sweetener as it is syrupy but you could omit sweetener completely if you wish. We don't recommend that you eat this for breakfast every day. Keep it to once or twice a week.

The weekly meal plans have included granola once a week. You should only need to make every two weeks as one batch is sufficient to last for the week after.

 *Servings: 6*

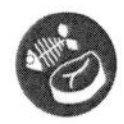 *Preparation Time: 10 minutes*

 *Cooking Time: 40 minutes*

 *Total Time: 50 minutes*

Ingredients

DRY INGREDIENTS

- 50g walnuts
- 50g cashews
- 50g flaked almonds
- 50g sunflower seeds
- 50g pumpkin seeds
- 50g ground almonds
- 30g coconut flakes
- 30g flaxseeds
- 30g dates
- 50g dried cranberries
- 2 tsp ground cinnamon

WET INGREDIENTS

- 2 tbsp raw honey
- 2 tbsp coconut oil
- 1 egg white
- 2 tbsp water

Preparation

1 Preheat the oven to 180C.
2 Mix all of the ingredients and spread it out on a large baking sheet.
3 Bake in the oven, stirring occasionally until everything is toasted.
4 Remove from the oven and allow to cool before packing into jars.
5 Serve with cold almond milk for breakfast or on its own as a snack.

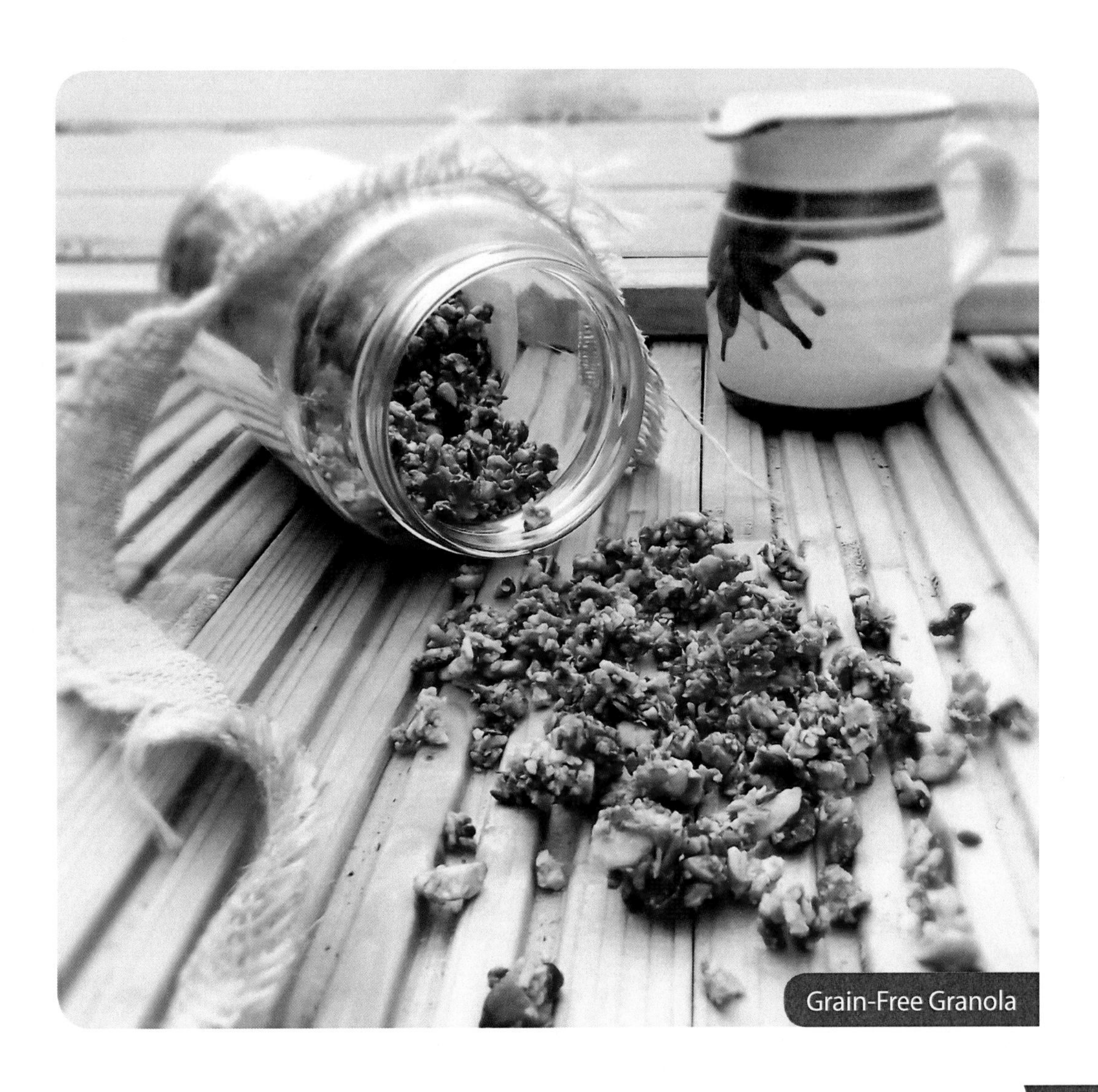
Grain-Free Granola

HAM AND TOMATO OMELETTE

 *Servings: 2*

 *Preparation Time: 5 minutes*

 *Cooking Time: 5 minutes*

 *Total Time: 10 minutes*

Ingredients

6 large eggs

2 tomatoes, chopped

1 pinch black pepper

200g baked ham, chopped

1 tbsp lard, dripping or goose fat

1 pinch paprika

Preparation

1. Beat the eggs together with the seasonings.
2. Heat a large skillet or non-stick frying pan over a medium heat and add the fat.
3. Add the eggs and scrape the sides into the middle, using a spatula, letting the runny eggs fill the spaces that you create.
4. Continue until the egg is almost set.
5. Add the ham and tomatoes on top and fold one half over.
6. Cut in half and serve on two plates.
7. Eat immediately.

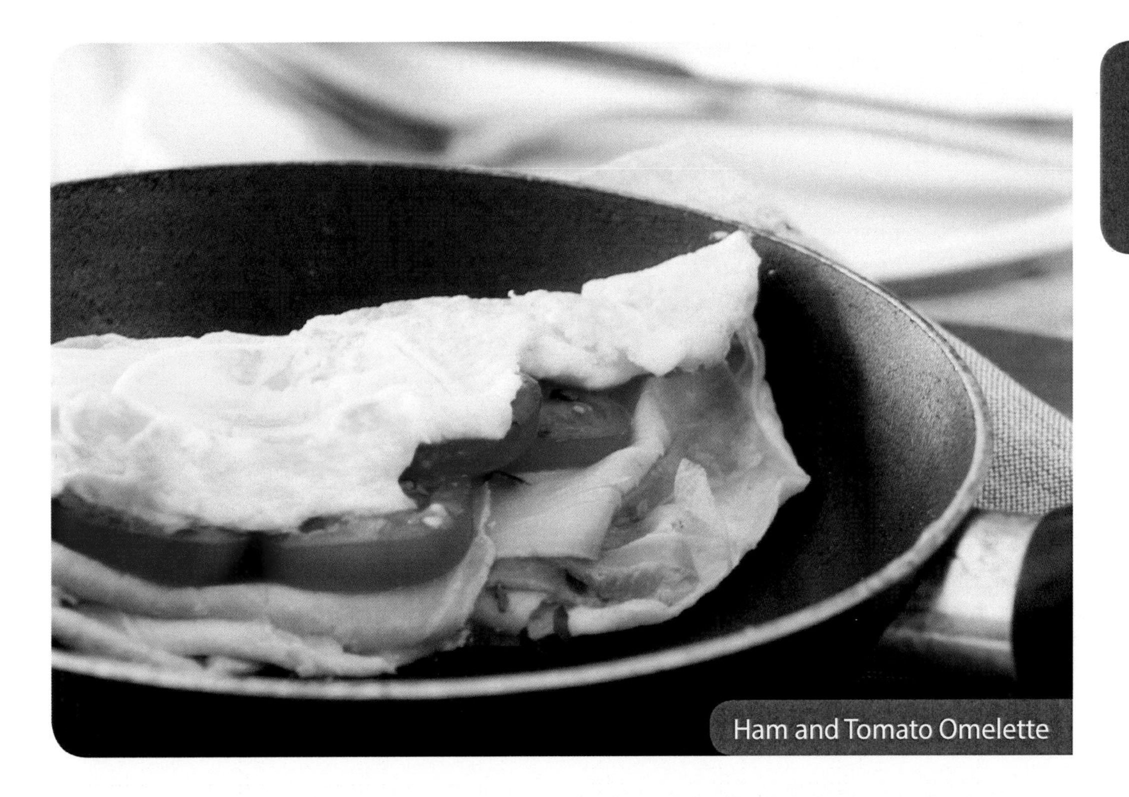

Ham and Tomato Omelette

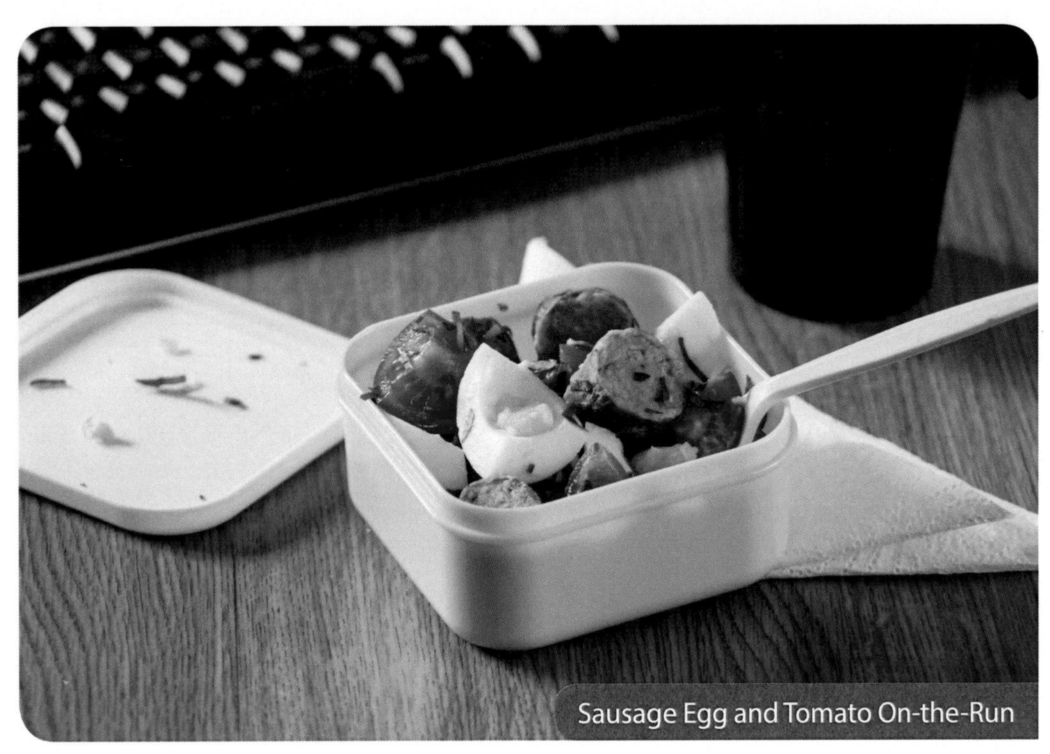

Sausage Egg and Tomato On-the-Run

SAUSAGE EGG AND TOMATO ON-THE-RUN

You can prepare this dish the night before so you can grab and go in the morning.

 *Servings: 2*

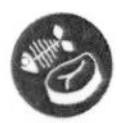 *Preparation Time: 10 minutes*

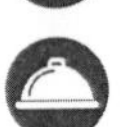 *Cooking Time: 40 minutes*

 *Total Time: 50 minutes*

Ingredients

4 large pork sausages

4 tomatoes, chopped

Sea salt

4 eggs

2 tbsp fresh parsley, chopped

Freshly ground black pepper

Preparation

1. Preheat the oven to 180C.
2. Cook the sausages for 40 minutes or longer depending how crispy you like the skin.
3. Place the eggs in a pan of cold water and bring it up to the boil.
4. Once the water has started to boil cook the eggs for 7-10 minutes (depending on how well you like your eggs done).
5. Whilst the eggs are boiling you can chop the tomatoes and parsley.
6. Once the sausages and eggs are cooled, chop into pieces and mix with the tomatoes and parsley and add seasoning to taste.

MUSHROOM OMELETTE

 *Servings: 2*

 *Preparation Time: 5 minutes*

 *Cooking Time: 5 minutes*

 *Total Time: 10 minutes*

Ingredients

6 eggs

1 tbsp lard, dripping or goose fat

1 pinch black pepper

150g mushrooms, sliced

1 pinch sea salt

1 pinch paprika

Preparation

1. Beat the eggs together with the seasonings.
2. Heat a large non-stick frying pan or skillet over a medium heat and add the fat.
3. Fry the mushrooms for a few minutes and set aside.
4. Add the eggs and scrape the sides into the middle, using a spatula, letting the runny eggs fill the spaces that you create.
5. Continue until the egg is almost set.
6. Add the mushrooms on top and fold one half over.
7. Cut in half and serve on two plates.
8. Eat immediately.

BREAKFAST

SCRAMBLED EGGS WITH MUSHROOM AND PEPPERS

 *Servings: 2*

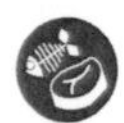 *Preparation Time: 5 minutes*

 *Cooking Time: 10 minutes*

 *Total Time: 15 minutes*

Ingredients

4 large eggs, beaten

6 mushrooms, sliced

1 pinch sea salt

1 pinch paprika

1 red pepper, thinly sliced

1 tbsp lard, dripping or goose fat

1 pinch black pepper

Preparation

1. Heat a non-stick frying pan over a medium heat and add the fat.
2. Gently fry the mushrooms and peppers until soft.
3. Beat the eggs together with the seasonings.
4. Add the eggs, stirring until just set.
5. Serve hot.

SCRAMBLED EGGS WITH SPINACH AND TOMATO

 *Servings: 2*

 *Preparation Time: 5 minutes*

 *Cooking Time: 10 minutes*

 *Total Time: 15 minutes*

Ingredients

6 eggs, beaten

1 pinch sea salt

4 tomatoes, chopped

1 tbsp olive oil

1 pinch freshly ground black pepper

100g baby spinach

Preparation

1. Heat the oil in a large saucepan and add the tomatoes with the spinach.
2. Stir until the spinach has wilted, add the eggs and seasoning.
3. Stir until the eggs are set.
4. Serve hot on warm plates.

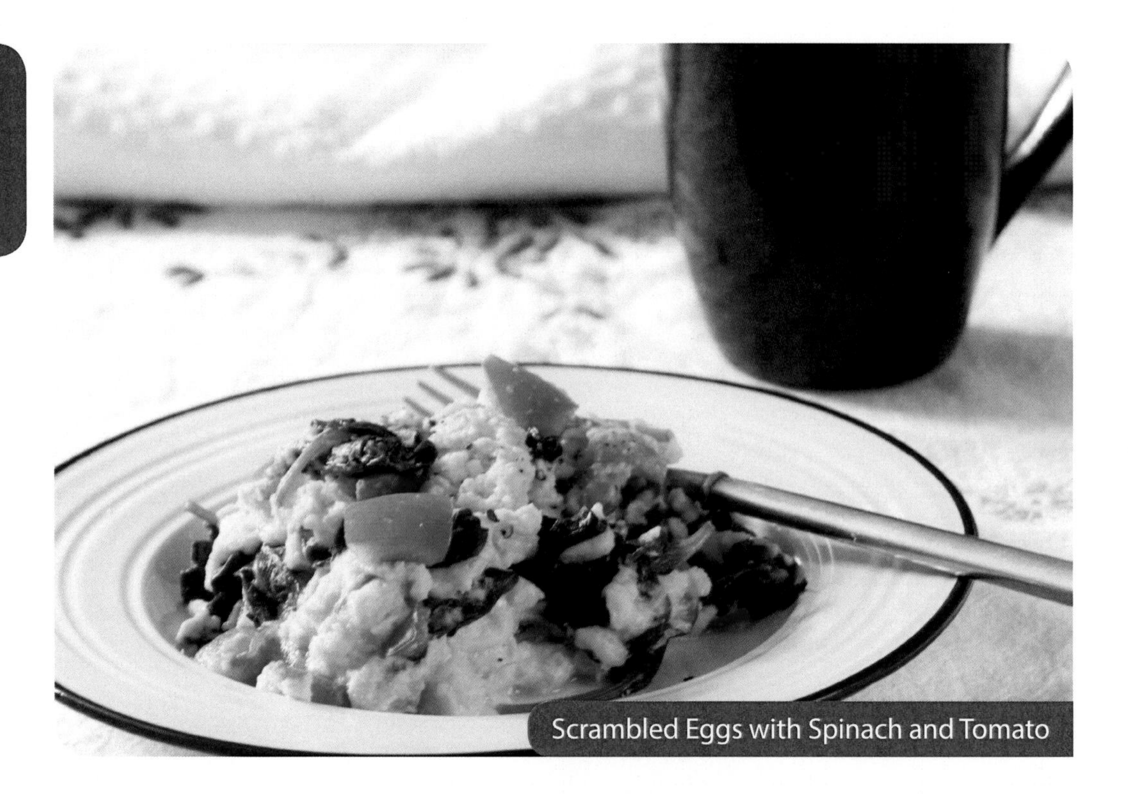

Scrambled Eggs with Spinach and Tomato

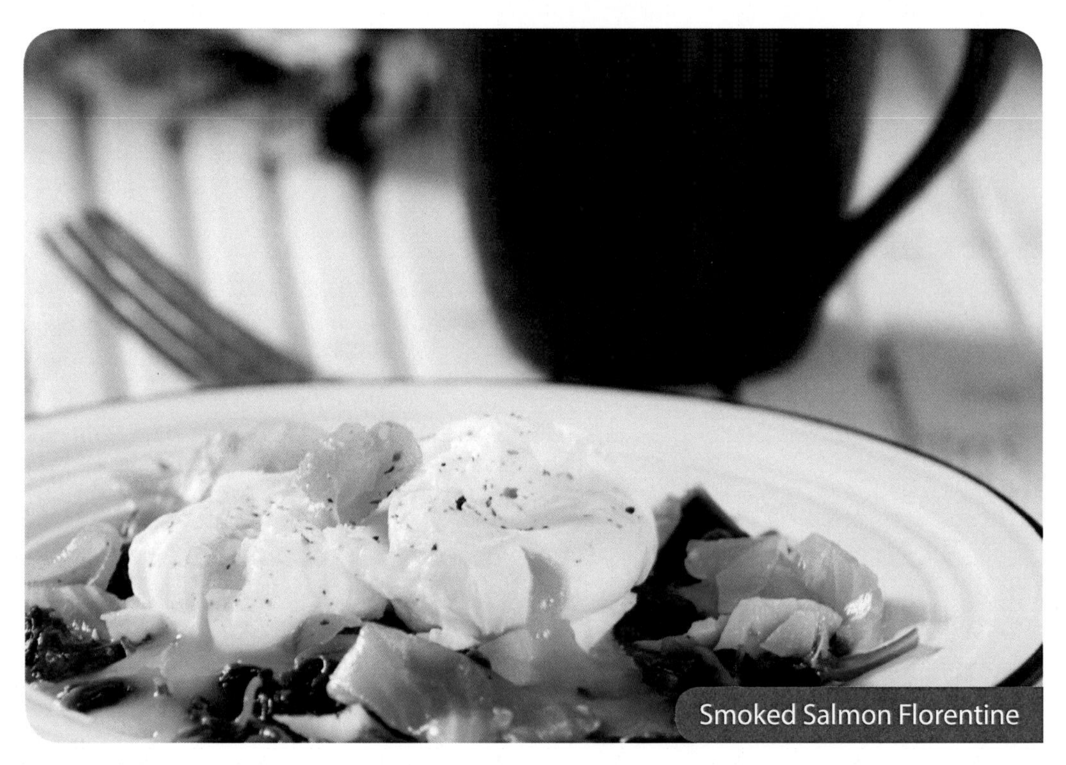

Smoked Salmon Florentine

SMOKED SALMON FLORENTINE

 *Servings: 2*

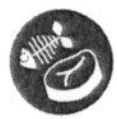 *Preparation Time: 5 minutes*

 *Cooking Time: 10 minutes*

 *Total Time: 15 minutes*

Ingredients

100g baby spinach leaves

4 eggs

Freshly ground black pepper

1 tbsp lemon juice, freshly squeezed

100g smoked salmon, chopped

1 tbsp white wine vinegar

1 tbsp olive oil

Preparation

1. Place a large pan of unsalted water on to boil.
2. Place the spinach in a frying pan with the olive oil and plenty of black pepper. Heat until it wilts and set aside.
3. Add the vinegar to the rapidly boiling water and place the eggs into the boiling water.
4. Remove the pan from the heat, put the lid on and set aside for 3 minutes.
5. Stir the smoked salmon into the warm spinach, dress with lemon, and divide between warm plates.
6. Top the salmon with the poached eggs and eat immediately.

WARM SPICED APRICOT COMPOTE WITH GRANOLA

 *Servings: 2*

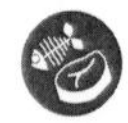 *Preparation Time: 5 minutes*

 *Cooking Time: 10 minutes*

 *Total Time: 15 minutes*

Ingredients

100g dried apricots

1 cinnamon stick

2 oranges, juice only

100ml water

You will also need a portion of the grain-free granola

Preparation

1. Place all the ingredients in a pan and simmer gently for about 5 minutes, until the liquid has reduced and the fruit is soft.
2. Serve warm or cold with the grain-free granola.

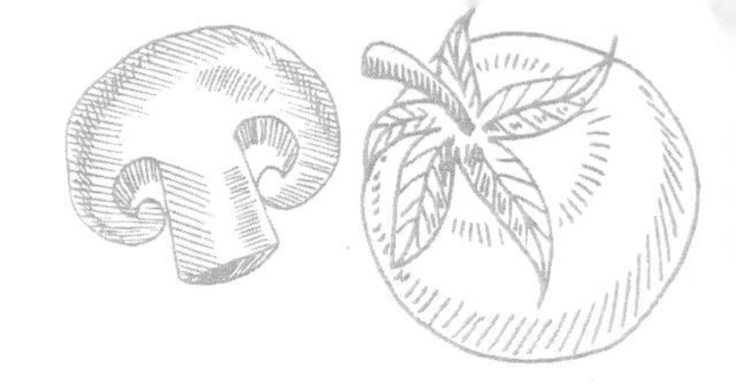

LUNCH

Lunch time is always the meal that people worry about when starting any diet as you will most likely have to eat away from the home which equals temptation. We know that lunches can be tricky for many so we have come up with a variety of recipes to keep your lunchtimes both tasty and varied.

Although all of our lunches are easy to prepare, we have where possible, tried to incorporate leftover ingredients to minimise on preparation time.

Try to get into a routine of preparing your lunch the night before and then it is all sorted and ready to go in the morning. By being prepared you will avoid the temptation of the work canteen or even worse the vending machine.

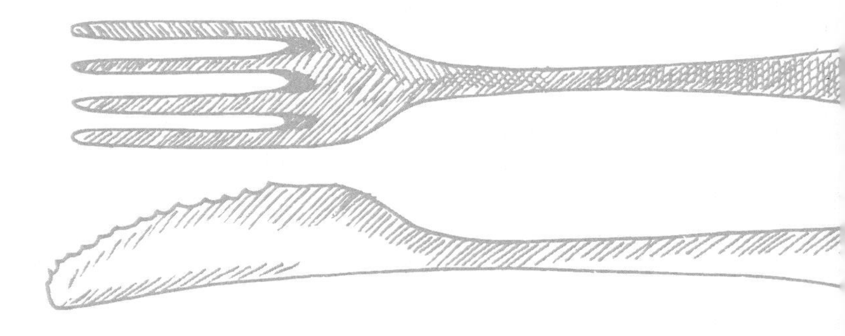

APPLE, HAM AND PARSLEY SALAD

 *Servings: 2*

 *Preparation Time: 15 minutes*

Ingredients

2 leftover gammon steaks, chopped

2 green apples, cored and chopped

4 tbsp fresh parsley, chopped

1 bag mixed salad leaf

½ red onion, thinly sliced

2 tomatoes, chopped

Preparation

1. Chop up the gammon steaks, apples, parsley, tomato and onion.
2. Place the chopped ingredients into a bowl with the mixed leaf salad and mix together.
3. Use some Mustard Vinaigrette to dress if desired.

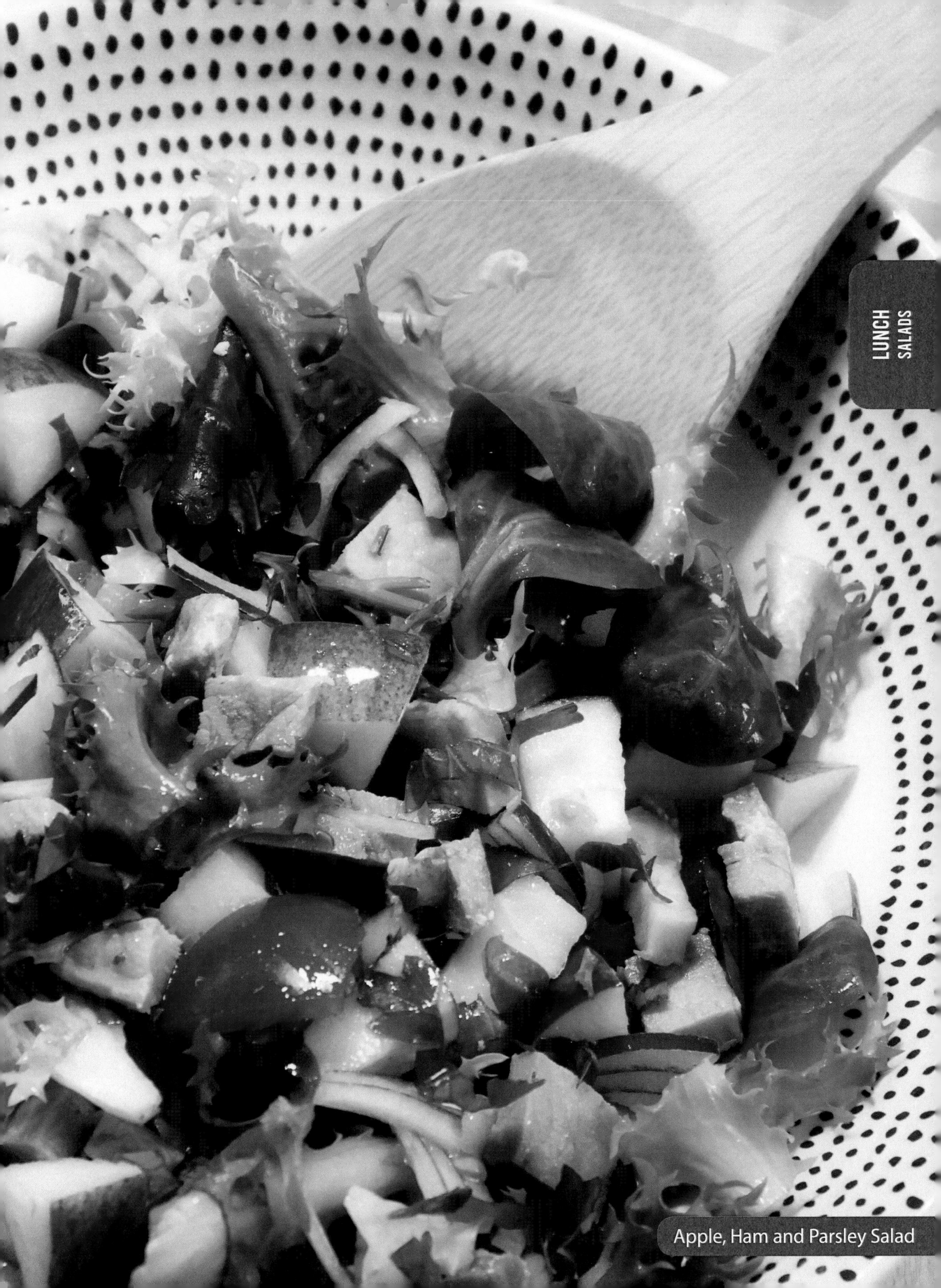

Apple, Ham and Parsley Salad

BEEF, HORSERADISH AND TOMATO SALAD

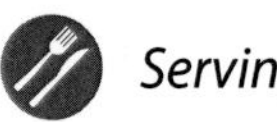 *Servings: 2*

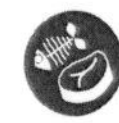 *Preparation Time: 10 minutes*

Ingredients

bag mixed salad leaf

large tomatoes, chopped

300g beef, cooked and chopped

½ red onion, sliced

FOR THE DRESSING

2 tsp horseradish

1 pinch sea salt

2 tbsp extra virgin olive oil

1 tbsp balsamic vinegar

Preparation

1 Make up the dressing by combining the ingredients in a small bowl/ramekin.
2 Toss together with the salad ingredients and serve.

CHICKEN, BACON AND MANGO SALAD

 *Servings: 2*

 *Preparation Time: 15 minutes*

Ingredients

4 rashers bacon, cooked, chopped

1 mango, diced

1 red chilli, chopped

300g cooked chicken, diced

1 bag mixed crisp salad leaves

12 walnuts, chopped

FOR THE DRESSING

2 tbsp walnut oil

Sea salt

½ orange, juice only

Preparation

1 Combine the dressing ingredients in a small bowl or ramekin.
2 Mix together all of the salad ingredients and dress with the oil and orange juice.
3 Check the seasoning and serve.

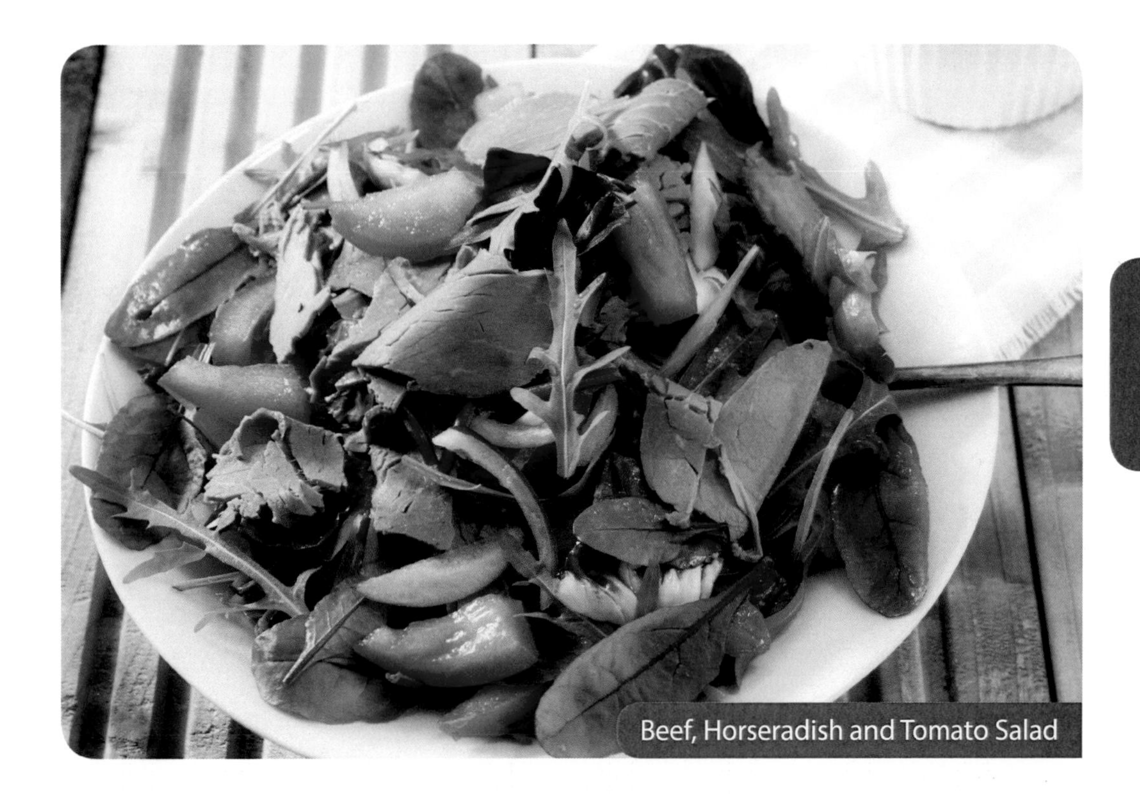

Beef, Horseradish and Tomato Salad

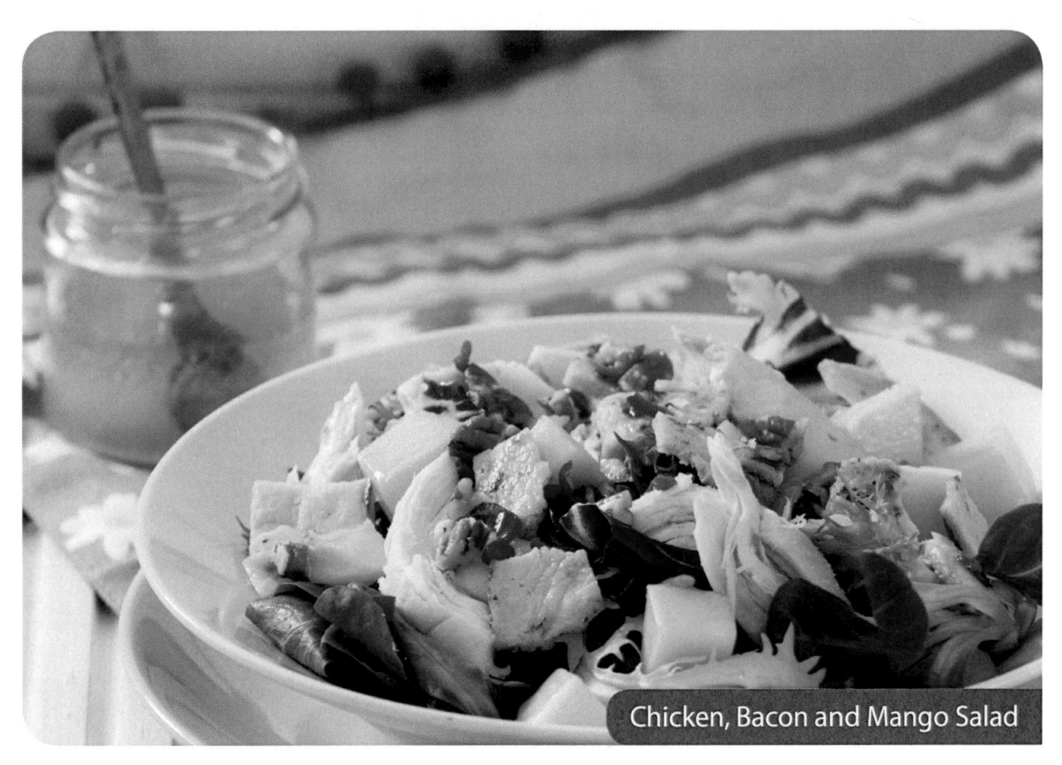

Chicken, Bacon and Mango Salad

AVOCADO, TOMATO AND BASIL SALAD

 *Servings: 2*

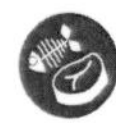 *Preparation Time: 10 minutes*

Ingredients

3 large ripe tomatoes, sliced

½ red onion, sliced thin

Olive oil

Freshly ground black pepper

6 fresh basil leaves, torn

2 avocado, sliced

Sea salt

LUNCH
SALADS

Preparation

1. Prepare the avocado, onion and tomatoes.
2. Arrange ingredients in alternating layers.
3. Season to taste and drizzle with good olive oil.

BACON AND FRISEE SALAD

 *Servings: 2*

 *Preparation Time: 2 minutes*

 *Cooking Time: 10 minutes*

 *Total Time: 12 minutes*

Ingredients

300g bacon, chopped

1 head endive, curly frisee type (or any type of salad leaf that you prefer)

Preparation

1. Fry the bacon until crisp and add to the frisee lettuce with the juices from the pan.
2. Incredibly simple but a great combo. You won't notice you only have two ingredients.

CHICKEN, SUN DRIED TOMATO, OLIVE AND HERB SALAD

 *Servings: 2*

 *Preparation Time: 15 minutes*

Ingredients

300g cooked chicken, diced

1 bag mixed crisp salad leaves

4 spring onions

2 tbsp coriander leaves

12 walnuts, chopped

1 tbsp balsamic vinegar

100g sun dried tomatoes, chopped

20 olives

2 tbsp parsley leaves

2 tbsp chopped chives

Sea salt

Preparation

1. Prepare the chicken, tomatoes, spring onions, herbs and walnuts.
2. Mix together all of the salad ingredients.
3. Dress with balsamic vinegar and some olive oil if you wish.
4. Season to taste and serve.

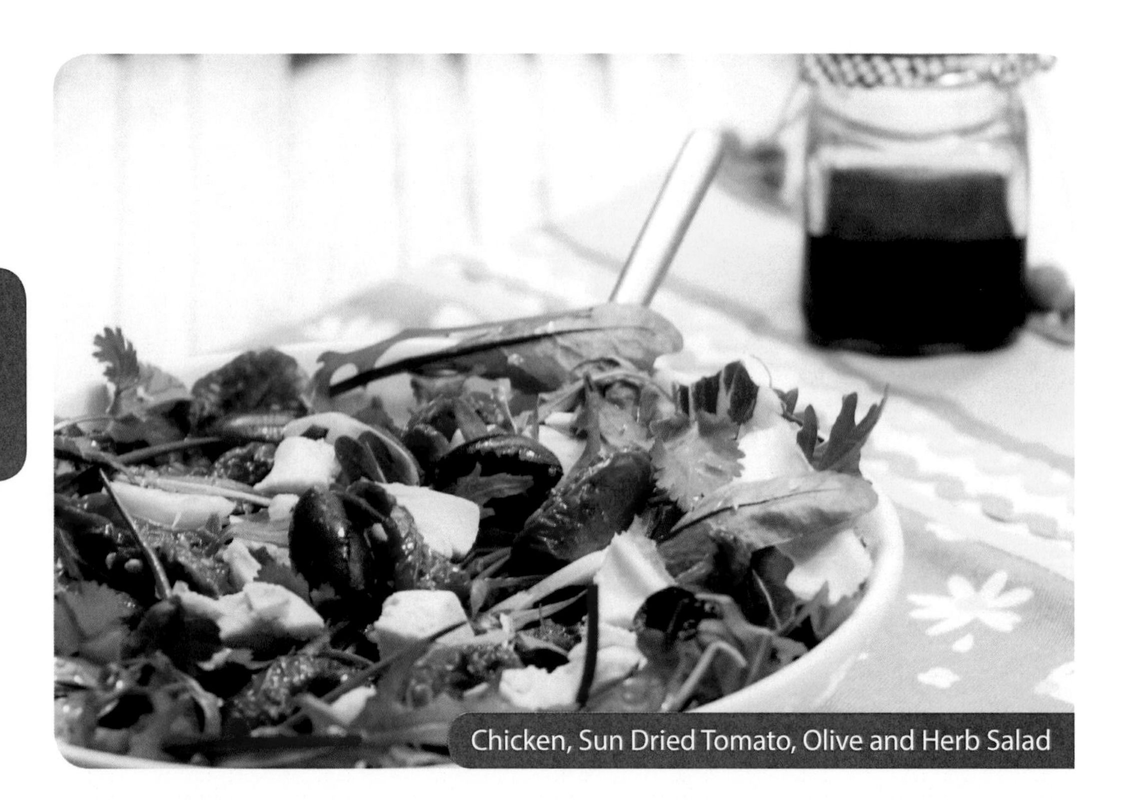

Chicken, Sun Dried Tomato, Olive and Herb Salad

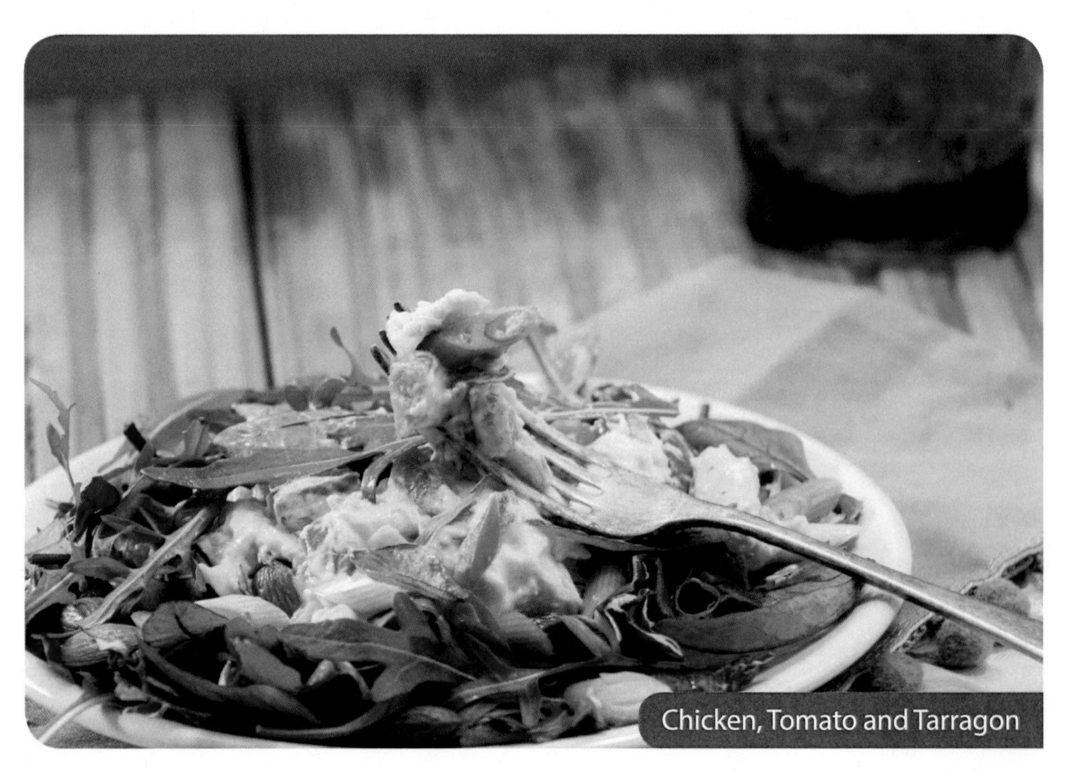

Chicken, Tomato and Tarragon

CHICKEN, TOMATO AND TARRAGON

This is a great dish for using up leftover meat from a Roast Chicken dinner. Once combined with the other ingredients, this becomes a fulfilling and tasty lunch as well as a real money saver.

 *Servings: 2*

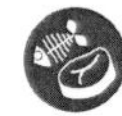 *Preparation Time: 10 minutes*

Ingredients

300g cooked chicken, chopped

1 tbsp fresh tarragon, chopped

2 large tomatoes, chopped

2 tbsp Paleo Mayonnaise

¼ red onion, finely chopped

2 portions of Simple Leaf Salad side dish

Preparation

1. Chop up the leftover chicken along with the onion, tomato and tarragon.
2. Mix all of the ingredients together.
3. Use as a topping for the Simple Leaf Salad side dish.

CHOPPED ITALIAN STYLE SALAD

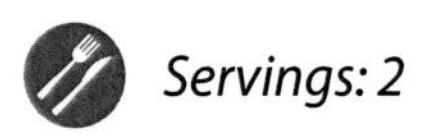 *Servings: 2*

 *Preparation Time: 15 minutes*

LUNCH
SALADS

Ingredients

300g cooked chicken, shredded

1 small bunch basil, torn

½ head Romaine lettuce, shredded

16 slices salami, chopped

50g sun dried tomatoes, chopped

1 avocado, chopped

12 black olives

8 artichoke hearts

½ red onion, thinly sliced

Preparation

1 Chop the avocado, artichoke, onion and the salami and place in a bowl.

2 Add the remaining ingredients and mix well.

3 Dress with some olive oil and balsamic vinegar if you wish.

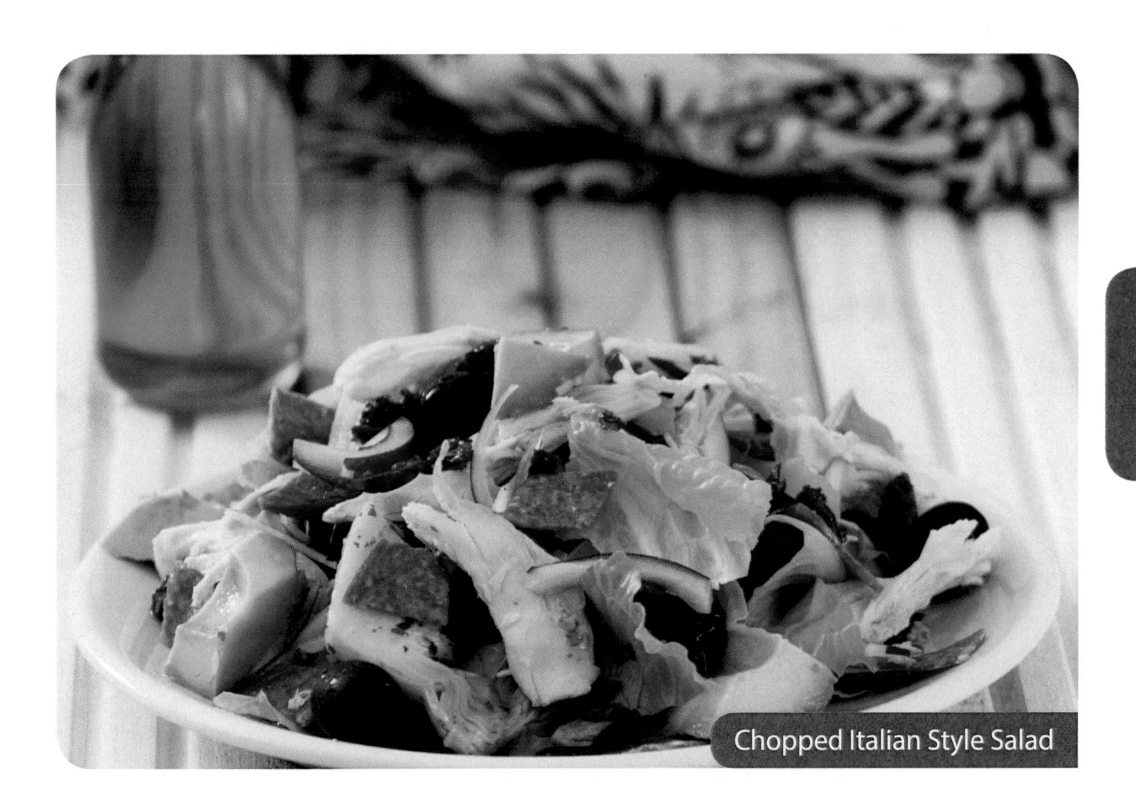

Chopped Italian Style Salad

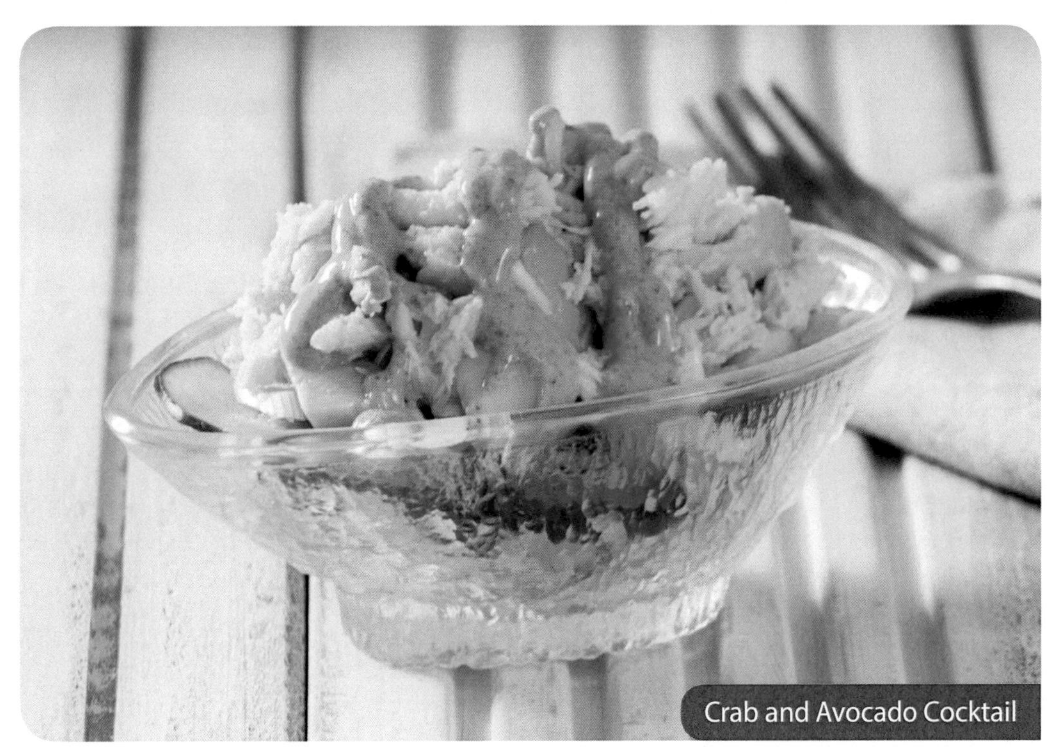

Crab and Avocado Cocktail

CRAB AND AVOCADO COCKTAIL

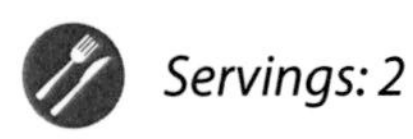

Servings: 2

Preparation Time: 20 minutes

Ingredients

200g white crab meat

2 tomatoes, thinly sliced

2 spring onions, finely chopped

2 ripe avocado, chopped

½ cucumber, thinly sliced

¼ iceberg lettuce, shredded

FOR THE SAUCE

4 tbsp Paleo Mayonnaise

1 lime, juice only

1 tsp paprika

Preparation

1. Prepare the avocado, tomatoes, cucumber, spring onion and lettuce.
2. Mix the sauce ingredients together.
3. Place the salad ingredients into bowls, or glasses, and place the crab meat on top.
4. Cover with the sauce.
5. Serve chilled.

CRAB, GRILLED GRAPEFRUIT AND ROCKET SALAD

You will need to prepare the grapefruit for this dish ahead of time; nobody wants to grill grapefruit at the crack of dawn.

 *Servings: 2*

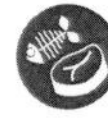 *Preparation Time: 10 minutes*

 *Cooking Time: 5 minutes*

 *Total Time: 15 minutes*

Ingredients

200g white crabmeat

100g rocket

4 basil leaves, torn

1 ruby grapefruit

2 tbsp walnut oil

Sea salt

Preparation

1. Peel the grapefruit and slice into thin rounds.
2. Heat a frying pan, no oil, and when smoking hot lay a few of the grapefruit slices in.
3. All that you want to do is char the fruit on either side to develop the flavours.
4. Do all of the grapefruit in this manner and slice into smaller pieces when ready.
5. Set aside the grapefruit and allow to cool.
6. Toss the grapefruit, crab meat, rocket, and basil in the oil and add a pinch of salt.
7. You do not need any sharpness to the dressing as the grapefruit already supplies it.

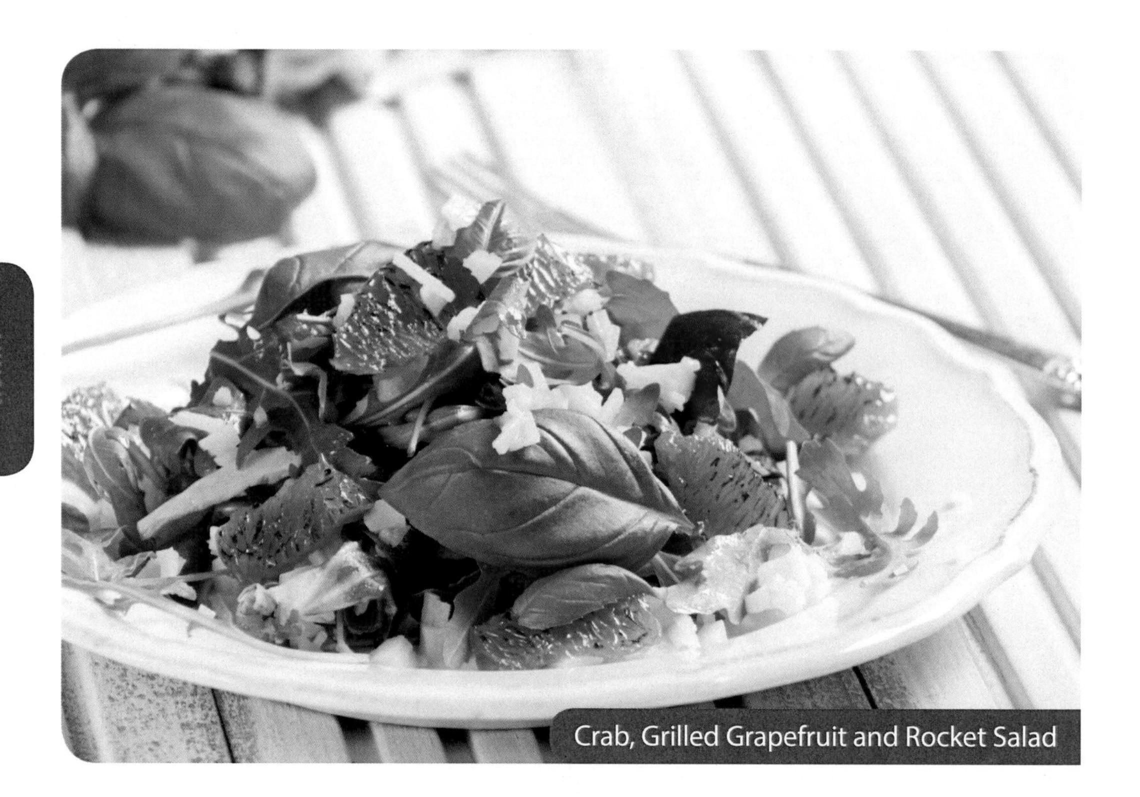

Crab, Grilled Grapefruit and Rocket Salad

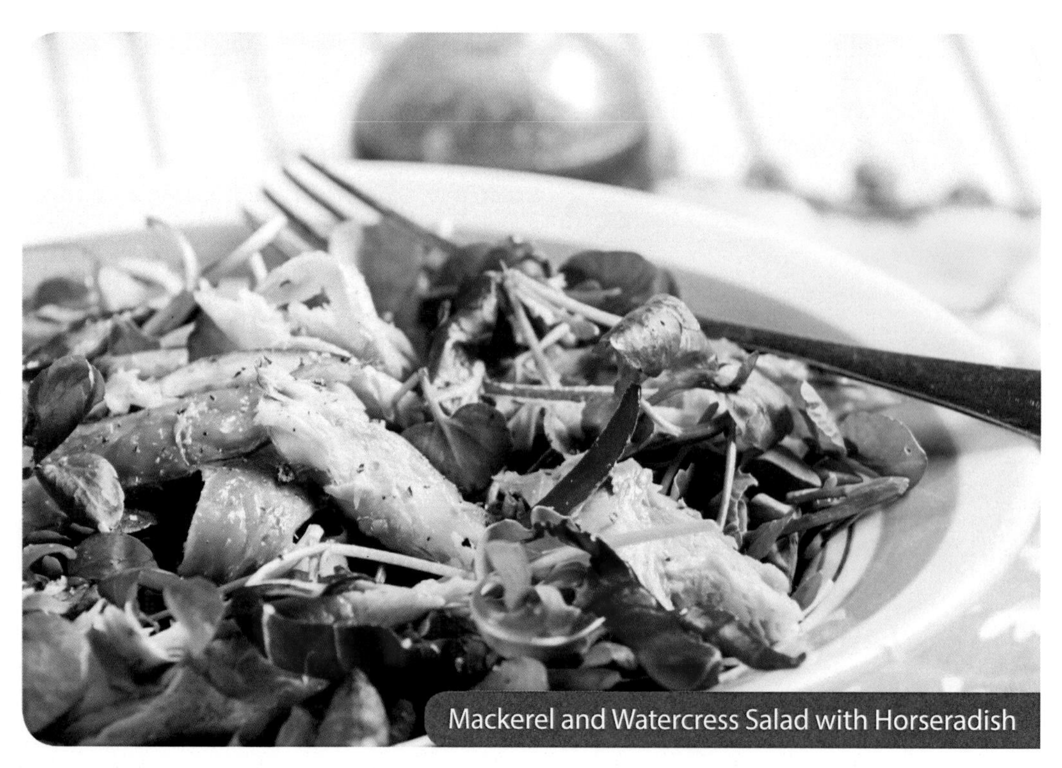

Mackerel and Watercress Salad with Horseradish

MACKEREL AND WATERCRESS SALAD WITH HORSERADISH

Carry the dressing separately if eating away from home and mix when ready to eat.

 *Servings: 2*

 *Preparation Time: 20 minutes*

Ingredients

2 fillets smoked mackerel

100g watercress or salad mix

1 green apple, chopped

1 red onion, finely sliced

FOR THE DRESSING

1 tbsp horseradish

1 tbsp balsamic vinegar

2 tbsp walnut oil

Freshly ground black pepper

Preparation

1. Prepare the apple and onion and mix with the watercress.
2. Break the smoked mackerel into pieces and add to the salad ingredients.
3. Mix the dressing in a bowl and toss with the salad ingredients.
4. Season to taste.

EGG SALAD

 *Servings: 2*

 *Preparation Time: 5 minutes*

 *Cooking Time: 20 minutes*

 *Total Time: 25 minutes*

Ingredients

1 bag rocket

4 hard boiled eggs

2 tbsp fresh dill, chopped

12 cherry tomatoes

½ cucumber, chopped

Sea salt

Preparation

1. Place the eggs into a pan and fill with cold water.
2. Place onto the heat and bring the pan to the boil.
3. Once the water starts to boil the eggs will take 7-10 minutes to cook.
4. Once you have cooked the eggs to your liking take off the heat and allow to cool under cold running water.
5. Once cooled remove the shells and chop or slice the eggs, as preferred.
6. Chop the tomatoes, cucumber and dill and mix all the ingredients together in a bowl.
7. Season to taste.

FIG, HAM AND PISTACHIO SALAD

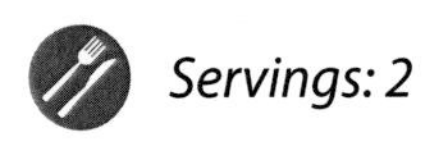
Servings: 2

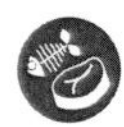
Preparation Time: 15 minutes

Ingredients

1 bag mixed salad greens
4 ripe figs, quartered
Sea salt
2 tbsp fresh parsley, chopped
200g sliced ham
2 tbsp pistachio nuts
Freshly ground black pepper

FOR THE DRESSING

1 tbsp extra virgin olive oil
1 tbsp balsamic vinegar

Preparation

1. Slice the ham and quarter the figs.
2. Place the salad ingredients into a bowl and mix together.
3. Mix together the dressing and pour onto the salad.
4. Season to taste and eat immediately.

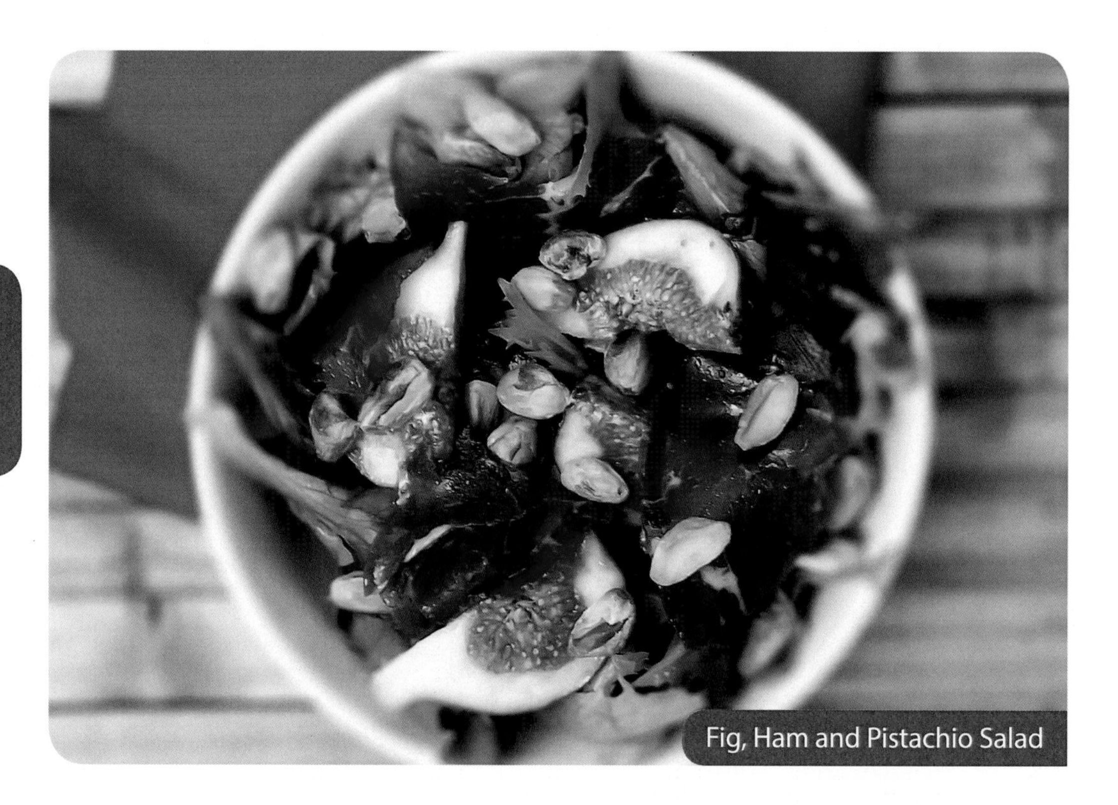
Fig, Ham and Pistachio Salad

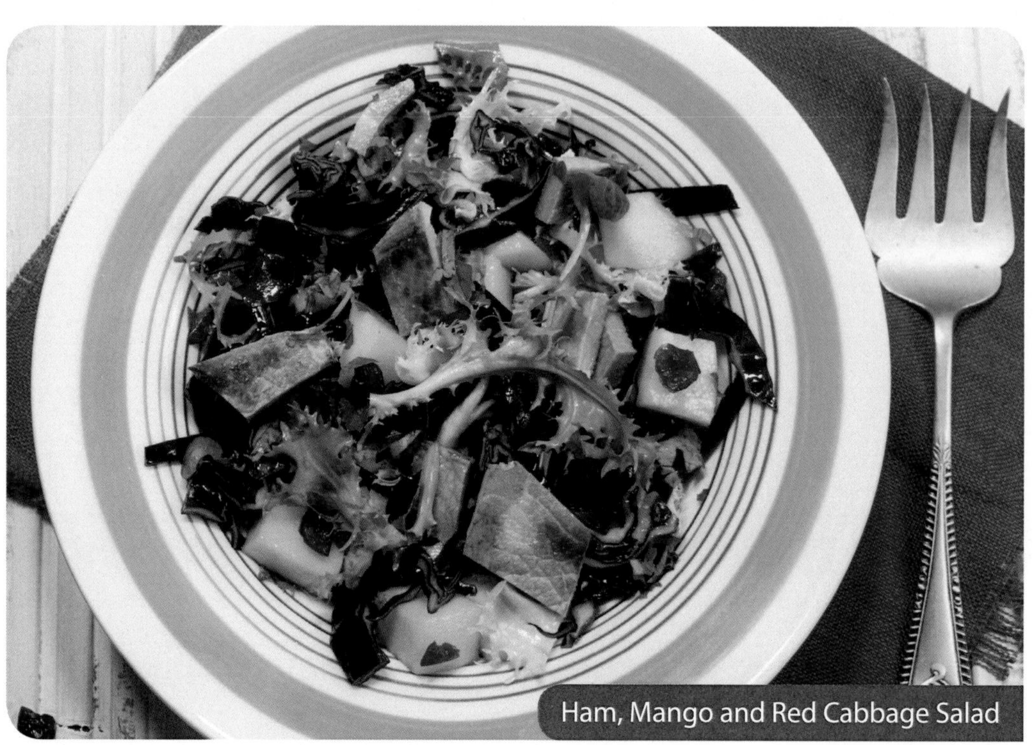
Ham, Mango and Red Cabbage Salad

HAM, MANGO AND RED CABBAGE SALAD

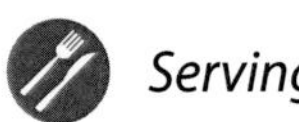 *Servings: 2*

 *Preparation Time: 15 minutes*

Ingredients

300g thick cut ham, chopped

½ bag mixed crisp salad leaves

30g dried cranberries

Sea salt

1 mango, diced

¼ head red cabbage, shredded

2 tbsp fresh parsley

FOR THE DRESSING

2 tbsp olive oil

1 orange, juice only

Preparation

1. Chop the ham, mango and cabbage.
2. Place in a bowl with the salad leaves, parsley and cranberries.
3. Mix together the dressing and toss with the salad mixture.
4. Season to taste.

MEDITERRANEAN VEGETABLE SALAD

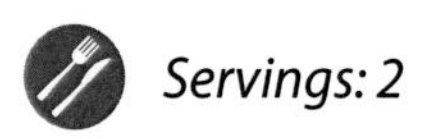
Servings: 2

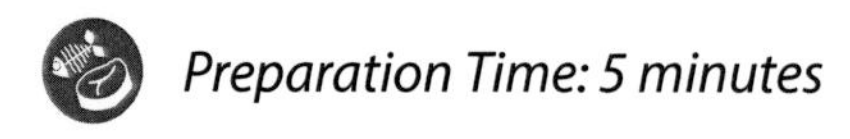
Preparation Time: 5 minutes

LUNCH
SALADS

Ingredients

1 bag mixed salad leaf

12 black olives

1 red pepper, chopped

Leftover Roasted Mediterranean Vegetables

1 tbsp balsamic vinegar

2 tbsp fresh parsley, chopped

Preparation

1 Chop the pepper and parsley.

2 Place all ingredients into a bowl and mix together.

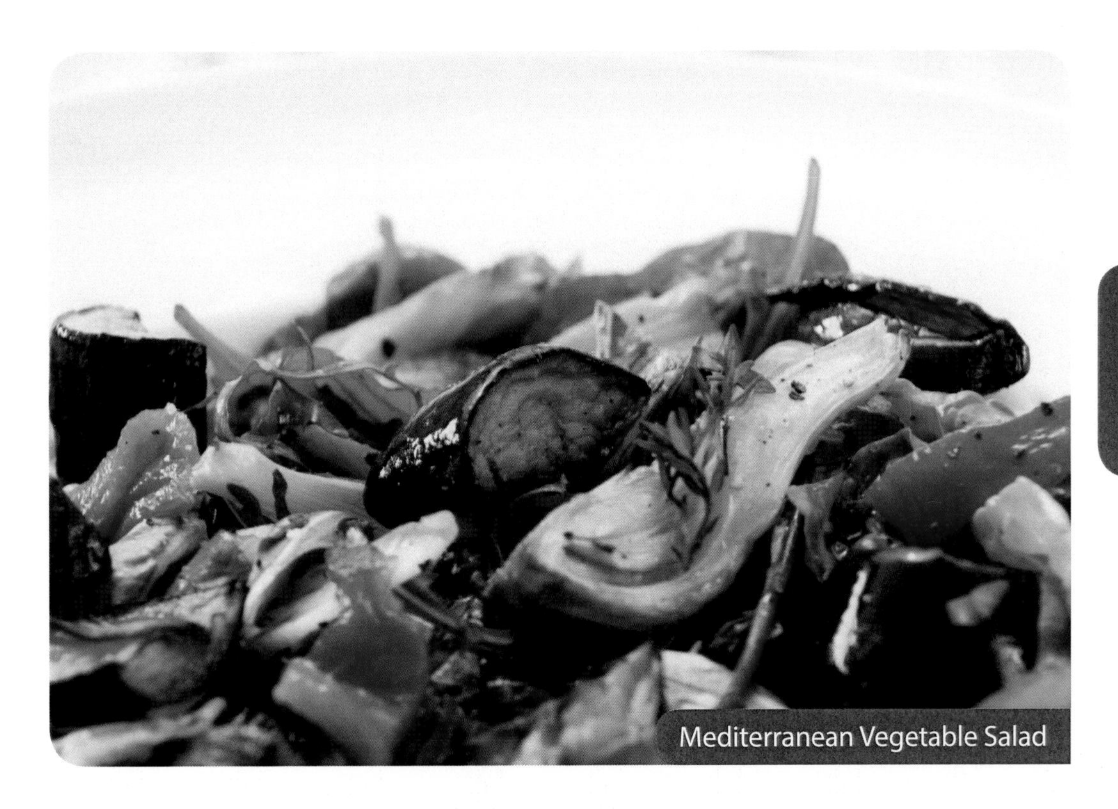

Mediterranean Vegetable Salad

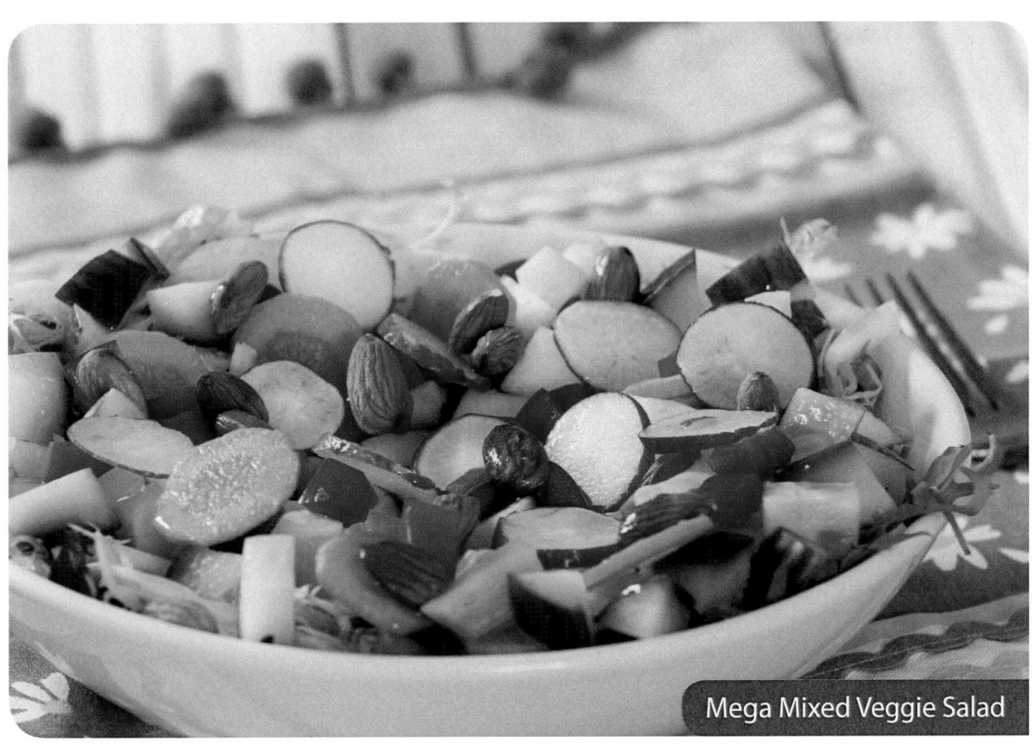

Mega Mixed Veggie Salad

MEGA MIXED VEGGIE SALAD

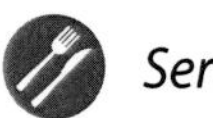 *Servings: 2*

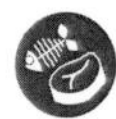 *Preparation Time: 10 minutes*

LUNCH
SALADS

Ingredients

1 bag crunchy salad leaf
1 apple, chopped
6 radishes, thinly sliced
½ yellow pepper, diced
½ red onion, sliced
Sea salt
Fresh parsley, chopped
½ cucumber, diced
1 fennel bulb, sliced
½ red pepper, diced
1 carrot, thinly sliced
20 whole almonds
Freshly ground black pepper
1 portion of Mustard Vinaigrette

Preparation

1. Prepare the cucumber, apple, fennel, radishes, peppers, carrot and red onion.
2. Place all the ingredients into a bowl and mix together well.
3. Serve with Mustard Vinaigrette.

MUSTARD CHICKEN SALAD

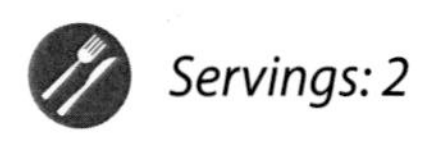
Servings: 2

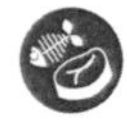
Preparation Time: 15 minutes

Ingredients

300g cooked chicken, chopped

¼ white cabbage, shredded

½ red onion, finely sliced

2 tbsp fresh parsley, chopped

Freshly ground black pepper

¼ head red cabbage, shredded

2 carrots, grated

50g gherkins, chopped

Sea salt

FOR THE DRESSING

2 tbsp extra virgin olive oil

1 tsp Dijon mustard

1 tbsp balsamic vinegar

Preparation

1 Make the dressing by mixing together the ingredients and set aside.

2 Toss together all the salad ingredients, ensuring evenly mixed through.

3 Add the dressing and season to taste before serving immediately.

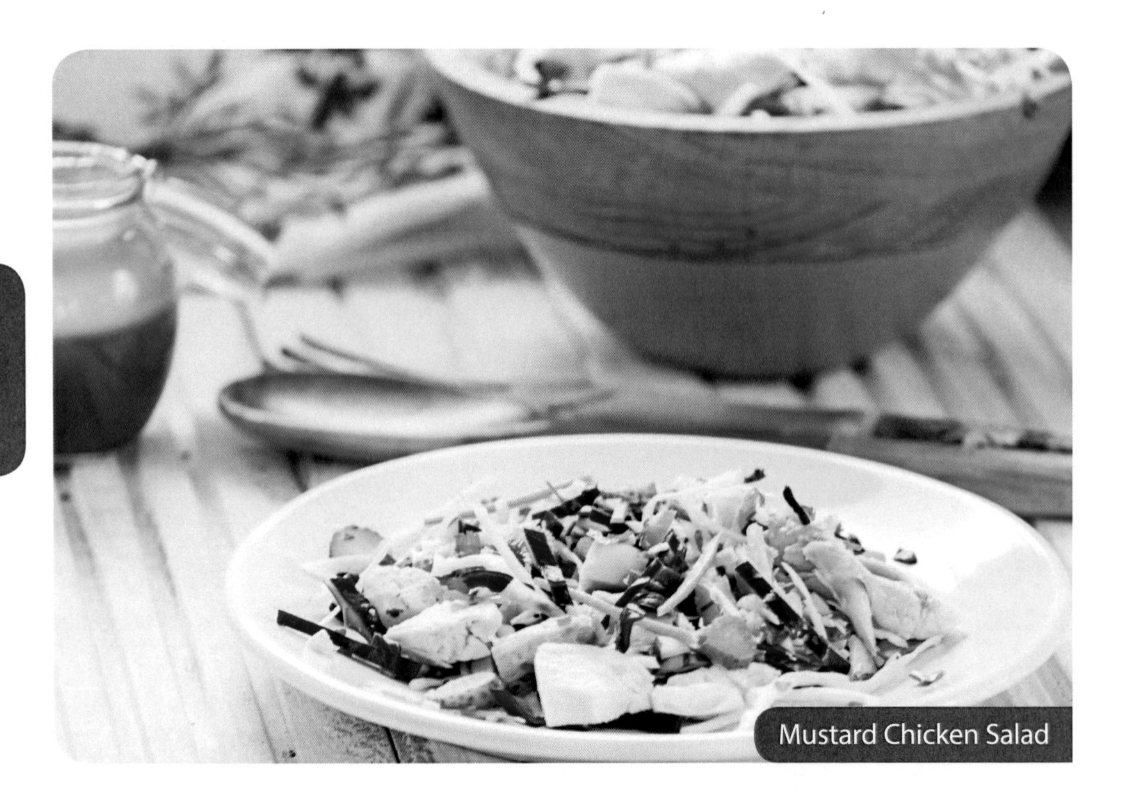

Mustard Chicken Salad

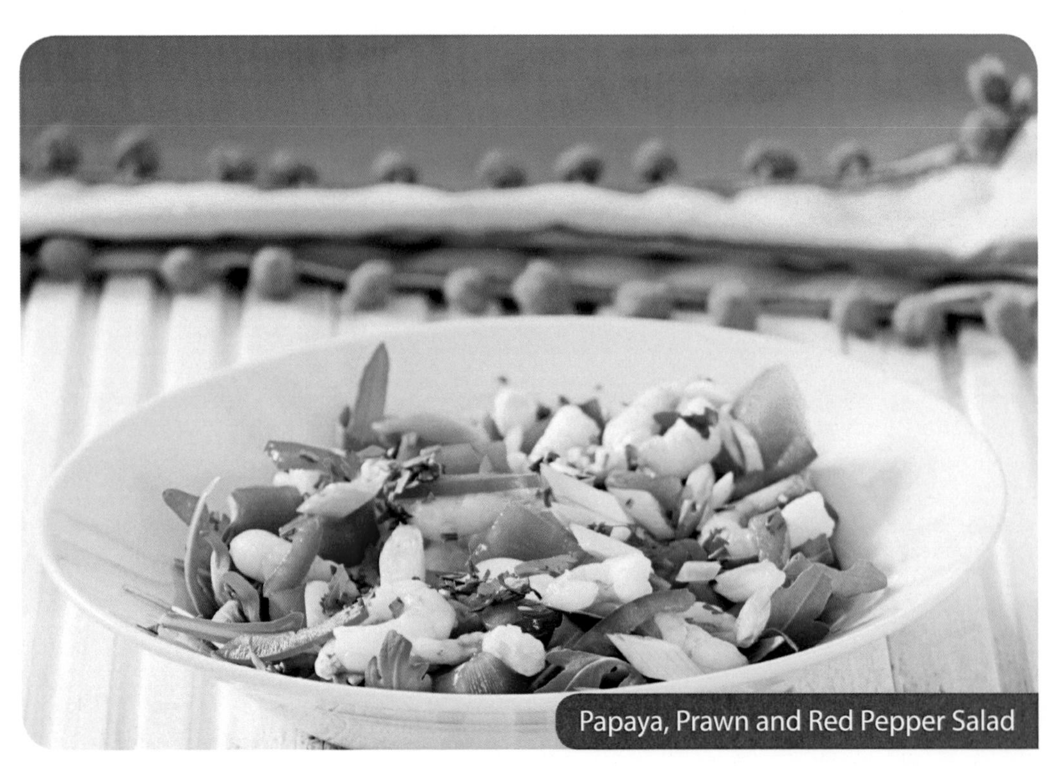

Papaya, Prawn and Red Pepper Salad

PAPAYA, PRAWN AND RED PEPPER SALAD

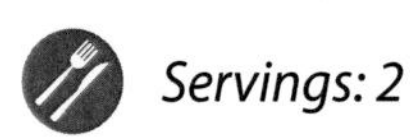
Servings: 2

Preparation Time: 15 minutes

Ingredients

2 papaya, chopped

4 spring onions, finely chopped

100g rocket

200g cooked prawns

½ red pepper, finely sliced

2 tbsp fresh coriander

FOR THE DRESSING

1 lime, juice only

2 tbsp walnut oil

Preparation

1. Prepare the papaya, spring onions and pepper.
2. Mix together all the salad ingredients.
3. Mix together the dressing and toss with the salad.
4. Season to taste.

PRAWN AND AVOCADO SALAD

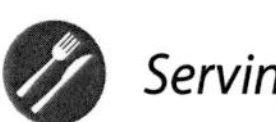 *Servings: 2*

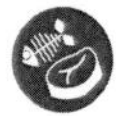 *Preparation Time: 10 minutes*

Ingredients

2 ripe avocado, chopped

½ cucumber, thinly sliced

1 bag mixed leaves

200g cooked prawns

FOR THE DRESSING

2 tbsp olive oil

Sea salt

1 lemon, juice only

Freshly ground black pepper

Ingredients

1. Prepare the avocado and cucumber and place into a bowl with the mixed salad leaves.
2. Add the prawns to the salad ingredients.
3. Mix the olive oil and lemon juice together and toss with the salad ingredients.
4. Season to taste.

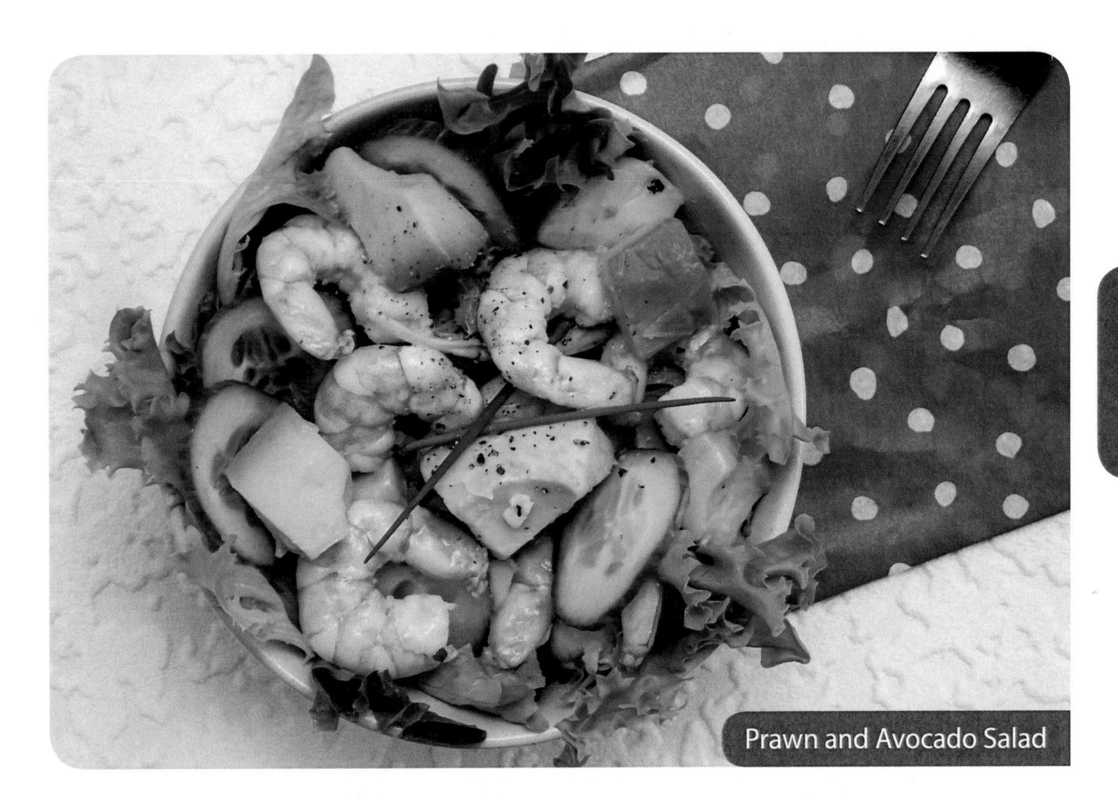

Prawn and Avocado Salad

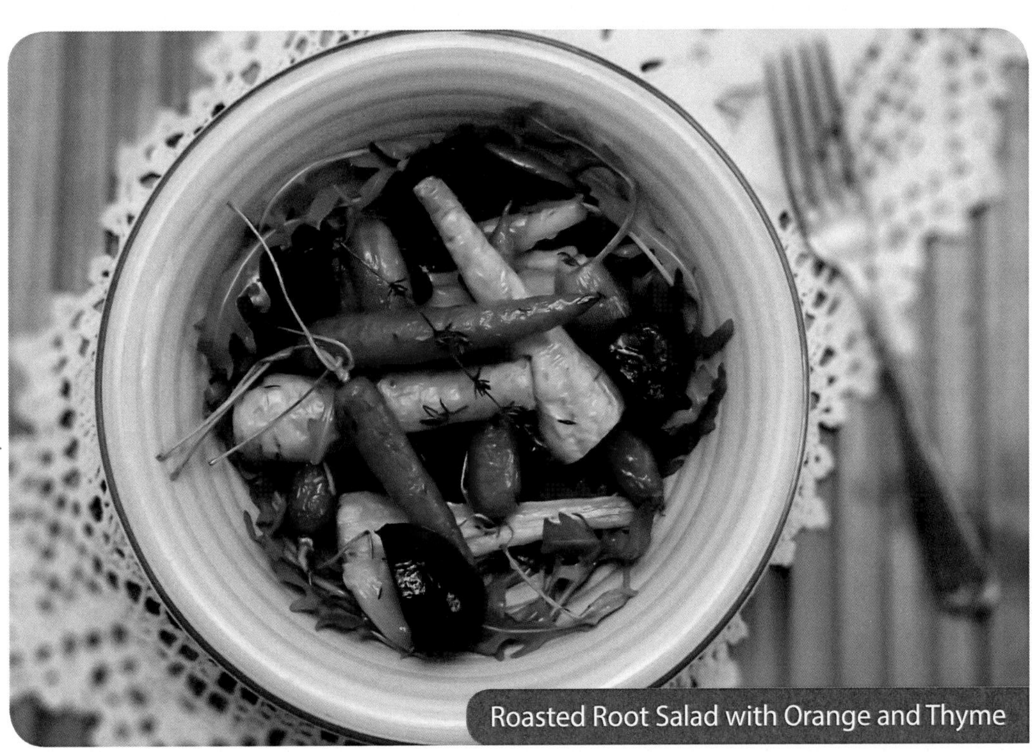

Roasted Root Salad with Orange and Thyme

SCALLOPS WITH FRISEE AND BACON

 *Servings: 2*

 *Preparation Time: 5 minutes*

 *Cooking Time: 10 minutes*

 *Total Time: 15 minutes*

Ingredients

10 fresh scallops, white meat only

100g frisee salad leaf
(or other salad leaf if you prefer)

100g streaky bacon lardons

FOR THE DRESSING

1 tbsp walnut oil

Sea salt

2 tbsp fresh parsley, chopped

1 tbsp balsamic vinegar

Freshly ground black pepper

Preparation

1. Heat a pan over a high heat and add the lardons. You should not need any cooking fat; the bacon should render enough oil to cook the remaining ingredients.
2. Cook for about 5 minutes or until the bacon is browned and crisp.
3. Remove from the pan and set to one side.
4. Add the scallops and sear for a minute or so on each side. They need to be cooked through, but overcook very easily. The scallops will be slightly firm to the touch, and opaque when done.
5. Season the scallops with salt and pepper then remove from the heat.
6. Allow to rest for a minute or two whilst you put the frisee in a big bowl.
7. Slice the scallops into thick slices and add to the frisee with the bacon.
8. Mix the oil and balsamic and toss with the frisee, bacon and scallops.
9. Serve in big bistro bowls and sprinkle the fresh parsley over the top.

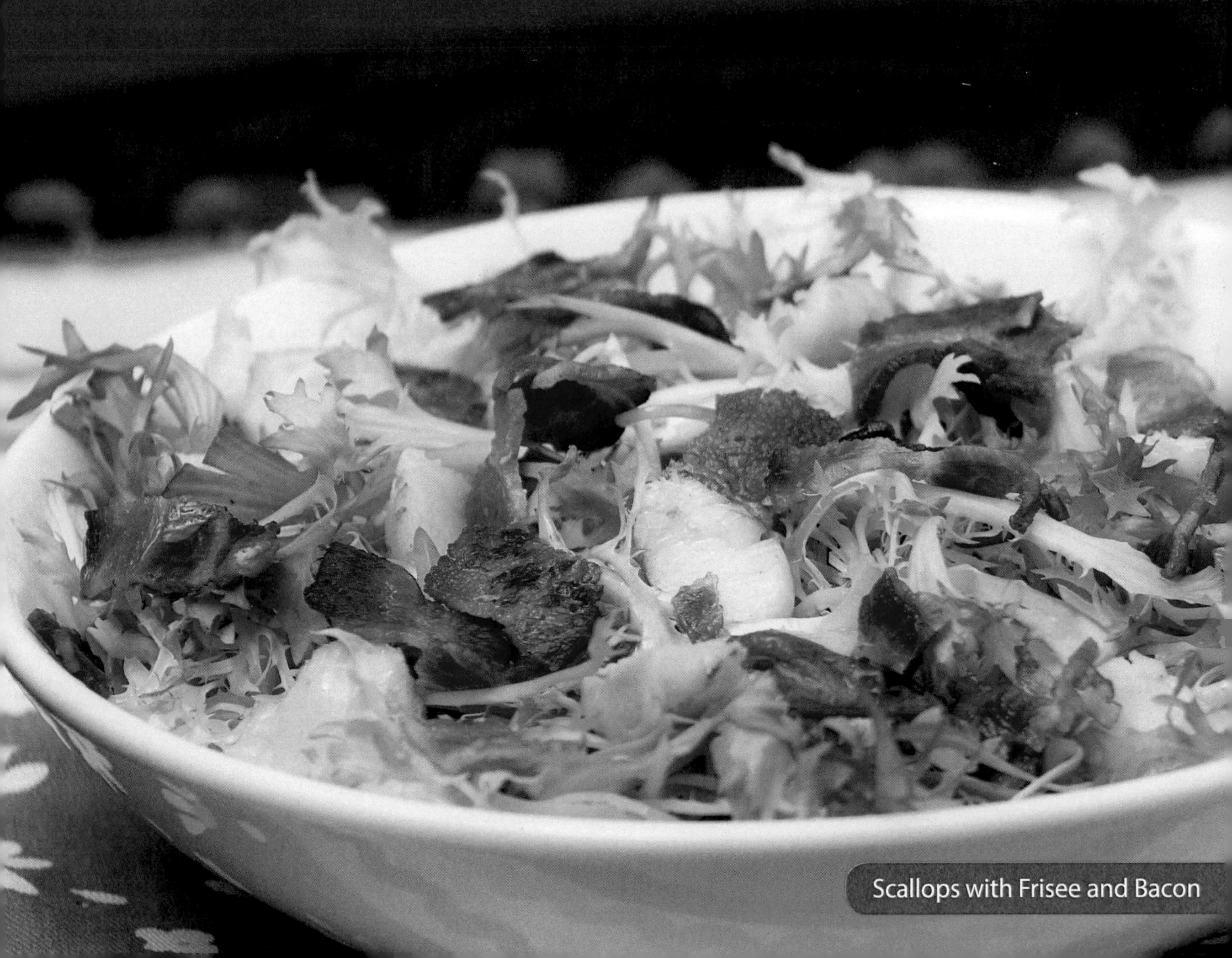

Scallops with Frisee and Bacon

ROASTED ROOT SALAD WITH ORANGE AND THYME

If you cannot get baby vegetables (you are looking for long skinny ones rather than tiny fat ones) use full sized ones and cut into thin wedges.

 *Servings: 2*

 *Preparation Time: 15 minutes*

 *Cooking Time: 40 minutes*

 *Total Time: 55 minutes*

Ingredients

2 tbsp lard, dripping or goose fat

150g baby parsnips

6 garlic cloves, smashed

4 sprigs fresh thyme

100g rocket

150g baby carrots

4 small beetroots, quartered

8 shallots, peeled and halved

Sea salt

FOR THE DRESSING

2 tbsp walnut oil

1 orange, juice only

Preparation

1. Preheat the oven to 200C.
2. Place the carrots, parsnips, beetroot and shallots onto a baking tray.
3. Evenly mix the fat, garlic and thyme within the vegetables.
4. Season well with sea salt and roast until tender and caramelised (30-40 minutes). You will need to move them around and turn them occasionally to prevent them sticking and burning.
5. Toss the rocket with the oil and orange juice, then top with the roasted roots.
6. Eat whilst still warm.

CARROT AND GINGER SOUP

 *Servings: 2*

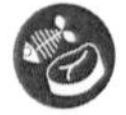 *Preparation Time: 20 minutes*

 *Cooking Time: 30 minutes*

 *Total Time: 50 minutes*

Ingredients

1 tbsp lard, dripping or goose fat

1 garlic clove, left whole

300g carrots, peeled and chopped

500ml vegetable stock or water

½ tsp allspice, ground

1 onion, chopped

2 inches fresh ginger, peeled and chopped

1 orange, juice only

Sea salt

Preparation

1. Prepare the onions, carrots and ginger.
2. Heat the fat in a large saucepan.
3. Add the onions with the clove of garlic and a pinch of salt.
4. Cook the onions down for about 5 minutes and then add the carrots with the ginger.
5. Cover, turn the heat down, and cook for about 10 minutes until the carrots begin to soften.
6. Add the stock or water with the orange juice and simmer for another 15 minutes until the carrots are soft.
7. Blend until smooth and season to taste.
8. Sprinkle a dash of allspice on top to serve.

CHORIZO AND SAVOY CABBAGE BROTH

 *Servings: 2*

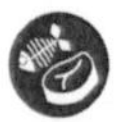 *Preparation Time: 10 minutes*

 *Cooking Time: 30 minutes*

 *Total Time: 40 minutes*

Ingredients

2 tbsp lard, dripping or goose fat

2 garlic cloves

1 tbsp tomato puree

500ml Chicken Stock

Sea salt

1 onion, chopped

150g chorizo, sliced

½ head Savoy cabbage, shredded

2 tbsp fresh parsley, chopped

Freshly ground black pepper

Preparation

1. Prepare the onion, chorizo, cabbage and parsley.
2. Over a medium flame, heat the fat in a large saucepan and fry the onion with the salt.
3. Cook the onions until they are soft and translucent.
4. Add the garlic, chorizo and tomato puree and stir. Then add the stock.
5. Add the cabbage and simmer for about 20 minutes or until the cabbage is tender.
6. Add the parsley, season to taste and serve hot.

CLEAR AND CALM SOUP

 *Servings: 2*

 *Preparation Time: 10 minutes*

 *Cooking Time: 20 minutes*

 *Total Time: 30 minutes*

Ingredients

1 litre Chicken Stock

1 stem lemongrass, finely chopped

2cm fresh ginger, grated

100g bok choi, shredded

2 red chilli, sliced finely

1 garlic clove, crushed

2 tbsp fresh coriander, chopped

1 pinch sea salt

Preparation

1. Prepare the chilli (deseed if you prefer less heat), lemongrass, garlic, ginger, coriander and bok choi.
2. Heat the Chicken Stock in a large saucepan over a medium heat.
3. Add all the ingredients except the coriander.
4. Bring almost to the boil, remove from the heat, cover and set aside.
5. Leave to infuse for ten minutes, add the coriander and serve hot.

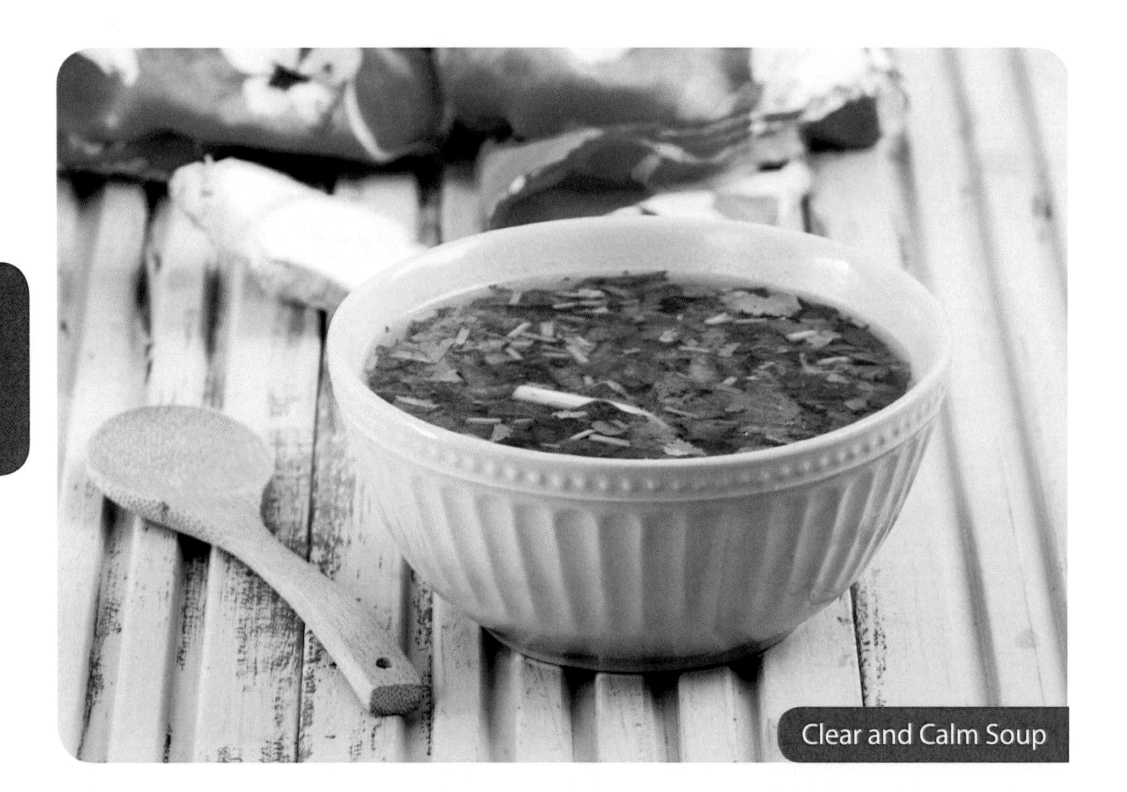

Clear and Calm Soup

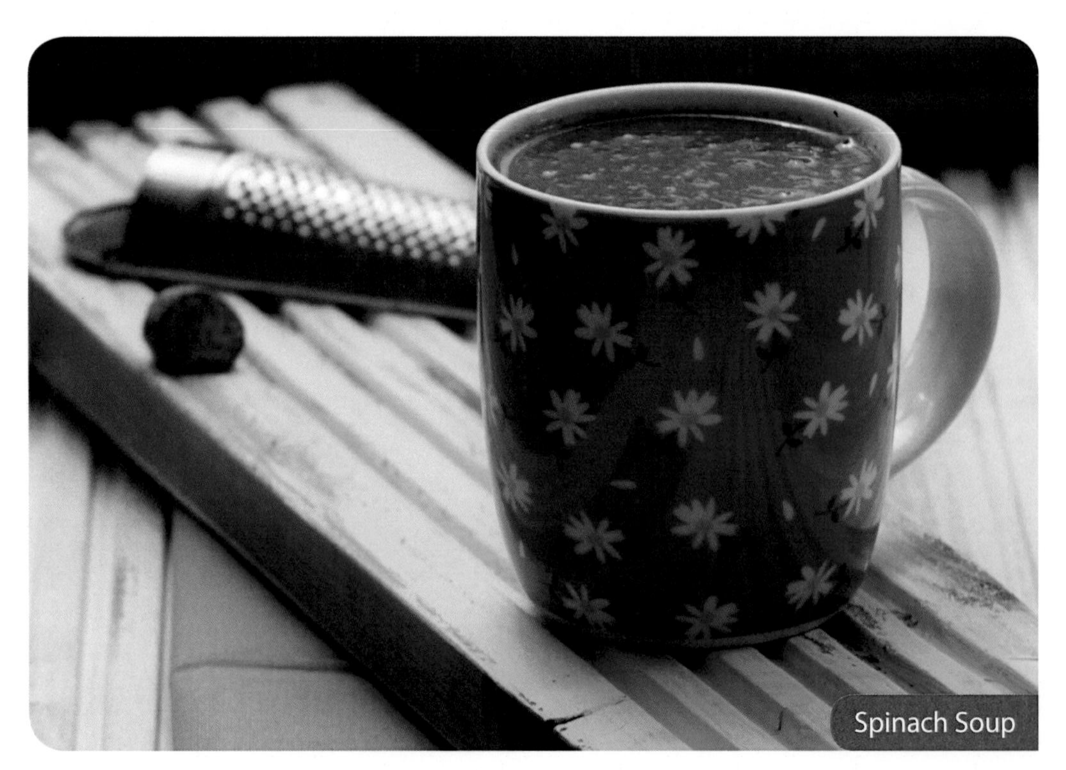

Spinach Soup

SPINACH SOUP

This soup really needs Chicken Stock to add depth of flavour.

 *Servings: 2*

 *Preparation Time: 5 minutes*

 *Cooking Time: 15 minutes*

 *Total Time: 20 minutes*

Ingredients

1 tbsp lard, dripping or goose fat

1 onion, finely chopped

500ml Chicken Stock

Sea salt

200g spinach

2 garlic cloves, crushed

Freshly grated nutmeg

Preparation

1. Prepare the onions and garlic.
2. Heat the fat in a large pan and cook the onions with a pinch of salt.
3. Lower the heat and allow to cook until soft and translucent; verging on golden even.
4. Add the garlic and spinach, closely followed by the chicken stock.
5. Simmer for about 10 minutes and blitz to smooth in a blender or processor.
6. Serve hot with a good grate of fresh nutmeg.

CURRIED CAULIFLOWER SOUP

 *Servings: 2*

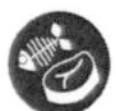 *Preparation Time: 10 minutes*

 *Cooking Time: 30 minutes*

 *Total Time: 40 minutes*

Ingredients

1 head cauliflower, in florets

1 onion, chopped

2 tsp curry powder

500ml Chicken Stock

1 garlic clove, crushed

2 tbsp lard, dripping or goose fat

Sea salt

Preparation

1. Prepare the cauliflower, onion and garlic.
2. Heat the fat in a sauce pan and add the onion, garlic, cauliflower, salt and spice.
3. Cover and cook for about 10 minutes.
4. Stir in the stock and simmer for about 20 minutes until the cauliflower is tender.
5. Blend until smooth adding seasoning to taste.
6. Serve hot.

LEEK AND BACON SOUP

 *Servings: 2*

 *Preparation Time: 10 minutes*

 *Cooking Time: 30 minutes*

 *Total Time: 40 minutes*

Ingredients

2 tbsp lard, dripping or goose fat

2 garlic cloves, crushed

2 large leeks, chopped

2 tbsp fresh parsley, chopped

Freshly ground black pepper

1 onion, chopped

150g bacon, sliced

500ml Chicken Stock

Sea salt

Preparation

1. Prepare the onion, bacon, leeks, parsley and garlic.
2. Heat the fat in a large saucepan and fry the onion and leeks with the salt.
3. Continue cooking until they are soft and translucent.
4. Add the garlic and bacon, stir, and then add the stock.
5. Simmer for about 20 minutes until the leeks are meltingly tender.
6. If you want a smooth soup then you can put into a blender or eat chunky as it is.
7. Season to taste and add the parsley.
8. Serve hot.

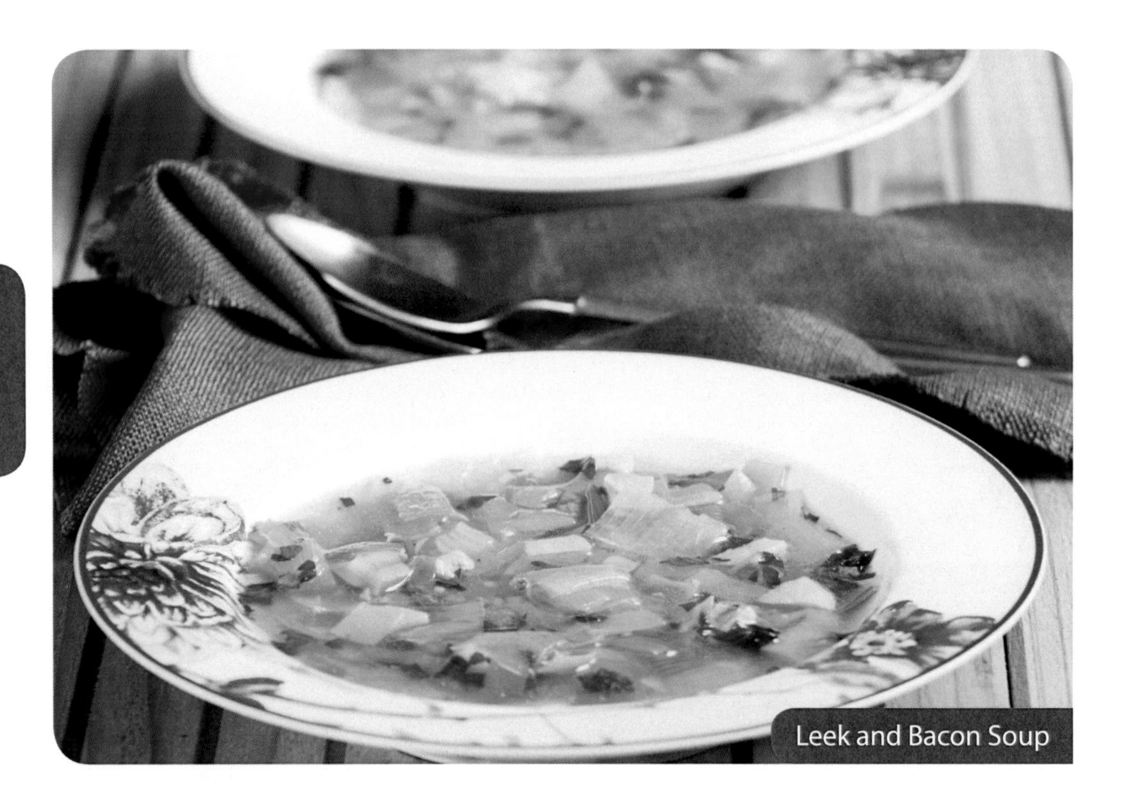
Leek and Bacon Soup

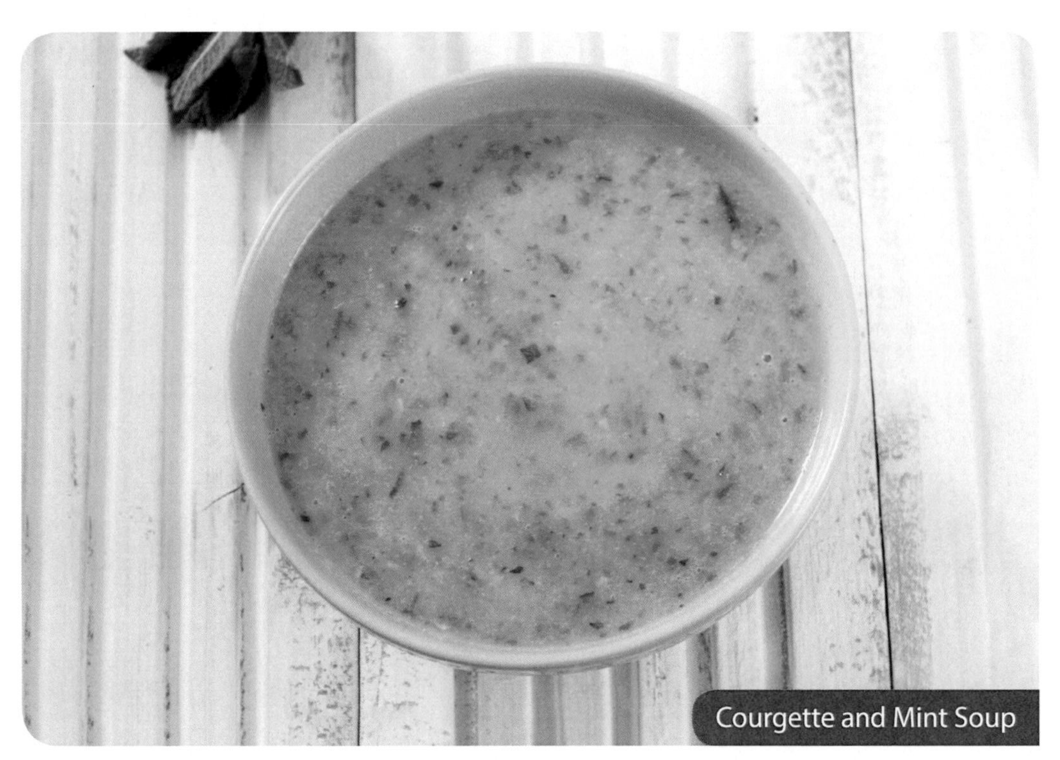
Courgette and Mint Soup

COURGETTE AND MINT SOUP

 *Servings: 2*

 *Preparation Time: 20 minutes*

 *Cooking Time: 30 minutes*

 *Total Time: 50 minutes*

Ingredients

4 large courgettes, chopped

2 tbsp lard, dripping or goose fat

500ml Chicken Stock

Sea salt

1 onion, diced

1 garlic clove, crushed

2 tbsp fresh mint, chopped

Freshly ground black pepper

Preparation

1. Prepare the courgettes, onion and mint.
2. Heat the fat in a saucepan and add the onions, courgette, and salt.
3. Cook over a low heat for about 10 minutes until the vegetables getting softer.
4. Add the garlic, followed by the Chicken Stock.
5. Simmer for 20 minutes until the courgette is tender.
6. Blitz in a blender, season to taste and add the fresh mint.
7. Serve hot.

LEEK AND CELERIAC SOUP

 *Servings: 2*

 *Preparation Time: 15 minutes*

 *Cooking Time: 30 minutes*

 *Total Time: 45 minutes*

Ingredients

1 tbsp lard, dripping or goose fat

½ celeriac, chopped

1 garlic clove, crushed

500ml Chicken Stock, or water

Sea salt

½ onion, chopped

2 leeks, chopped

1 tsp allspice

Freshly ground black pepper

Preparation

1 Heat the fat in a large saucepan and add the onions, leeks and celeriac with a pinch of salt and the allspice.

2 Stir to combine and cover. Cook over a gentle heat, stirring occasionally until the vegetables begin to soften.

3 Add the stock or water and simmer gently for about 20 minutes, or until the celeriac is soft.

4 Puree the soup in a blender and season to taste.

MEXICAN CHICKEN SOUP

 *Servings: 4*

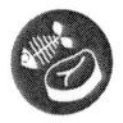 *Preparation Time: 30 minutes*

 *Cooking Time: 2 hours*

 *Total Time: 2 hours, 30 minutes*

Ingredients

1 small whole chicken
2 tbsp lard, dripping or goose fat
4 green chillies (fat jalapenos), finely chopped
1 tsp dried oregano
400g tinned chopped tomatoes
1 small bunch fresh coriander, finely chopped
Sea salt
1 red onion, diced
2 garlic cloves, finely chopped
1 tsp cumin
1 tbsp smoked paprika
1 lime, in quarters
1 small bunch fresh mint, finely chopped
Freshly ground black pepper

Preparation

1. Prepare the onion, garlic, chillies and herbs. Deseed the chillies for a milder soup.
2. Heat the fat in a pan large enough to take the chicken.
3. Fry the onion with the cumin and paprika.
4. Add the garlic, half of the herbs and the chillies.
5. Add the tinned tomatoes, the lime pieces and the chicken.
6. Season and cover with cold water and bring to the boil.
7. Simmer for two hours, until the chicken falls from the bone.
8. Serve in soup bowls with the rest of the herbs for garnish.

SQUASH AND BACON SOUP

 *Servings: 2*

 *Preparation Time: 10 minutes*

 *Cooking Time: 30 minutes*

 *Total Time: 40 minutes*

Ingredients

½ butternut squash, peeled and cut into 1-inch cubes

1 large onion, finely chopped

1 tsp lard, dripping or goose fat

100g smoked bacon, chopped

Freshly ground black pepper

Freshly grated nutmeg

8 pecan nuts, crumbled

500ml Chicken Stock, or water

Preparation

1. Melt the fat in a large saucepan and add the squash, bacon and onion. Cook over a low heat for about 5 minutes.
2. Add the nutmeg and the chicken stock; simmer gently until the squash is soft.
3. Season with black pepper and process in a blender just enough to break down the squash but leave bits of bacon.
4. Serve with crumbled pecans on top.

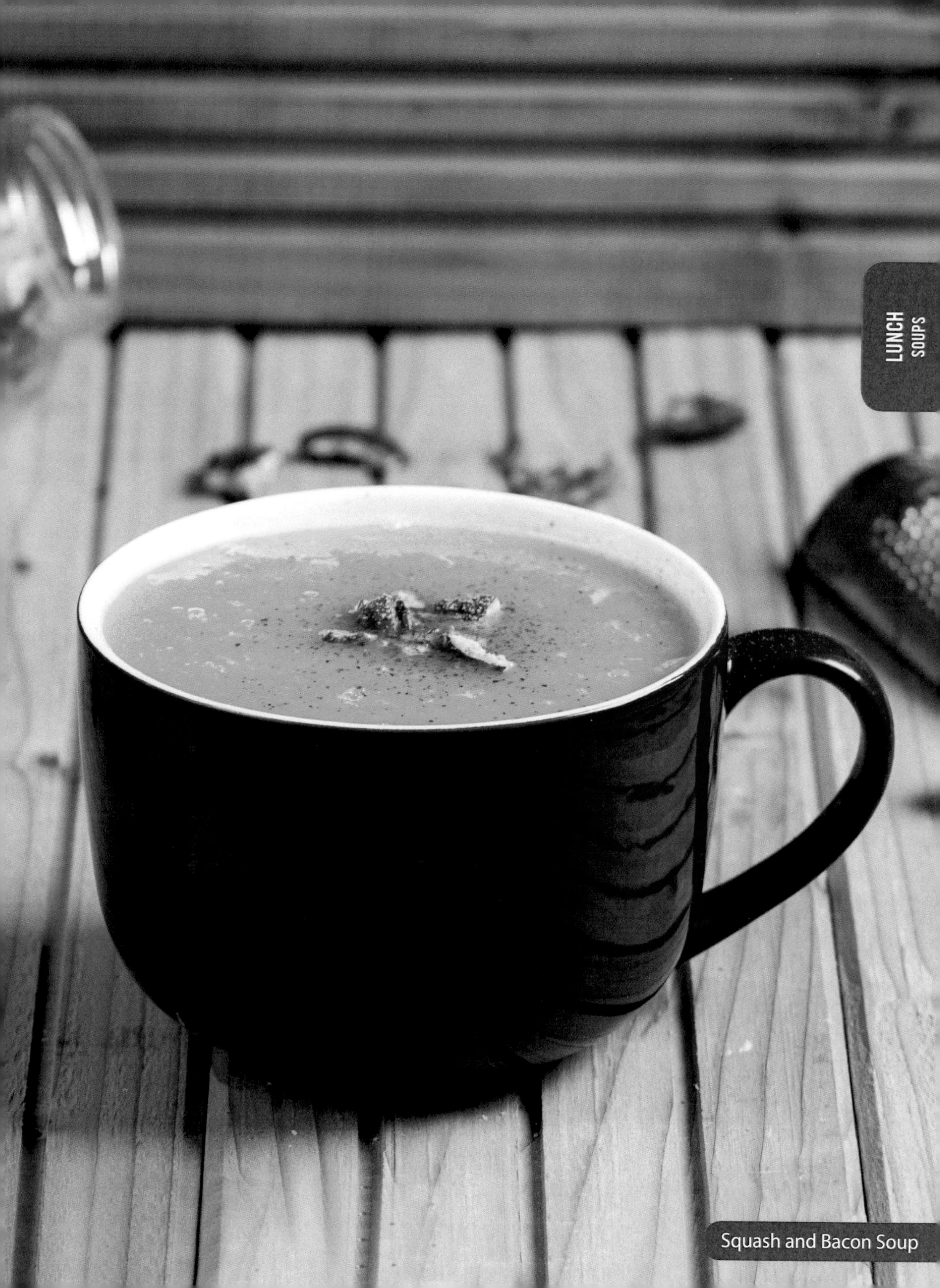

Squash and Bacon Soup

SPINACH AND SQUASH SOUP

 *Servings: 2*

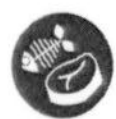 *Preparation Time: 10 minutes*

 *Cooking Time: 30 minutes*

 *Total Time: 40 minutes*

Ingredients

½ large butternut squash, peeled and cubed

1 small garlic clove, crushed

2 tbsp coconut oil

1 tsp ground allspice

1 large onion, coarsely chopped

150g spinach

1 pinch sea salt

300ml Chicken Stock (or water)

Preparation

1. Prepare the butternut squash, onion and garlic.
2. Heat the oil in a large saucepan over a medium heat.
3. Add the butternut squash, garlic, onion, allspice, and salt.
4. Stir to combine and cook gently for 5 to 10 minutes until everything begins to soften.
5. Pour in the cold stock, add the spinach and simmer gently until the squash is soft.
6. Blitz in a food processor, just to break it down slightly.
7. Season to taste.
8. Serve hot.

CHILLI CHICKEN STIR FRIED GREENS

 *Servings: 2*

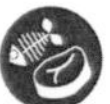 *Preparation Time: 15 minutes*

 *Cooking Time: 10 minutes*

 *Total Time: 25 minutes*

Ingredients

1 tbsp coconut oil

½ red onion, diced

1 inch ginger, grated

4 large bok choi

Sea salt

2 chicken breasts, chopped

2 red chillies, sliced

2 garlic cloves, minced

2 limes, juice only

Preparation

1. Heat the coconut oil in a wok or frying pan over a high heat and add the chicken with the onions and chillies and a pinch of salt.
2. Cook, stirring occasionally, until the chicken is cooked through and the onions are soft.
3. Add the bok choi with the ginger, garlic and lime juice. Cook for only a minute; you want the greens just wilting and those aromatic flavours really clean and fresh.
4. Tip into bowls and serve hot.

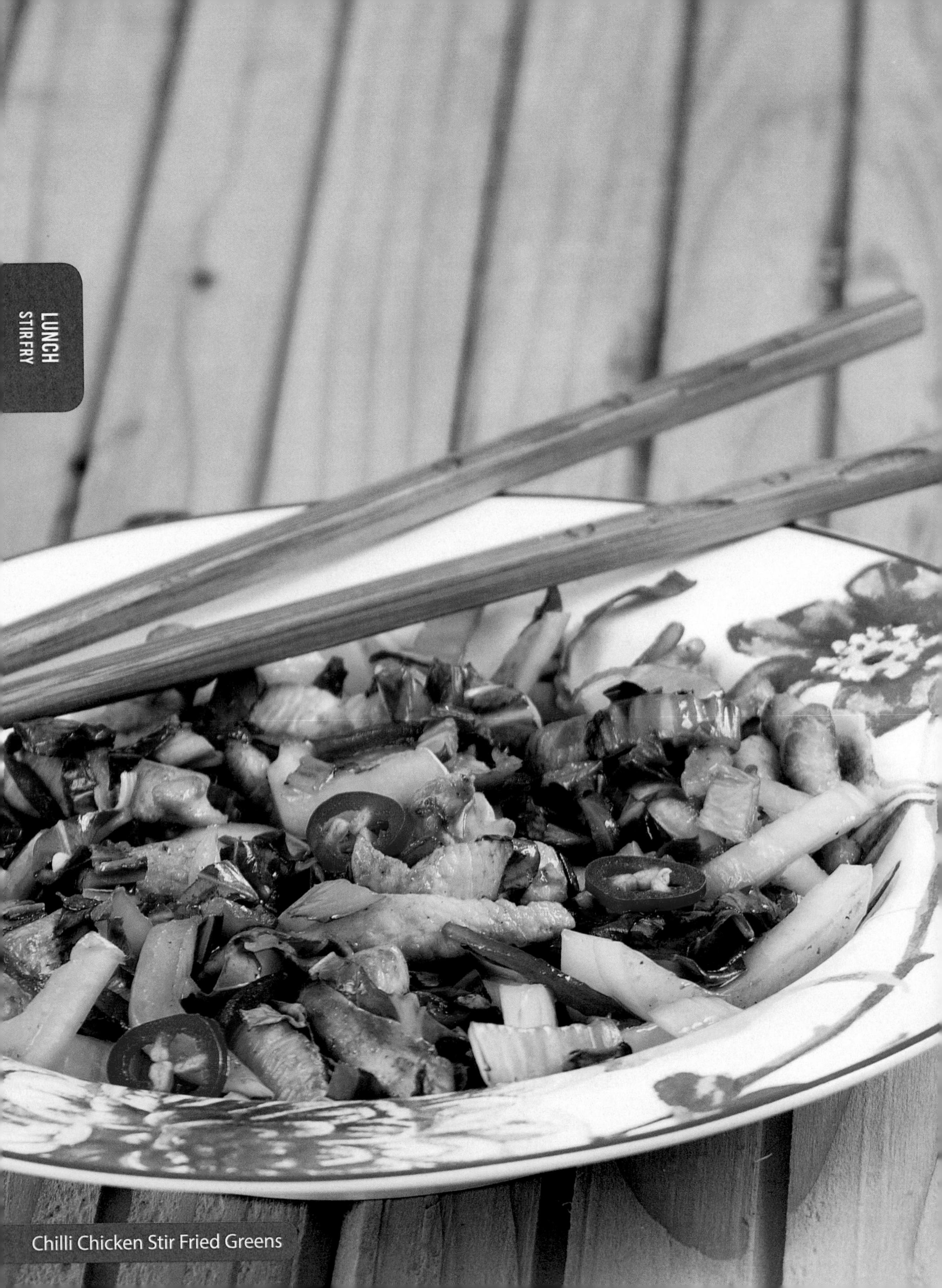

Chilli Chicken Stir Fried Greens

WRAPS

ASIAN TUNA WRAP

Make sure you buy tuna in brine, spring water or olive oil and avoid those tinned with Sunflower Oil.

 *Servings: 2*

 *Preparation Time: 10 minutes*

Ingredients

8 large iceberg lettuce leaves

1 handful beansprouts

2 spring onions, thinly sliced

¼ cucumber, thinly sliced

1 tin tuna, drained

1 carrot, grated

1 tbsp sesame oil

Preparation

1. Prepare the carrot, cucumber and spring onions.
2. Drain the tuna and place into a bowl with all of the ingredients except for the lettuce.
3. Mix all the ingredients together and then share evenly between the 8 lettuce leaves. Roll into wraps.

AVOCADO AND BACON WRAP

 *Servings: 2*

 *Preparation Time: 5 minutes*

 *Cooking Time: 10 minutes*

 *Total Time: 15 minutes*

Ingredients

8 large iceberg lettuce leaves

8 rashers bacon, cooked

2 avocado, sliced

Preparation

1. Place the bacon into a non-stick frying pan and cook until it is as crispy as you desire.
2. Whilst the bacon is cooking slice the avocado.
3. Once the bacon is cooked, chop and add to the avocado.
4. Place the fillings into each lettuce leaf and use as a wrap.

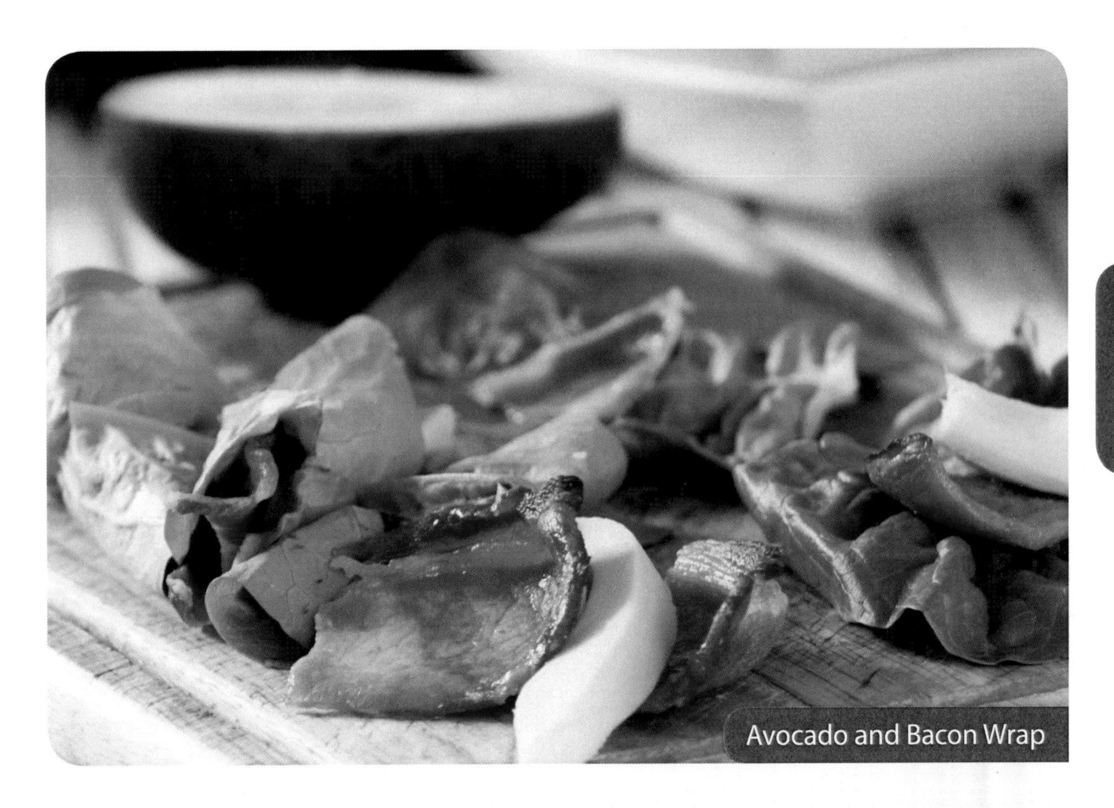

Avocado and Bacon Wrap

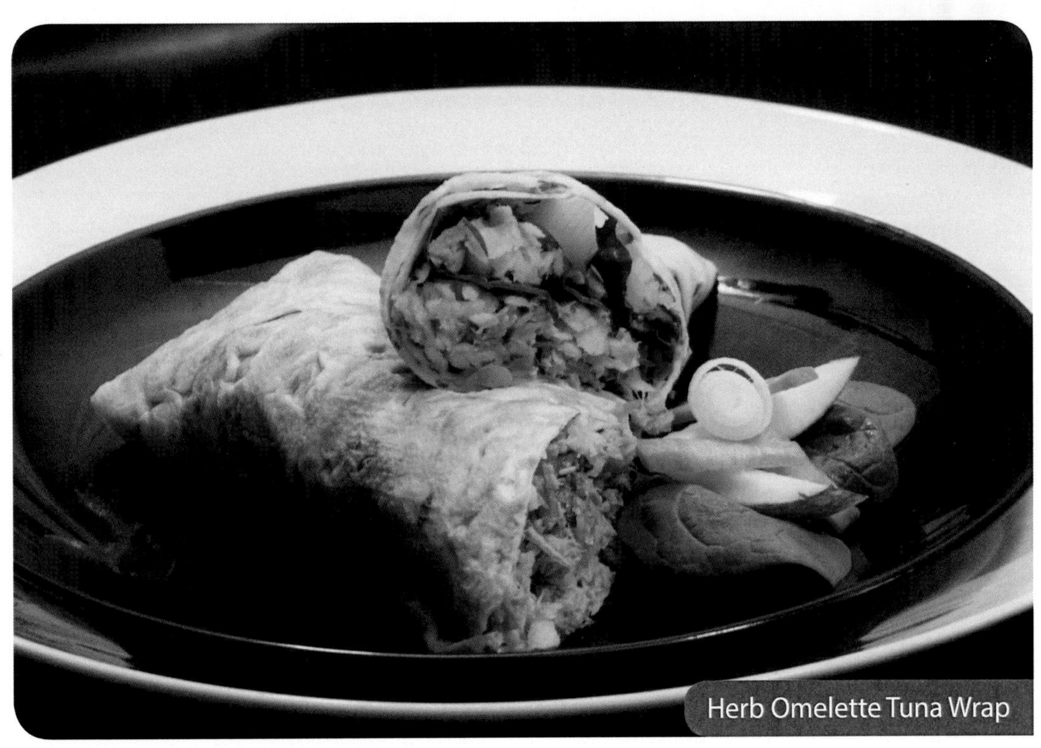

Herb Omelette Tuna Wrap

HERB OMELETTE TUNA WRAP

These thin omelettes make an excellent Paleo wrapper and can be served either hot or cold so are a good idea for a packed lunch.

 *Servings: 2*

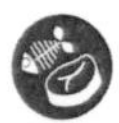 *Preparation Time: 20 minutes*

 *Cooking Time: 10 minutes*

 *Total Time: 30 minutes*

Ingredients

FOR THE OMELETTE

3 large eggs

1 tbsp parsley, finely chopped

1 pinch freshly ground black pepper

1 tbsp water

1 pinch sea salt

1 tsp lard, dripping or goose fat

FOR THE FILLING

1 tin tuna, drained

1 large carrot, grated

1 green apple, grated

2 spring onions, finely chopped

1 handful baby spinach leaves

Preparation

1. Prepare the parsley, onions, carrot and apple.
2. Drain the tuna and mix with the spring onions, carrot, spinach and apple.
3. Set the mixture aside. You could add a drop of olive oil if it needs moistening.
4. Beat the eggs with the water, salt and parsley.
5. Heat the fat in a frying pan.
6. When the pan is smoking hot, add enough of the egg mixture and tilt the pan so that the egg covers the surface in a thin layer. How many you get will depend on the size of your pan; aim for either 2 large or 4 small pancake-like omelettes.
7. Allow to cook for 2 or 3 minutes until golden on the bottom surface and then slide out onto a plate. There is no need to flip as it cooked through already.
8. Cook each omelette wrap in the same way and once all cooked leave to cool.
9. Place the filling inside the omelette as you would a wrap, pack it up and go.

BLT WRAP

 *Servings: 2*

 *Preparation Time: 5 minutes*

 *Cooking Time: 10 minutes*

 *Total Time: 15 minutes*

Ingredients

8 large iceberg lettuce leaves

8 rashers bacon

4 tomatoes

½ bag rocket

Paleo Mayonnaise (optional)

Preparation

1. Cook the bacon to your liking in a skillet or non-stick frying pan. Add some olive oil or coconut oil if needed.
2. While the bacon is cooking slice the tomatoes and make the Mayonnaise if you wish to use this.
3. Place the bacon, tomatoes and rocket inside each lettuce leaf and wrap.

ITALIAN WRAP

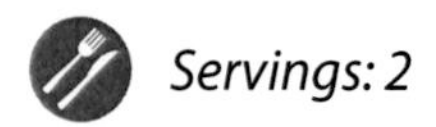

Servings: 2

Preparation Time: 10 minutes

Ingredients

8 large iceberg lettuce leaves

2 tomatoes, sliced

½ small jar artichoke hearts, sliced

½ small jar roasted red bell pepper, seeded and julienned

8 slices salami, very thinly sliced

12 black olives

1 handful rocket

Preparation

1 Prepare the salami, tomatoes, peppers and artichoke and place in a bowl.

2 Add the olives and the rocket and mix well together.

3 Place the filling inside the lettuce leaf as use as a wrap.

SALMON, SPRING ONION AND CUCUMBER WRAP

 *Servings: 2*

 *Preparation Time: 10 minutes*

Ingredients

8 large iceberg lettuce leaves

1 apple, sliced

¼ cucumber, sliced

1 tin of salmon, drained

½ bag rocket

4 spring onions, finely chopped

Preparation

1. Prepare the apple, cucumber and the spring onions and drain the salmon.
2. Mix all the ingredients, except the lettuce, into a bowl and season to taste.
3. Wrap the fillings inside each lettuce leaf, using it as a wrap.

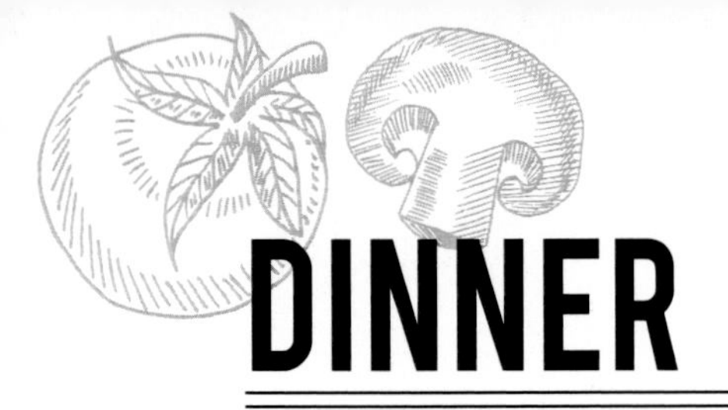

DINNER

For most people this is the main meal of the day and our recipes will not disappoint. We have created over 60 recipes based on a variety of ingredients including beef, pork, lamb, chicken, turkey, duck and fish so there will be something for everyone. It includes favourites such as steak and burgers and even a Shepherds Pie for times when comfort food is needed. The variety is amazing and the taste superb. You will not be going hungry!

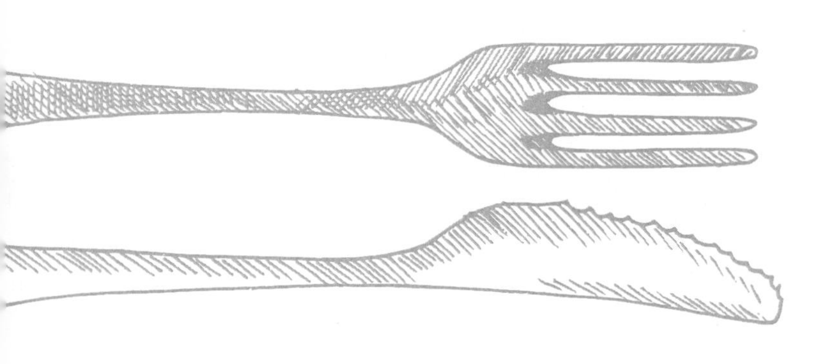

BEEF

BEANLESS BEEF CHILLI

The cooking time of this chilli is simmering time to get a really good texture and flavour. If you are in a hurry, omit the water and turn the heat up. Everyone's palate for chilli is different so alter the heat as you wish; you could provide a bowl of chopped fresh chillies on the side for those who really like the spice.

 *Servings: 4*

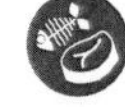 *Preparation Time: 20 minutes*

 *Cooking Time: 1 hour*

 *Total Time:1 hour, 20 minutes*

DINNER BEEF

Ingredients

½ tbsp lard, beef dripping or goose fat

1 yellow pepper, chopped

2 garlic cloves, crushed

1 tsp paprika

1 pinch oregano

2 tbsp tomato puree

200ml water

2 tbsp fresh coriander, chopped

1 red onion, finely chopped

1 onion, chopped

800g beef mince

1 tsp cumin

½ tsp chilli powder

1 pinch flaked sea salt

400g chopped tinned tomatoes

1 pinch freshly ground black pepper

1 large tomato, finely chopped

Preparation

1. Prepare the vegetables.
2. Heat the fat in a large saucepan over a medium heat.
3. Add the chopped onion, peppers and mince.
4. Keep stirring until the vegetables are soft and the mince has coloured.
5. Add the garlic, salt and spices; stirring to combine.

6 Add the tomato puree, stir, and then add tinned tomatoes and water.
7 Turn the heat to medium-low and simmer for about an hour until thick and glossy.
8 Check your seasoning and adjust as necessary.
9 Top with the coriander, chopped onion and tomato to serve.
10 Serve with Baked Sweet Potato and Tomato and Spring Onion Salad.

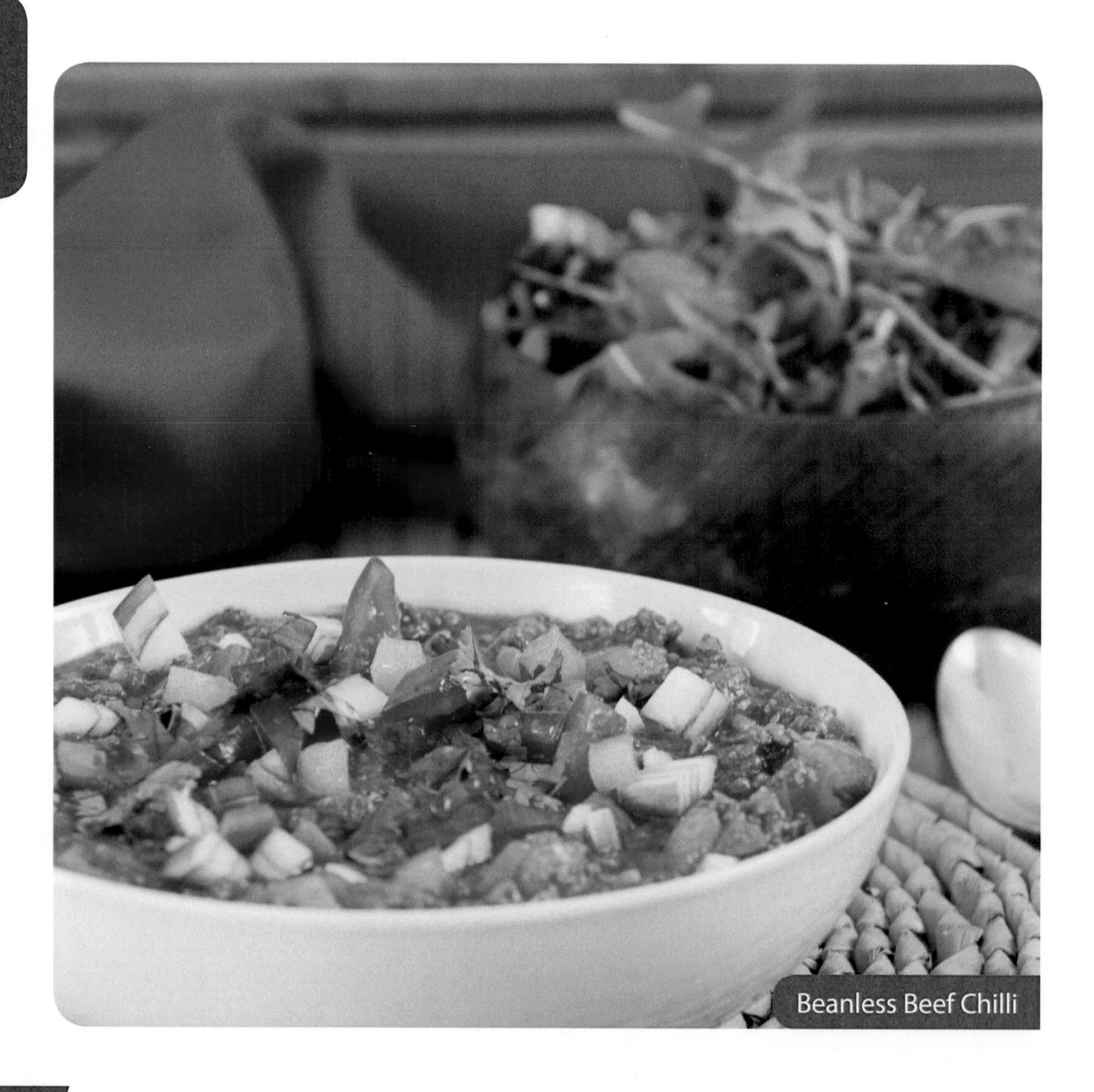

Beanless Beef Chilli

BEEF BOURGUIGNON

 *Servings: 4*

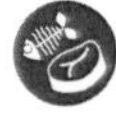 *Preparation Time: 15 minutes*

 *Cooking Time: 2 hours*

 *Total Time: 2 hours, 15 minutes*

Ingredients

500g stewing beef, cut in 2-inch cubes

1 carrot, thickly sliced

200g streaky bacon, chopped

1 tsp dried thyme

2 garlic cloves, crushed

1 tbsp tomato paste

1 pinch sea salt

2 tbsp lard, dripping or goose fat

1 onion, thickly sliced

1 bay leaf

20 small shallots, peeled

300ml red wine

1 lb mushrooms, quarters

1 pinch freshly ground black pepper

Preparation

1. Preheat your oven to 150C.
2. Prepare the beef, carrot, onion, bacon, shallots, garlic and mushrooms.
3. Heat the fat in a large casserole dish.
4. Brown the beef, bacon, onions and carrots with the herbs and a pinch of salt.
5. Add the tomato paste with the garlic, shallots, bayleaf and thyme and stir in the wine.
6. Season, cover and place in the oven for about 90 minutes.
7. Once the meat is falling apart add the mushrooms.
8. Place back in the oven for a further 30 minutes.
9. Serve hot with Pan Steamed Broccoli.

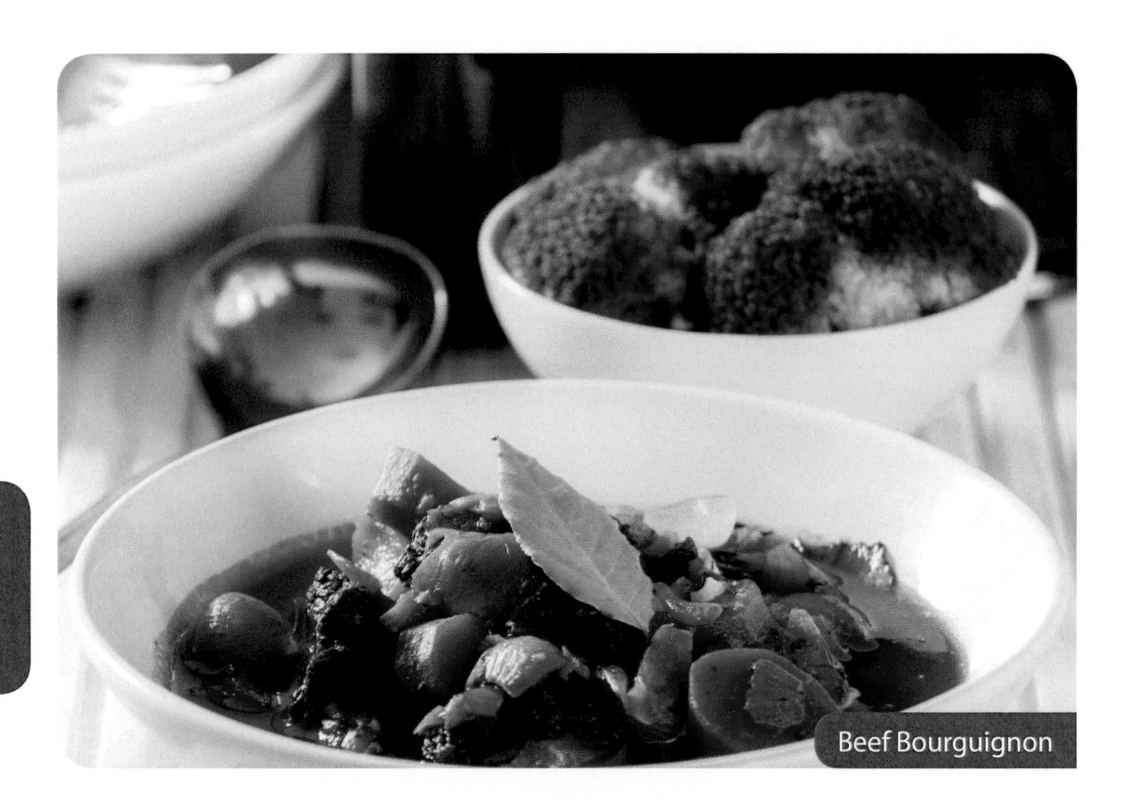
Beef Bourguignon

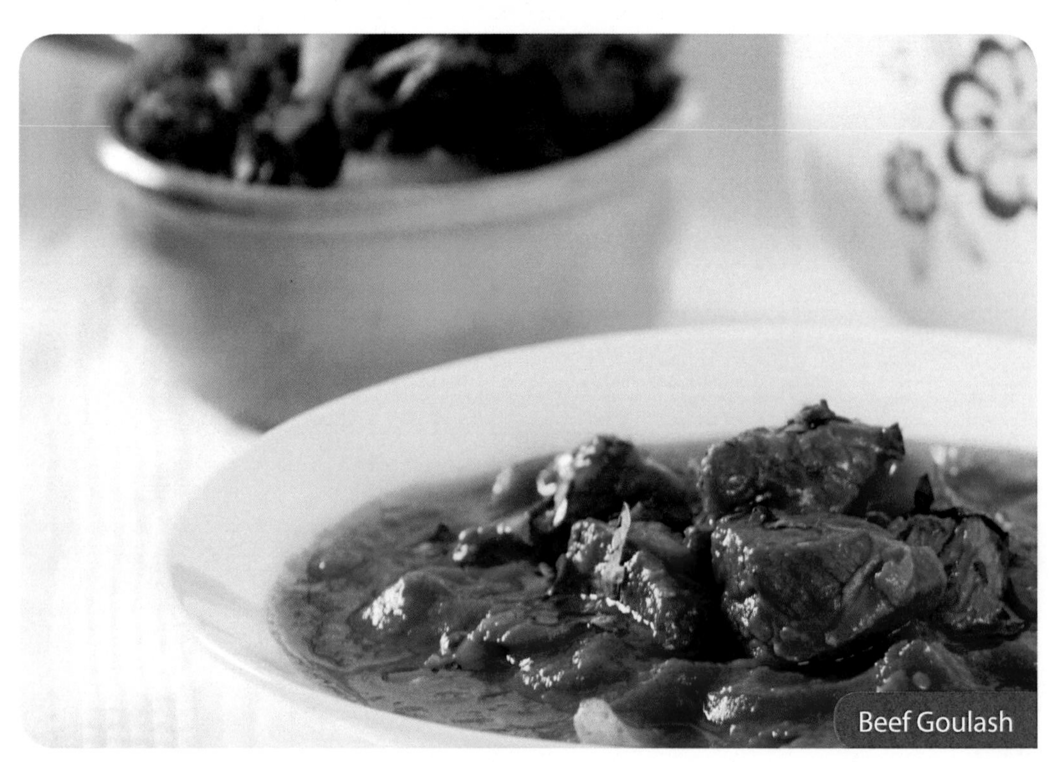
Beef Goulash

BEEF GOULASH

If you can find a good source of spices, go for Hungarian paprika for this dish; it is different to Spanish paprika in that it lacks in robustness but makes up for it in fragrant delicate flavour. Use a good braising steak for this dish.

 *Servings: 4*

 *Preparation Time: 20 minutes*

 *Cooking Time: 1 hour*

 *Total Time: 1 hour, 20 minutes*

DINNER BEEF

Ingredients

1 tbsp lard, dripping or goose fat

800g braising steak, cubed

2 red peppers, thickly sliced

2 onions, thickly sliced

2 garlic cloves, crushed

2 tbsp paprika

1 tbsp tomato purée

2 bay leaves

200ml cold water

400g chopped tomatoes

Freshly ground black pepper

Sea salt

Preparation

1. Preheat the oven to 180C.
2. Prepare the steak, peppers, onions and garlic.
3. Heat the fat in a large casserole dish and add the steak, peppers and onions.
4. Cook until the steak is browned and the vegetables soft.
5. Add the garlic, paprika and seasoning.
6. Stir in the tomato puree, add the bay leaf then pour in the tomatoes with the water.
7. Cover with foil or tight fitting lid.
8. Transfer to the oven for about an hour until the steak is tender and the sauce reduced.
9. Serve hot with the side dishes set out in your weekly meal planner.

BURGER WITH WATERCRESS SAUCE AND BUTTERNUT SQUASH

A simply seasoned steak burger, topped with a tangy watercress mayonnaise and served with sweet creamy butternut squash. We have deliberately kept the flavours simple; use great quality ingredients and let them speak for themselves. Do not use lean mince for this dish as you will need the fat for flavour and to keep the burgers moist.

 *Servings: 2*

 *Preparation Time: 30 minutes*

 *Cooking Time: 30 minutes*

 *Total Time: 1 hour*

Ingredients

FOR THE BURGER

500g steak mince

1 tsp dried mixed herbs

FOR THE SQUASH

1 butternut squash, peeled and cut into 1-inch cubes

2 tbsp lard, dripping or goose fat

FOR THE SAUCE

1 small bunch watercress

½ small onion

4 tbsp Paleo Mayonnaise

SEASONINGS

Sea salt

Freshly ground black pepper

Preparation

1. Preheat the oven to 180C.
2. Prepare the butternut squash.
3. Mix the steak mince with salt and a good amount of black pepper.

4. Create 2 or 4 burgers from the mixture depending how big you like your burgers.
5. Put the fat with the butternut on a roasting tray with a generous amount of seasoning.
6. Roast in the oven for about 30 minutes until soft.
7. In a food processor, blend the Mayonnaise with the watercress and the onion.
8. Grill or fry the burgers as you like them.
9. Serve the burgers with the butternut squash and top with the watercress sauce.

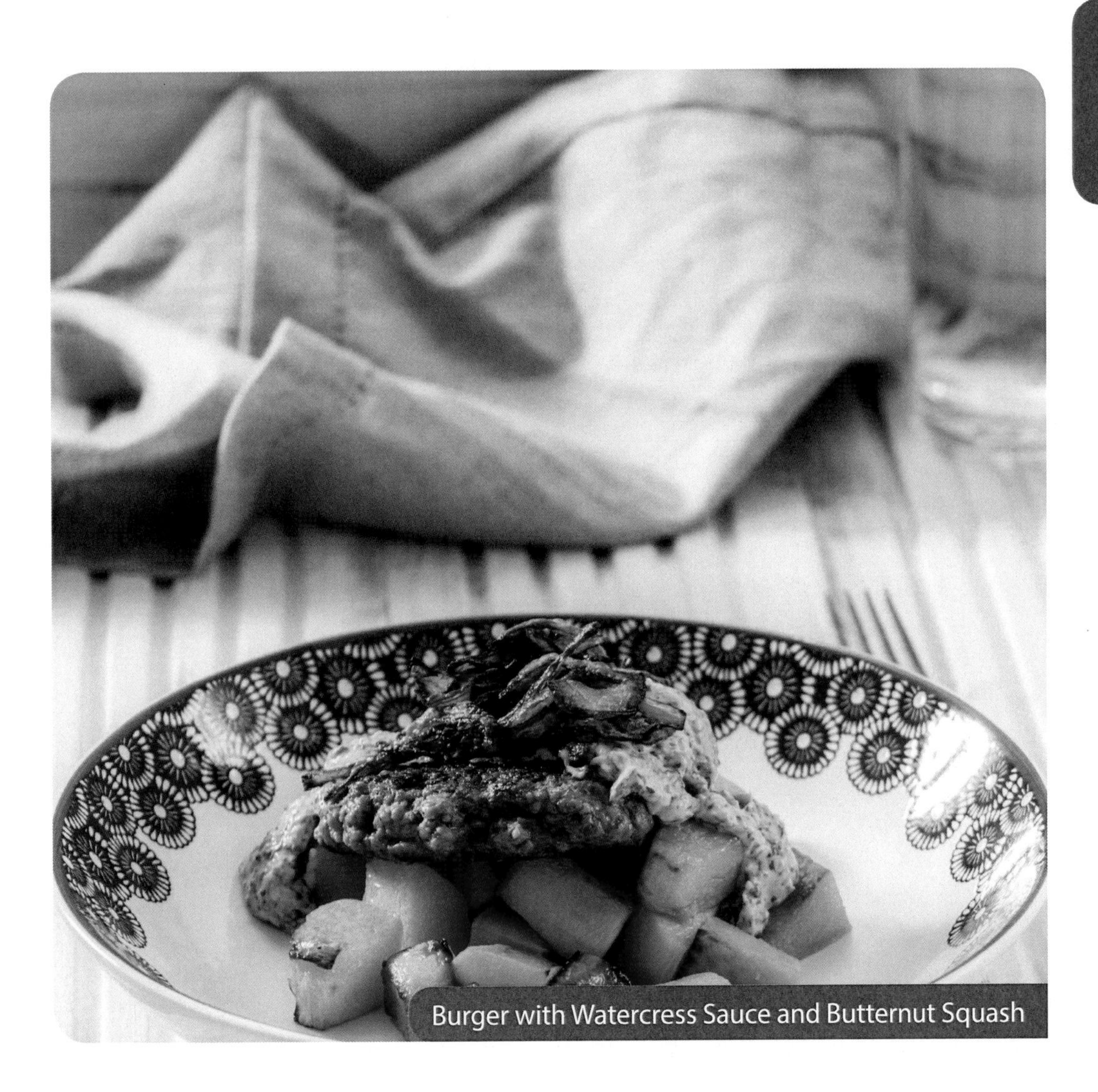
Burger with Watercress Sauce and Butternut Squash

CARNE ASADA

Carne Asada is simply a Mexican style marinated steak. Many recipes will tell you to slice the meat before marinating but steak should be sliced after grilling to get the best texture. Marinade overnight for the flavours to develop. The recipe makes enough for a cold lunch another day.

 *Servings: 2 (plus leftovers for 2)*

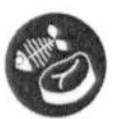 *Preparation Time: 10 minutes*

 *Cooking Time: 10 minutes*

 *Inactive Time: 24 hours*

 *Total Time: 24 hours, 20 minutes*

Ingredients

3 rib eye steaks (200-250g each)

1 tsp lard, dripping or goose fat

FOR THE MARINADE

4 garlic cloves, crushed

2 red chilli peppers, finely chopped

4 tbsp fresh coriander, chopped

1 tsp cumin

1 tsp paprika

1 tsp allspice

1 tsp oregano

2 limes, juice only

1 orange, juice only

Preparation

1. Prepare the marinade ingredients and then mix together. If you prefer less heat, deseed the chillies.
2. Submerge the steaks into the marinade and leave overnight if possible.
3. When you are ready to cook, drain the marinade from the meat and pat dry.
4. Allow the steak to reach room temperature before cooking.
5. Heat a large frying pan over a high heat and add the fat.
6. Add a pinch of salt to one side of the steaks and place in the pan, salted side down. Once cooked halfway, salt the other side and turn.

7 Your average steak should take roughly 2 minutes on each side for rare, 3 minutes for medium or 4/5 minutes for well done.

8 Leave the steaks to rest for 5 minutes before slicing thinly.

9 Serve hot with the side dishes set out in your weekly meal planner.

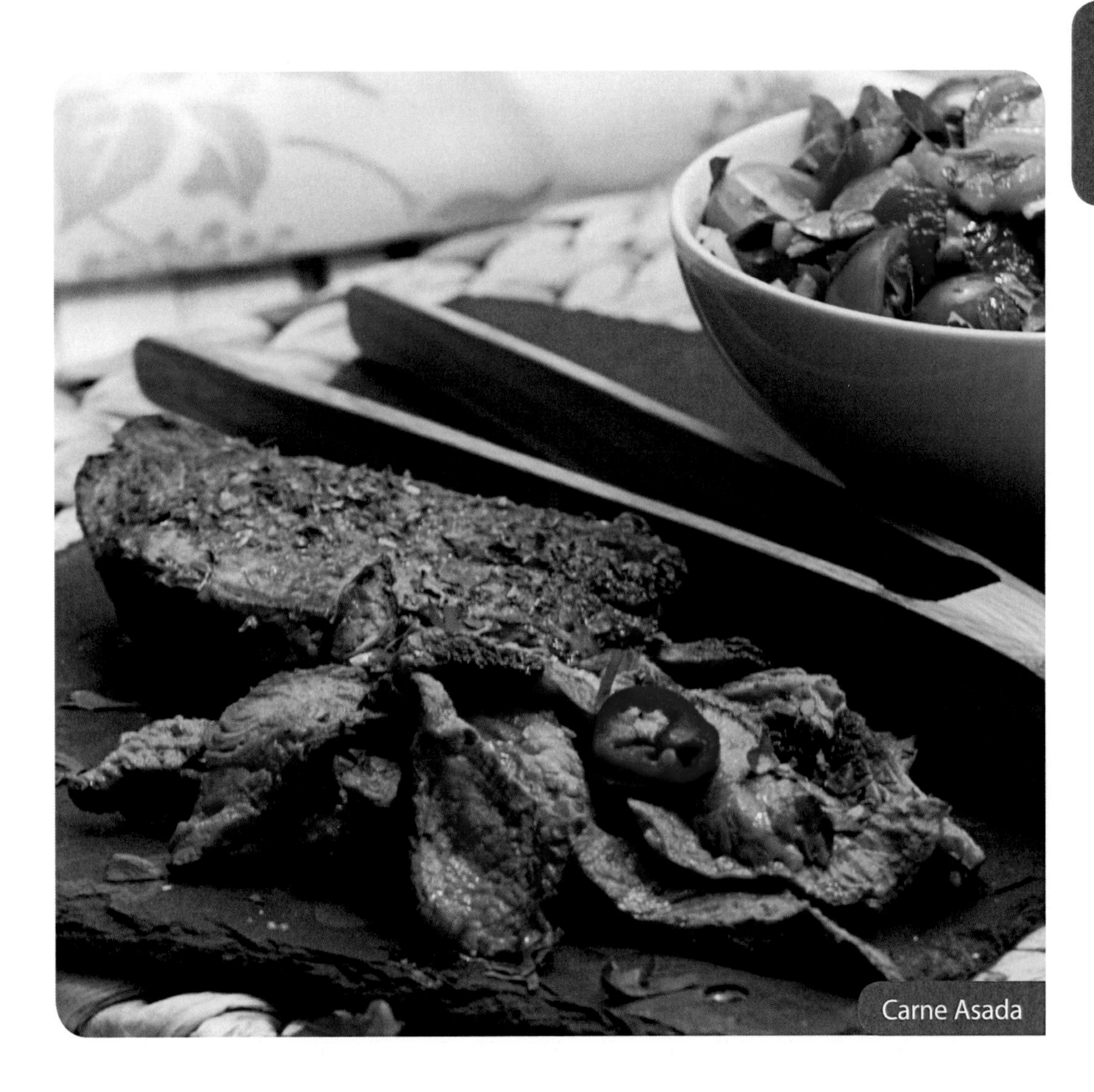

Carne Asada

CLASSIC BEEF STEW

A classic beef stew full of root vegetables and tender meat. Brisket is a great choice for this dish, though a good local butcher can guide you if in doubt. Choose any variation of vegetables that you like and play with the flavours too.

Bay leaves freeze exceptionally well. Get a big pack of fresh bay leaves if you can and freeze it; that way you will always have a ready supply of fresh bay leaves.

 *Servings: 4-6*

 *Preparation Time: 30 minutes*

 *Cooking Time: 1 hr, 30 minutes*

 *Total Time: 2 hours*

Ingredients

800g beef brisket, chopped in 2 inch chunks
2 tbsp lard, dripping or goose fat
4 carrots, in large chunks
4 parsnips, in large chunks
2 leeks, in large chunks
2 onions, chopped
2 garlic cloves, peeled but whole
2 bay leaves
2 tbsp tomato puree
1 tbsp paprika
Sea salt
Freshly ground black pepper
Fresh parsley, chopped (for garnish)

Preparation

1. Prepare the beef, carrots, parsnips, leeks, onions and garlic.
2. Heat the fat in a large saucepan and add the beef with the onions and garlic.
3. Cook until brown, stirring occasionally.
4. Add the tomato puree, paprika, bay leaves and seasoning.
5. Add all of the vegetables, stir to combine.
6. Add cold water. The water should just cover the meat and vegetable mix.
7. Turn the heat down to medium low and simmer for about 90 minutes.
8. The beef should be tender and the sauce thick and broth like (satisfying yet light).
9. Serve hot with Roasted Roots and Simple Kale.

COCOA STEAK

Cooking times will vary according to the thickness of the steak but as a rough guide you need 2 minutes on each side for rare, 3 minutes for medium or 4/5 minutes for well done.

 *Servings: 2*

 *Preparation Time: 15 minutes*

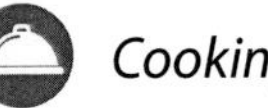 *Cooking Time: 10 minutes*

 *Total Time: 25 minutes*

Ingredients

2 sirloin or rib eye steaks, 200-250g

1 tsp olive oil

1 tsp unsweetened cocoa powder

¼ tsp paprika

¼ tsp pepper

¼ tsp sea salt

Preparation

1. Bring the steaks to room temperature and rub with the oil, then cocoa, paprika and pepper.
2. Heat a frying pan over a high heat.
3. Lay the steaks in the smoking hot pan and season with salt. Your average steak should take roughly 2 minutes on each side for rare, 3 minutes for medium or 4/5 minutes for well done.
4. When the steaks are done, leave to rest for 5 minutes to tenderise.
5. Serve hot with the side dishes set out in your weekly meal planner.

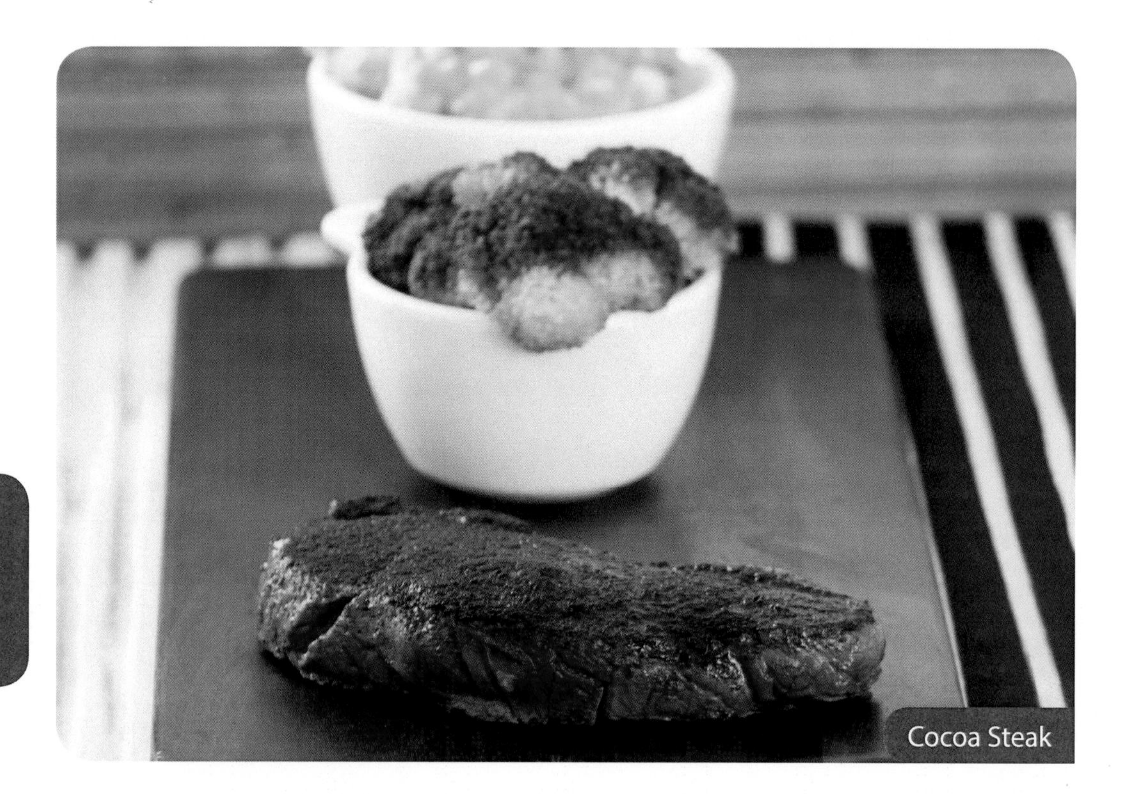

Cocoa Steak

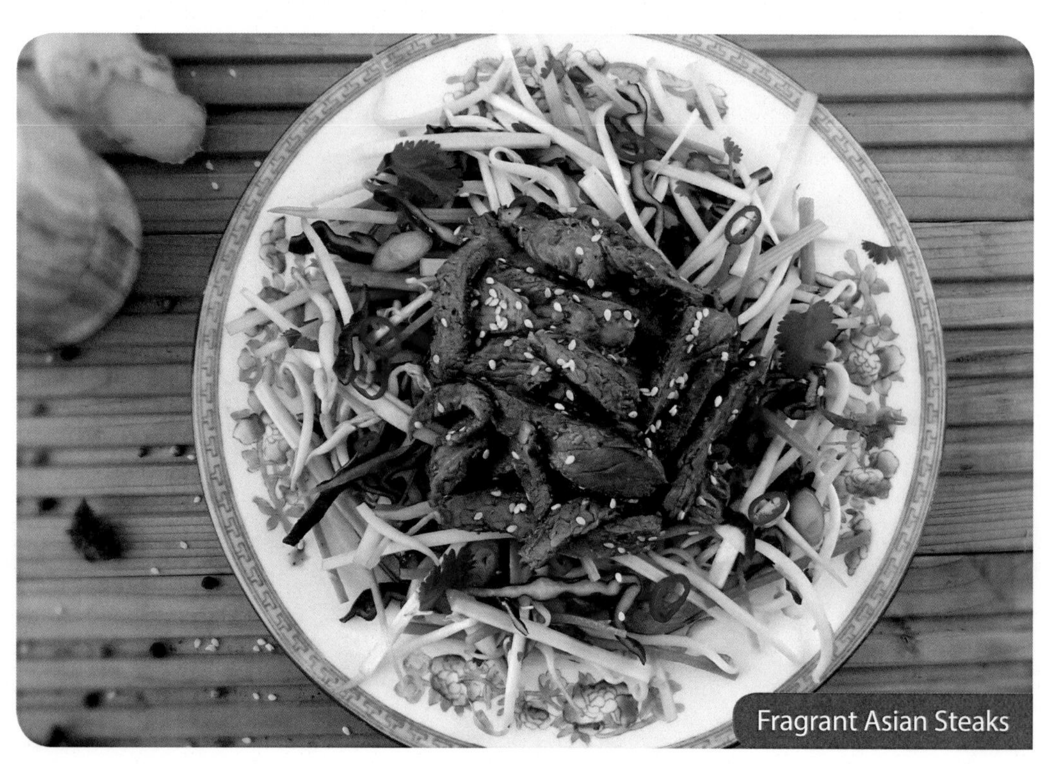

Fragrant Asian Steaks

FRAGRANT ASIAN STEAKS

Contrary to popular belief, you won't spend every day chowing down on steaks, but grass fed beef is a source of important protein and nutrients on a Paleo diet so a weekly fix of steak is a great idea that you will find you are more than ready for. Here, we mix it up a little with a quick rub of sesame oil; once cooked, the steak is thinly sliced and tossed in a fragrant blend of aromatic spices.

Serve with our crunchy Sharp Asian Slaw and coconut aminos; an acceptable Paleo substitute for soy sauce and a very useful kitchen staple. You can find coconut aminos in your local health food store or online. The spices are best when freshly ground, but ready ground is an acceptable alternative.

 *Servings: 2*

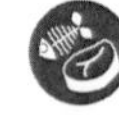 *Preparation Time: 10 minutes*

 *Cooking Time: 10 minutes*

 *Total Time: 20 minutes*

Ingredients

2 sirloin steaks (200-250g)

1 tsp black peppercorns

1 tsp coriander seeds

1 tbsp coconut aminos

1 tsp sesame oil

½ tbsp star anise

1 tsp sesame seeds

Preparation

1. Bring the steaks to room temperature and rub each side with a touch of sesame oil.
2. Heat a large frying pan over a high heat and add the steaks.
3. Your average steak should take roughly 2 minutes on each side for rare, 3 minutes for medium or 4/5 minutes for well done.
4. Allow the steaks to rest for 5 minutes.
5. Whilst the steaks are resting crush the remainder of the ingredients and mix together.
6. Once the steaks have rested slice thinly and mix with the other ingredients.
7. Serve over our Sharp Asian Slaw.

GARLIC STEAK

Always go for quality over quantity with steak. Thick steaks tend to work better for this recipe, unless you like yours well done.

 *Servings: 2*

 *Preparation Time: 10 minutes*

 *Cooking Time: 10 minutes*

 *Total Time: 20 minutes*

Ingredients

2 sirloin steaks (200-250g each)

1 tbsp olive oil

2 garlic cloves, crushed

2 tbsp fresh parsley, chopped

Sea salt

Freshly ground black pepper

Preparation

1. Bring the steaks to room temperature.
2. Rub each steak with oil and season with pepper only.
3. Heat a large frying pan until it is smoking hot.
4. Salt the side of the meant that will touch the pan first and place in the hot pan.
5. Your average steak should take roughly 2 minutes on each side for rare, 3 minutes for medium or 4/5 for well done.
6. Before you turn the steak, salt the upper surface and turn the steak over.
7. Cook until ready and then turn off the heat.
8. Add the garlic and the parsley to the steak and shake the pan. Remove from the pan and allow the steak to rest for 5 minutes.
9. Serve with Red Salad and Mustard Vinaigrette.

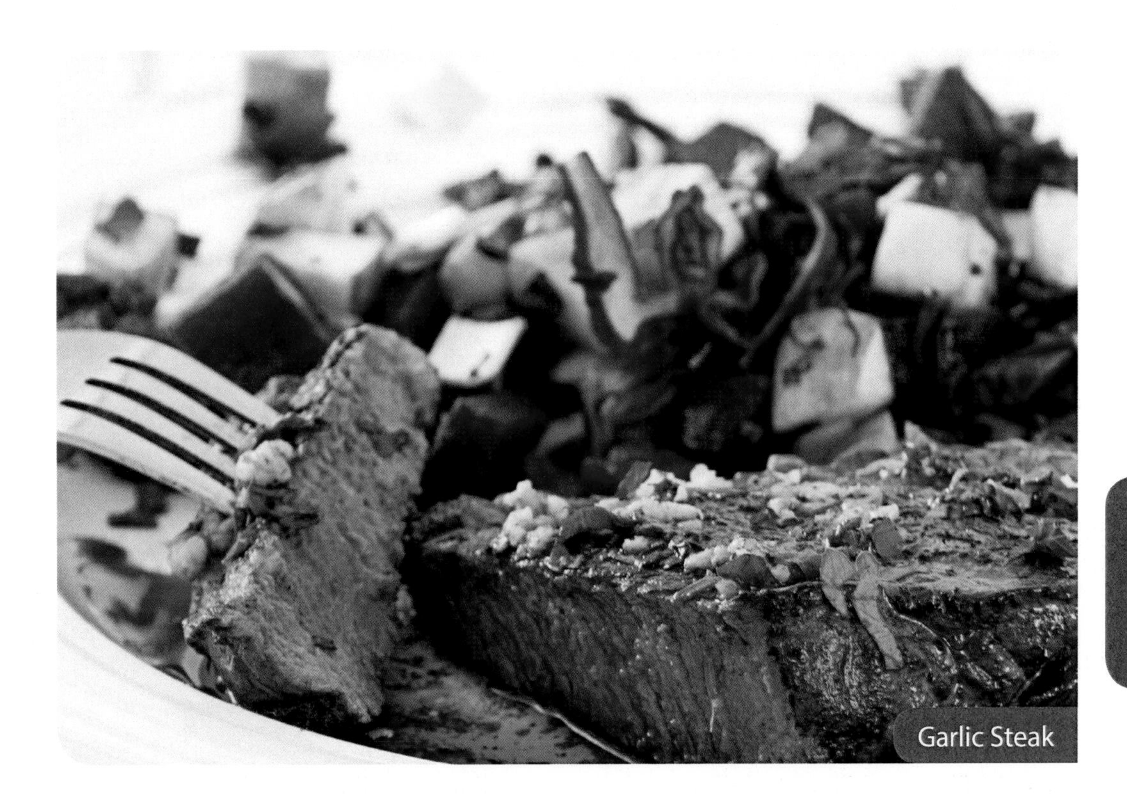
Garlic Steak

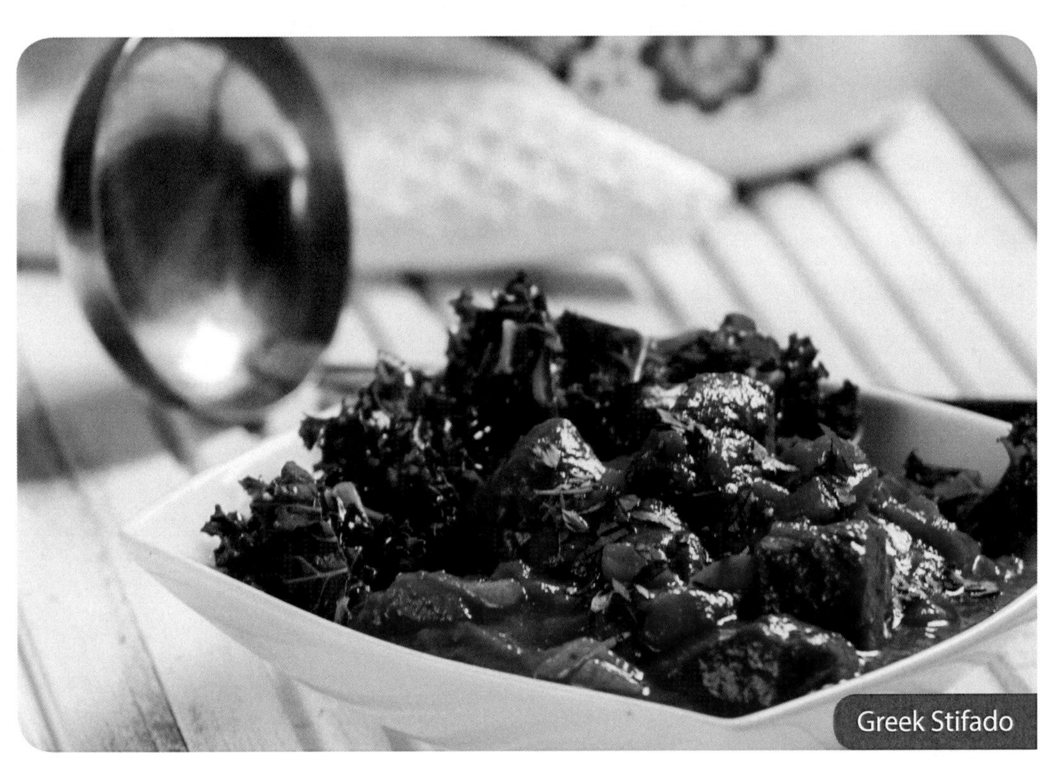
Greek Stifado

GREEK STIFADO

A Greek classic stew; rich with tomatoes and meat, fragrant with cinnamon and an unusual sweet sharpness from the addition of vinegar. It needs a good slow simmer to get the best from the textures and flavours.

 *Servings: 4*

 *Preparation Time: 20 minutes*

 *Cooking Time: 1 hr, 30 minutes*

 *Total Time: 1 hr, 50 minutes*

Ingredients

1 tbsp lard, dripping or goose fat

4 onions, sliced

1 tbsp ground cinnamon

200ml red wine

400g tin chopped tomatoes

1 pinch sea salt

800g braising steak, in large cubes

2 garlic cloves, crushed

1 tbsp tomato puree

4 tbsp red wine vinegar

2 bay leaves

1 pinch freshly ground black pepper

Preparation

1. Prepare the steak, onions and garlic.
2. Heat the fat in a large pan over a medium heat.
3. Add the steak with the onions and cook to brown.
4. Add the garlic, stir for a minute.
5. Add the cinnamon and stir for a further minute.
6. Season to taste and stir in the tomato puree and cook for 1 minute.
7. Pour in the chopped tomatoes, wine, bay leaf and vinegar.
8. Turn the heat down low and simmer for about 90 minutes.
9. The steak should be meltingly tender and the sauce thick and glossy.
10. Add lots of black pepper and season to taste.
11. Serve hot with the side dishes set out in your weekly meal planner.

HORSERADISH AND PARSLEY BURGER

Do not use lean mince for this recipe as you will want the fat for both flavour and moistness of the steak patties.

 *Servings: 4*

 *Preparation Time: 10 minutes*

 *Cooking Time: 15 minutes*

 *Total Time: 25 minutes*

Ingredients

500g beef mince

1 tbsp horseradish

4 tbsp fresh parsley, chopped

1 garlic clove, crushed

1 pinch sea salt

1 pinch freshly ground black pepper

Preparation

1. Mix all of the ingredients thoroughly. We do ours by hand, but you can use a food processor if you prefer.
2. Form into 4 patties and fry or grill for about 4-6 minutes on each side, depending on how well done you like your burgers.
3. Serve hot with Simple Leaf Salad and Sweet Potato Fries.

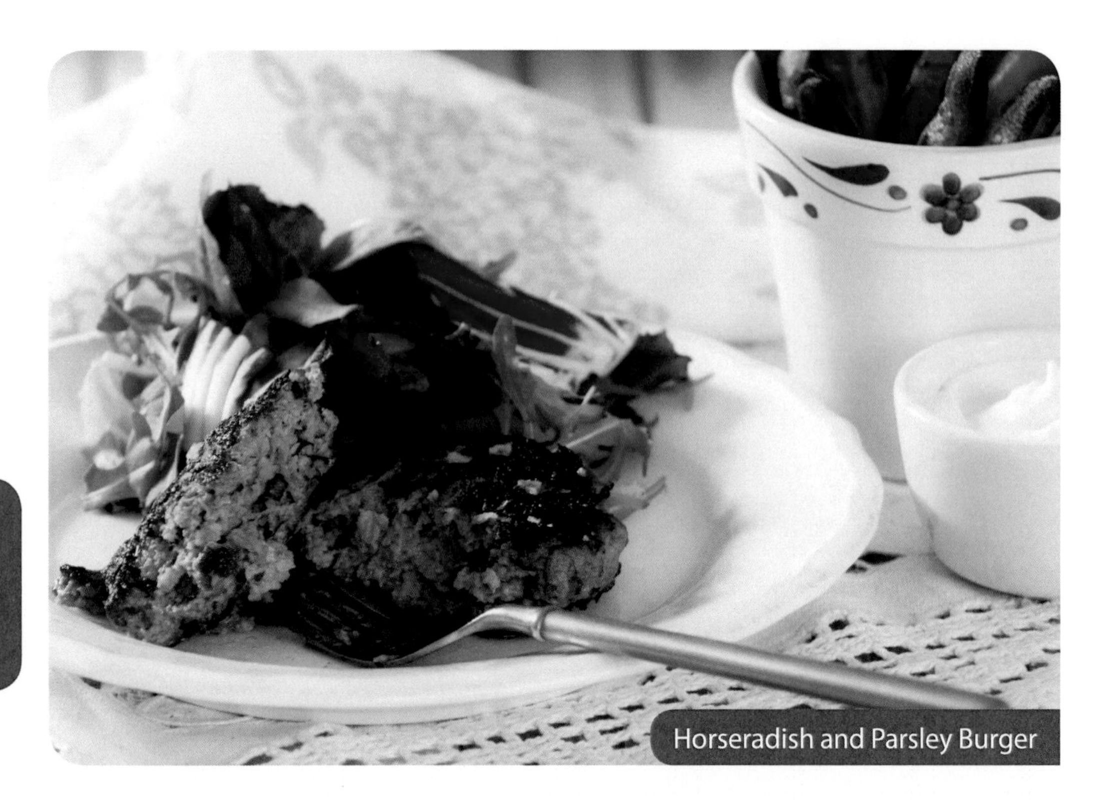

Horseradish and Parsley Burger

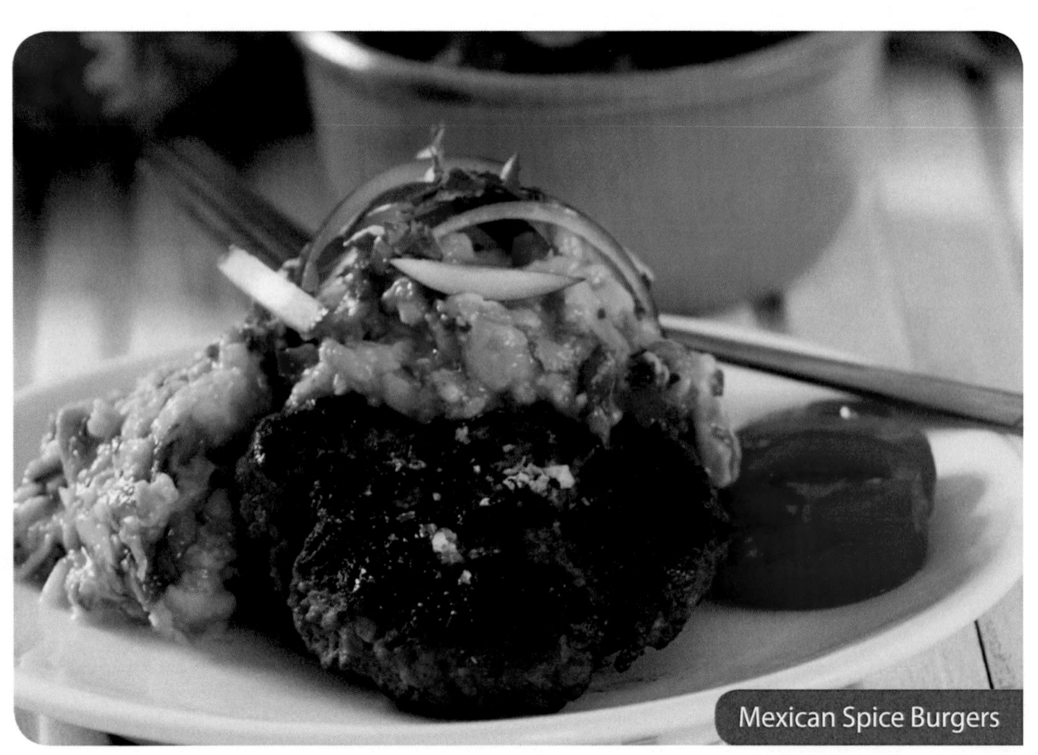

Mexican Spice Burgers

MEXICAN SPICE BURGERS

 *Servings: 4*

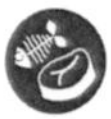 *Preparation Time: 10 minutes*

 *Cooking Time: 15 minutes*

 *Total Time: 25 minutes*

Ingredients

500g beef mince

1 garlic clove, chopped

½ tsp ground cumin

¼ tsp paprika

2 jalapeno peppers, seeded and finely chopped

1 onion, roughly chopped

2 tbsp olive oil

1 tsp dried oregano

¼ tsp sea salt

Preparation

1 Chop the onion, garlic and jalapeno peppers.

2 Mix all of the ingredients together to form the burger mix and shape into 4 patties.

3 Grill or pan fry (using olive oil) for 4-6 minutes on each side until cooked through.

4 Serve hot with Guacamole and Simple Raw Slaw.

MUSHROOM AND PEPPER BURGER

Use regular beef mince for this recipe. Lean mince will lack flavour and will be dry due to the lack of natural fats.

 *Servings: 4*

 *Preparation Time: 10 minutes*

 *Cooking Time: 20 minutes*

 *Total Time: 30 minutes*

DINNER
BEEF

Ingredients

500g beef mince

4 large Portabello mushrooms

1 pinch sea salt

4 eggs

1 red pepper, sliced

2 tbsp lard, dripping or goose fat

1 pinch freshly ground black pepper

Preparation

1. Preheat the oven to 120C.
2. Prepare the peppers.
3. Mix the mince with sea salt and black pepper and shape into 4 even patties.
4. Heat some of the fat in a frying pan over a medium heat.
5. Add the peppers with a pinch of salt. Cook the peppers until soft.
6. Add the mushrooms and cook all the way through, adding more fat or oil in needed.
7. When the peppers and mushrooms are cooked place in the oven to keep warm.
8. Add the burgers to the frying pan and cook for 4-6 minutes on each side.
9. Fry the eggs in a clean pan.
10. Stack the burgers with the mushrooms and peppers and top with a fried egg.
11. Serve with our Simple Leaf Salad to cut through the rich flavours.

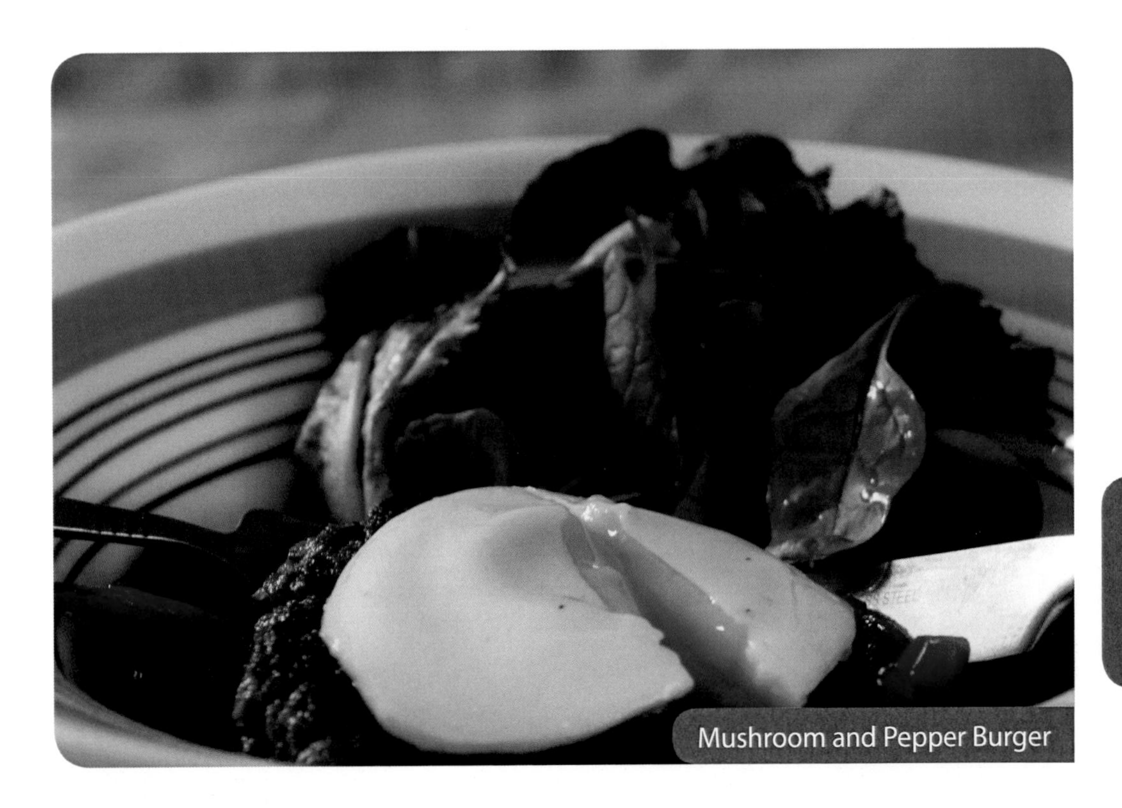
Mushroom and Pepper Burger

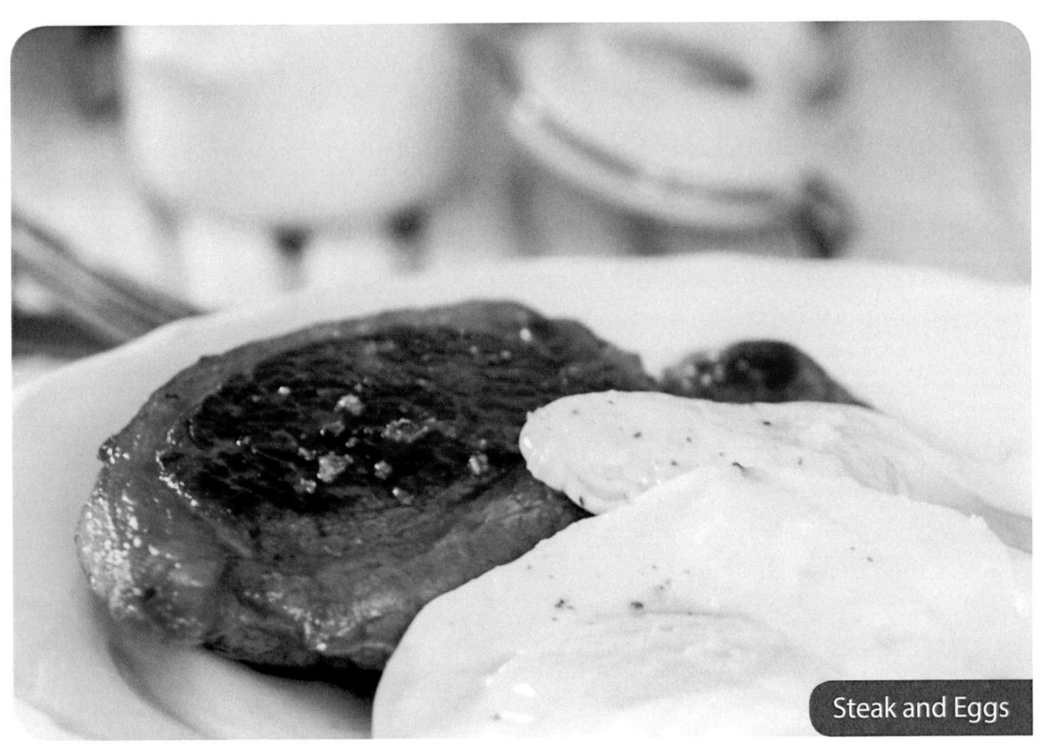
Steak and Eggs

STEAK WITH MIXED PEPPERCORNS

 *Servings: 2*

 *Preparation Time: 5 minutes*

 *Cooking Time: 10 minutes*

 *Total Time: 15 minutes*

Ingredients

2 Sirloin steaks (200-250g each)

2 tsp Black peppercorns, freshly cracked

1 tsp Green peppercorns, freshly cracked

1 pinch flaked sea salt

1 tbsp olive oil

1 tsp White peppercorns, freshly cracked

1 tsp Pink peppercorns, freshly cracked

Preparation

1. Bring the steaks to room temperature.
2. Prepare the peppercorns by crushing/cracking and mixing together. To do this you can use a pestle and mortar or by placing the corns inside a clean tea towel and crushing with the end of a rolling pin.
3. Rub the steaks with the oil and coat with the peppercorns on either side.
4. Place an unoiled frying pan over a high heat and leave until smoking.
5. Put the steaks into the pan.
6. Your average steak should take roughly 2 minutes on each side for rare, 3 minutes for medium or 4/5 minutes for well done.
7. Take the steaks from the pan and rest for 5 minutes.
8. Sprinkle the steaks with a little salt and serve with Avocado and Apple Salad.

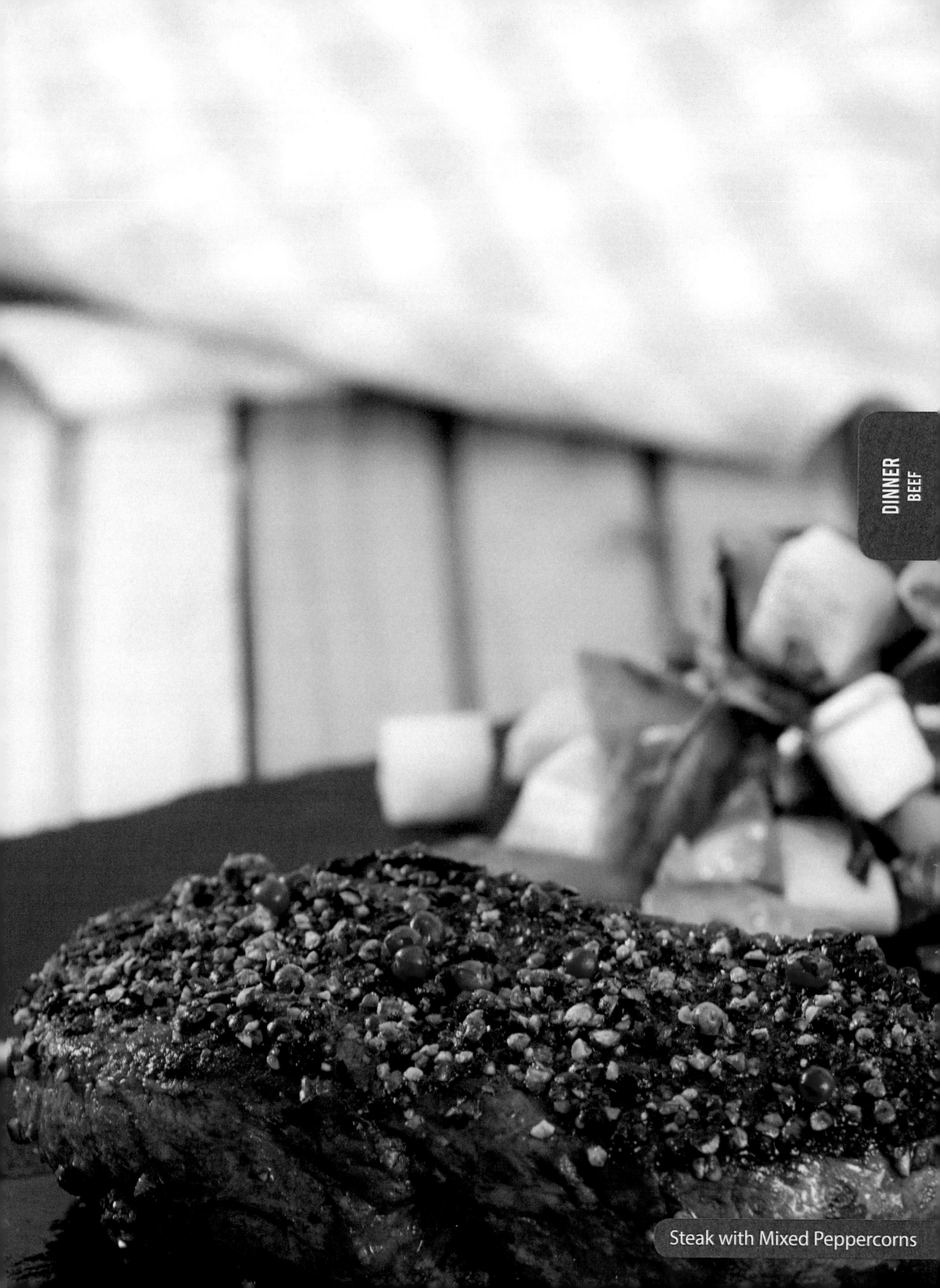

Steak with Mixed Peppercorns

STEAK AND EGGS

 *Servings: 2*

 *Preparation Time: 10 minutes*

 *Cooking Time: 15 minutes*

 *Total Time: 25 minutes*

Ingredients

2 sirloin steaks (200-250g each)

2 tbsp lard

1 pinch sea salt

1 pinch black pepper

1 tsp olive oil

4 eggs

1 pinch paprika

Preparation

1. Bring the steak to room temperature before cooking.
2. Rub the steaks with olive oil and black pepper. Sprinkle salt on one side.
3. Heat the pan to smoking hot, add the steaks salt side down.
4. Cook to your desired taste; 2 minutes each side for rare, 3 for medium, 4/5 for well done.
5. Remove the steak from the pan, set aside and lower the temperature.
6. Add the fat and crack in the eggs.
7. Cover, season to taste with some paprika, salt and pepper.
8. Cook until the whites are just set.
9. Serve the steak with the eggs and a side dish of Sweet Potato Fries.

POULTRY

BAKED ITALIAN CHICKEN

A one pot dish for the oven. Tender chicken pieces with rich tomato sauce, herbs and olives. You could bulk it out with onions and peppers if you wish; even mushrooms. Keep half for a left over lunch later in the week.

 *Servings: 4*

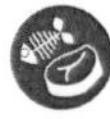 *Preparation Time: 10 minutes*

 *Cooking Time: 30 minutes*

 *Total Time: 40 minutes*

Ingredients

8 chicken thighs

1 tbsp olive oil

100g Kalamata olives

2 sprigs fresh oregano

Freshly ground black pepper

8 chicken drumsticks

½ recipe Basic Tomato Sauce

2 sprigs fresh thyme

Sea salt

Preparation

1. Preheat the oven to 180C.
2. Place the chicken pieces, skin side up, in a roasting tray. Season and drizzle with oil.
3. Pour the tomato sauce around the chicken, not over the skin, so that the pieces can brown.
4. Throw on the herbs and olives then bake for about 30 minutes until the chicken is tender and the skin is crisp.
5. Serve hot and enjoy with the side dishes set out in your weekly meal planner.

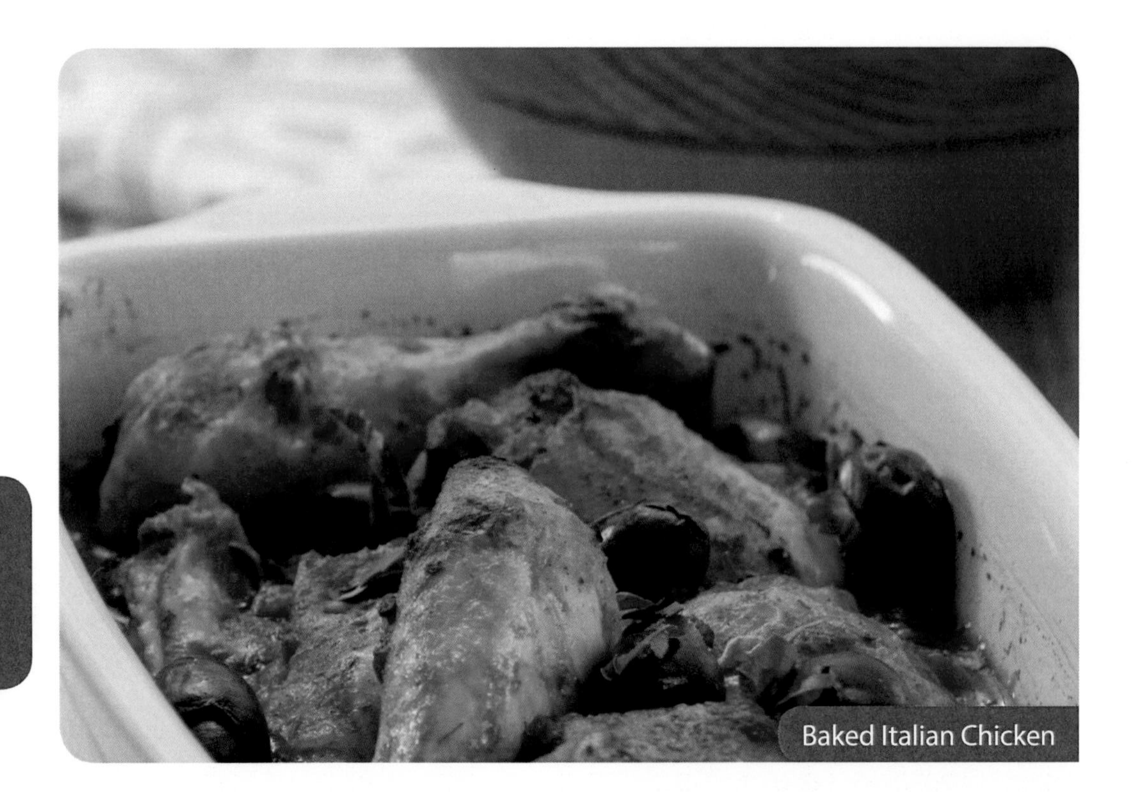
Baked Italian Chicken

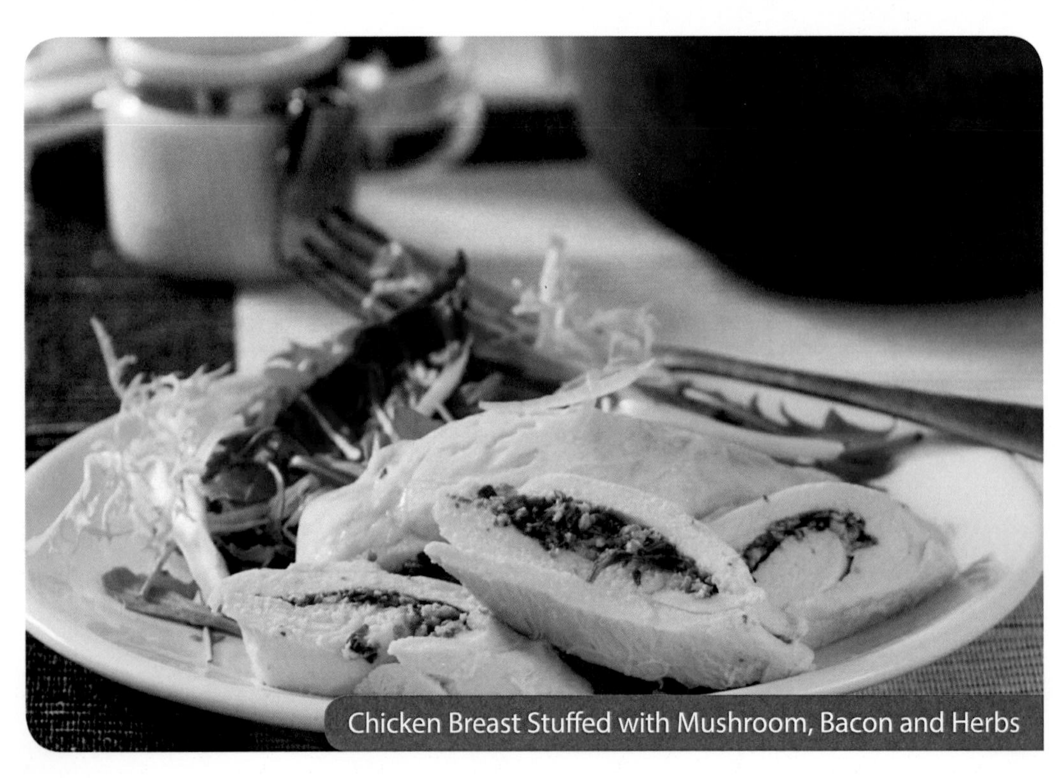
Chicken Breast Stuffed with Mushroom, Bacon and Herbs

CHICKEN BREAST STUFFED WITH MUSHROOM, BACON AND HERBS

Flattened chicken breasts are filled with mushroom bacon and herb stuffing then rolled and baked. The recipe doubles up to make a cold lunch that can be eaten with salad.

 *Servings: 4*

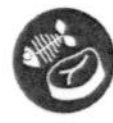 *Preparation Time: 20 minutes*

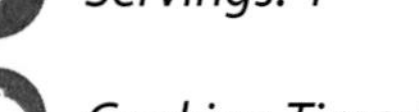 *Cooking Time: 20 minutes*

 *Total Time: 40 minutes*

Ingredients

4 chicken breast fillets

FOR THE FILLING

10 button mushrooms, cleaned

4 rashers streaky bacon, chopped

Freshly ground black pepper

1 garlic clove, crushed

½ bunch fresh parsley

½ lemon, juice only

Preparation

1. Preheat the oven to 200C.
2. To flatten the chicken breasts, cut through each sideways stopping before you get to the far edge so you can open the breast out into a heart shaped piece of chicken.
3. Lay the chicken between two pieces of cling film and then hit it with the base of a frying pan or a rolling pin to flatten out.
4. You should now have a large thin (about 3-5mm thick) chicken breast that will stuff and roll beautifully.
5. Put the ingredients for the filling in a food processor and blend to a coarse paste.
6. Spread the filling over the chicken breasts and roll up to form a spiral tube.
7. Lay the rolled chicken parcels on a baking tray and add 1 tbsp of water.
8. Cover the tray with foil and bake in the oven for about 20 minutes or until the chicken and filling are cooked through.
9. Serve hot with Simple Leaf Salad.

CINNAMON AND BLACK PEPPER CHICKEN

A moist one pot chicken dish that requires very little in the way of hard work; pop in the oven after work and have a sit down.

 *Servings: 4*

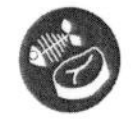 *Preparation Time: 10 minutes*

 *Cooking Time: 40 minutes*

 *Total Time: 50 minutes*

Ingredients

8 chicken thighs

2 onions, sliced

2 tsp cinnamon

1 tsp paprika

1 tbsp olive oil

8 chicken drumsticks

2 tsp freshly ground black pepper

2 garlic cloves, minced

Sea salt

200ml water

Preparation

1. Preheat the oven to 200C.
2. Prepare the onion and garlic.
3. Mix the onions and chicken pieces together with the spices, garlic and salt.
4. Place the water and oil in a roasting pan.
5. Add the chicken pieces with the onion and spices.
6. Cover with foil and bake for about 30 minutes until the chicken is moist and tender.
7. Serve hot and enjoy with the side dishes set out in your weekly meal planner.

CHICKEN FAJITA BOWL

Fajitas have become as ubiquitous in the British household as bangers and mash or shepherds pie but you don't have to go without just because you no longer eat tortillas. The recipe makes double so there will be leftovers for lunch. Instead of making guacamole or salsa, just add all of the flavours directly to the bowl.

 *Servings: 4*

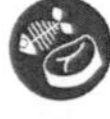 *Preparation Time: 15 minutes*

 *Cooking Time: 15 minutes*

 *Total Time: 30 minutes*

Ingredients

2 tbsp coconut oil

2 red peppers, thinly sliced

4 chicken breasts, cut in thin strips

2 onions, thinly sliced

FOR THE SPICE BLEND

1 tbsp ground coriander

1 tsp ground cumin

1 tsp garlic powder

1 tbsp paprika

1 tsp chilli powder

Sea salt

FOR THE TOPPINGS

2 tomatoes, chopped

2 ripe avocado, chopped

2 limes, juice only

1 red onion, finely chopped

2 tbsp fresh coriander, chopped

Preparation

1. Prepare the chicken, pepper, onions, tomatoes and avocado.
2. Heat the coconut oil in a large frying pan or wok and add the chicken, peppers and onions.
3. Cook over a medium heat until the chicken is cooked and the peppers are soft.
4. Add the spices and stir for another minute.
5. Set half of the mixture aside (to be used as left overs).
6. Serve the rest in bowls with desired toppings.

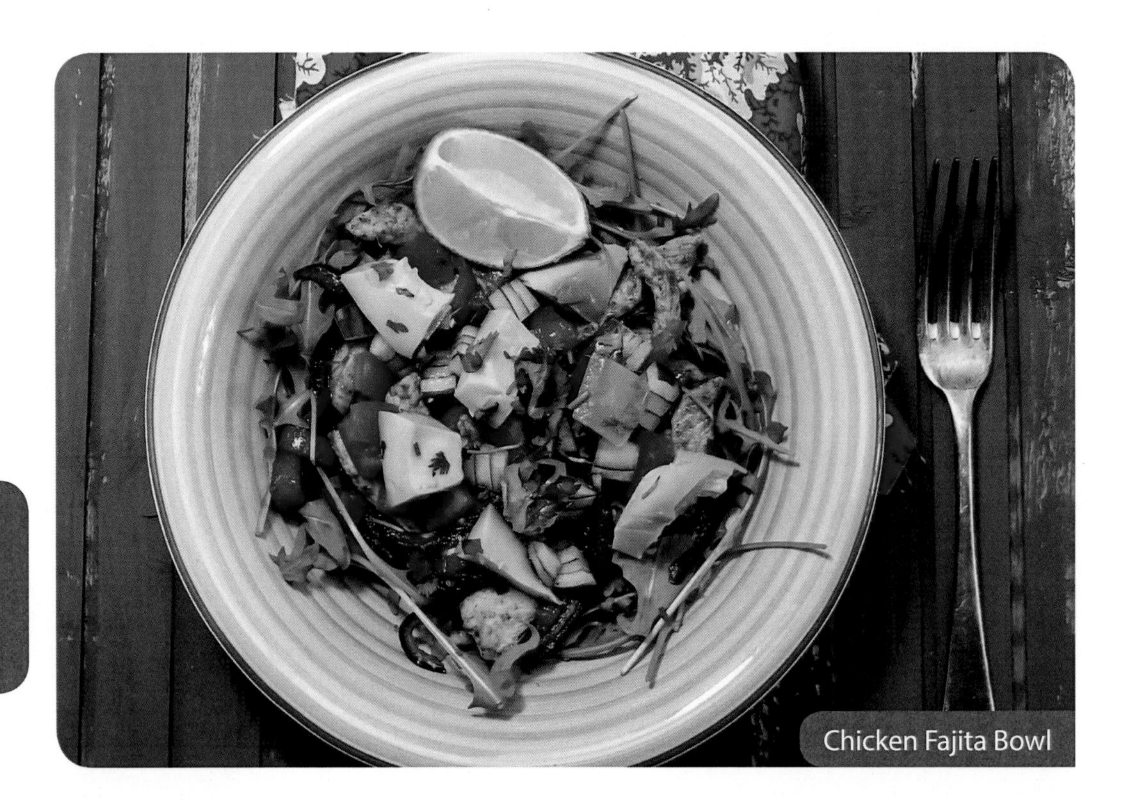

Chicken Fajita Bowl

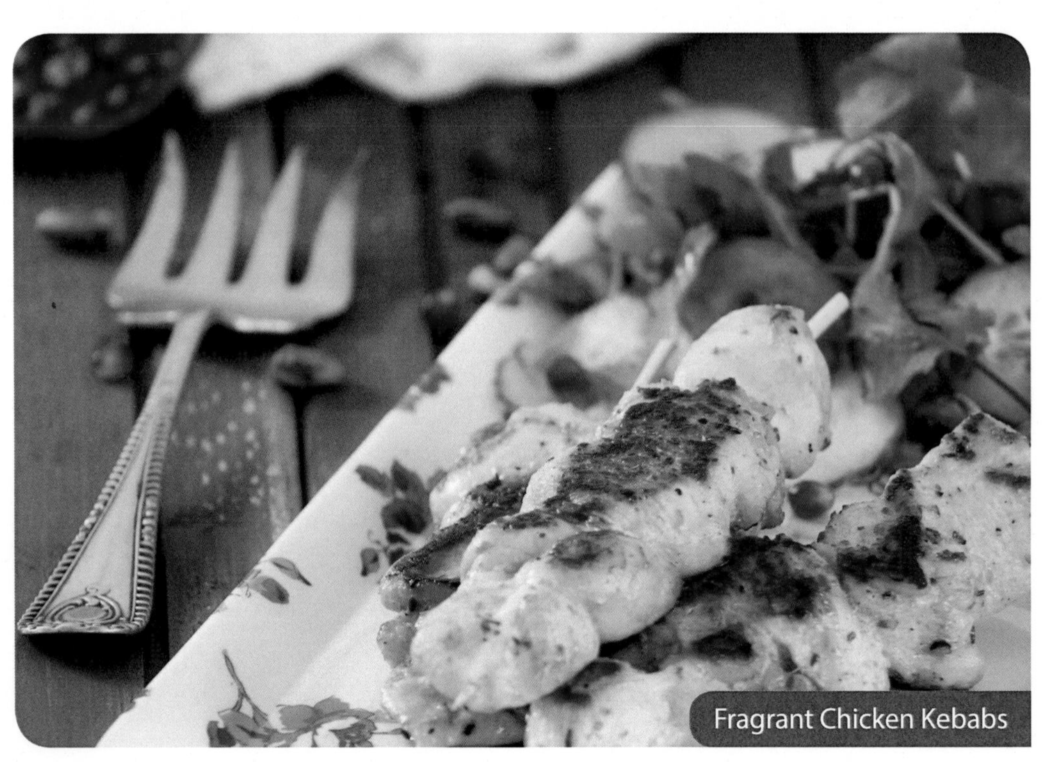

Fragrant Chicken Kebabs

FRAGRANT CHICKEN KEBABS

Succulent chicken breast with fragrant spices threaded onto skewers for quick and easy cooking.

 *Servings: 2*

 *Preparation Time: 15 minutes*

 *Cooking Time: 15 minutes*

 *Inactive Time: 24 hours*

 *Total Time: 24 hours, 30 minutes*

Ingredients

8 boneless chicken thighs, halved

½ tsp turmeric

½ tsp ground ginger

1 garlic clove, minced

½ tsp garlic powder

½ tsp black pepper

½ tsp ground coriander

2 tbsp apple cider vinegar

Preparation

1. You will need metal or wooden skewers that have been soaked for 30-60 minutes in cold water.
2. In a baking dish, mix the seasonings, garlic, and vinegar.
3. Add the chicken to seasonings and toss well to coat.
4. Cover and refrigerate for as long as you can, ideally 24 hours but at least 4 hours. The longer you marinade, the bolder the flavour.
5. Preheat the grill to a medium heat.
6. Thread the chicken onto skewers.
7. Grill the chicken for 3-5 minutes on each side or until cooked through.
8. Remove the chicken from the skewers before eating and serve with Rocket, Cucumber, Pistachio and Pomegranate Salad.

FRAGRANT HERB CHICKEN CURRY

 *Servings: 2*

 *Preparation Time: 10 minutes*

 *Cooking Time: 30 minutes*

 *Total Time: 40 minutes*

Ingredients

8 boneless chicken thighs, cut into 1inch pieces

1 tbsp coconut oil

½ tsp cinnamon

1 tsp turmeric

½ lemon, juice only

1 bunch fresh coriander, chopped

1 pinch sea salt

1 onion, finely chopped

1 inch fresh ginger, grated

2 green chilli, chopped

3 garlic cloves, crushed

200ml coconut milk

1 bunch fresh mint, chopped

1 pinch freshly ground black pepper

Preparation

1. Melt the coconut oil in a large frying pan and add the onion with a pinch of salt. Cook gently for a few minutes until it begins to soften.
2. Stir in the ginger, chillies, garlic and spices.
3. Add the chicken. Stir for a minute or so to colour the chicken.
4. Add the lemon juice. Cook for about 10 minutes.
5. Add the coconut milk, season well, turn the heat down low and cook for about 20 minutes until the chicken is cooked through.
6. Stir in the fresh herbs and serve hot with Cauliflower Rice.

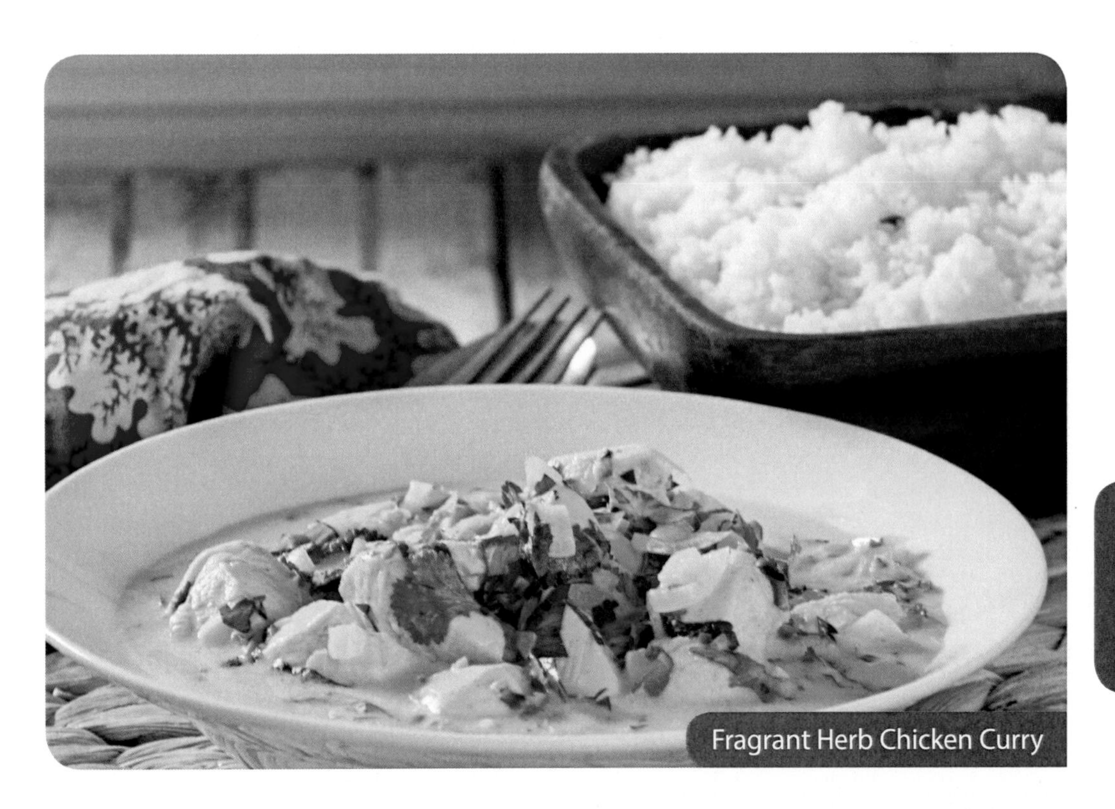

Fragrant Herb Chicken Curry

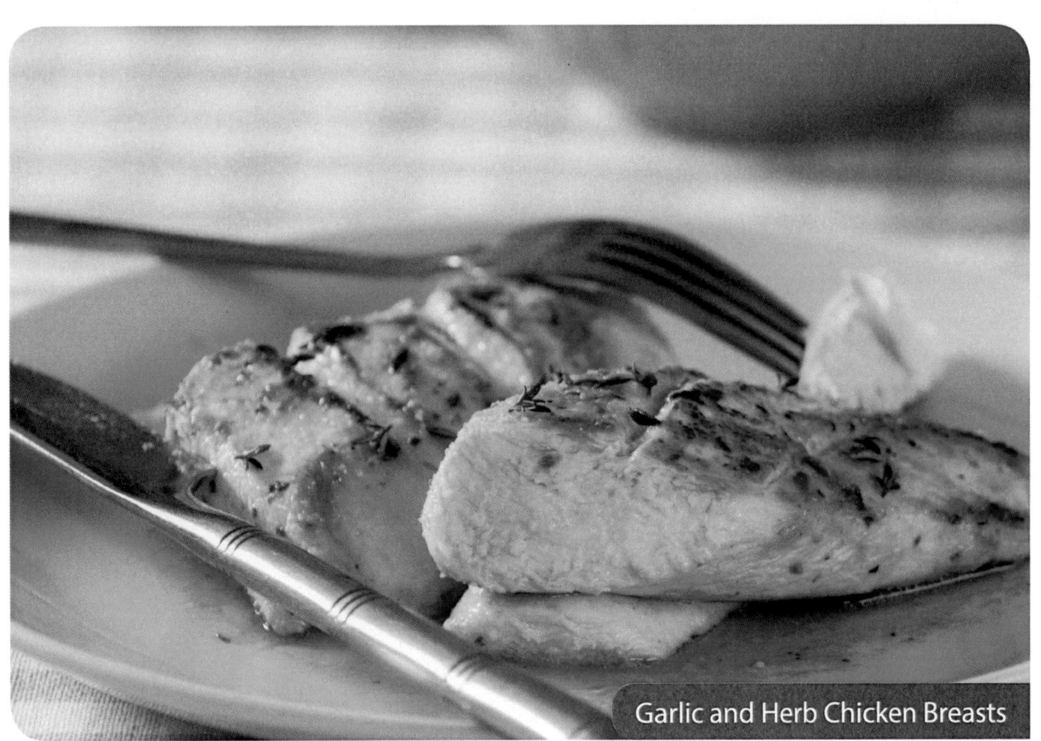

Garlic and Herb Chicken Breasts

GARLIC AND HERB CHICKEN BREASTS

We use garlic powder in this recipe as fresh garlic burns easily.

 *Servings: 2*

 *Preparation Time: 10 minutes*

 *Cooking Time: 20 minutes*

 *Inactive Time: 15 minutes*

 *Total Time: 45 minutes*

Ingredients

2 chicken breasts

1 tbsp olive oil

1 tsp ground oregano, chopped

Sea salt

1 tsp garlic powder

1 tsp ground thyme, chopped

1 lemon, juice only

Freshly ground black pepper

Preparation

1. Slash the chicken breasts diagonally and marinade with the garlic, oil and herbs.
2. Leave to rest for 15 minutes.
3. Heat a frying pan or skillet over a medium heat and add the chicken breasts.
4. Brown on both sides and then turn down the heat.
5. Squeeze over the lemon to create a little moisture, season, and cover the pan.
6. Cook for a further 5 minutes and then remove from the heat.
7. Leave the chicken to continue steaming off the heat.
8. Check to see if it is done after 5 minutes.
9. Serve with Simple Leaf Salad and the pan juices poured over the chicken.

JAMAICAN JERK CHICKEN

Unless it is mid-summer and you happen to be lighting the barbecue then cook this chicken in the oven or over an indoor grill. Barbecue is really best as you get the classic charred flavour from the coals. Feel free to use a Paleo friendly jerk spice but do make the actual paste fresh as it is all about the spring onions. Do try to use habanero chilli (fresh or dried) as it is a different experience from regular chilli.

 *Servings: 4*

 *Preparation Time: 15 minutes*

 *Cooking Time: 45 minutes*

 *Inactive Time: 24 hours*

 *Total Time: 25 hours*

Ingredients

8 chicken drumsticks

8 chicken thighs

FOR THE JERK PASTE

1 tbsp olive oil1 bunch spring onions

1 inch ginger

2 garlic cloves

2 tsp habanero powder

1 tsp dried thyme

1 tbsp allspice

1 lime, juice only

Sea salt

FOR THE GARNISH

2 tbsp fresh coriander, chopped

½ bunch spring onions, chopped

4 tomatoes, chopped

Preparation

1. Preheat the oven to 200C (unless using the barbeque for cooking).
2. Cut slits into the chicken for the marinade to infuse.
3. Blitz all of the ingredients for the jerk paste in a food processor.
4. Rub the paste into the chicken and place it all into a freezer bag.
5. Leave the chicken to marinate for as long as possible, ideally 24 hours.

6 Remove from the bag and place on a baking tray. Cook in the oven for about 45 minutes.
7 Garnish with coriander, chopped spring onions and tomatoes.
8 Serve hot with Fennel, Almond and Pomegranate Salad.
9 Remember to save any leftovers for lunch!

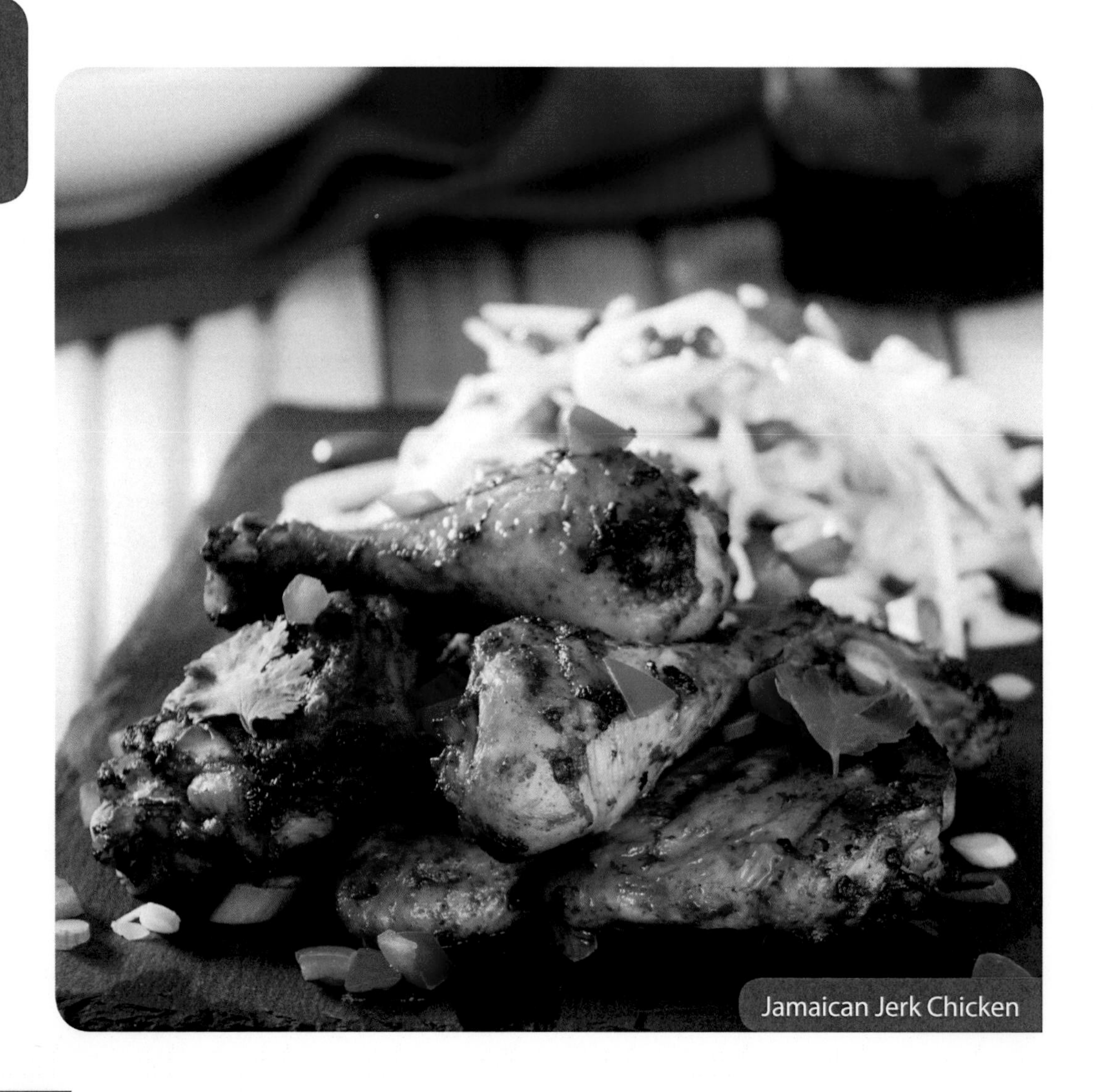
Jamaican Jerk Chicken

OLIVE, GARLIC & LEMON CHICKEN

Another variation of moist pan fried chicken thighs, this time with plenty of sharp lemon and garlic and the salted edge of green olives. Excellent served hot or cold and the double recipe caters for both.

 *Servings: 4*

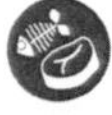 *Preparation Time: 20 minutes*

 *Cooking Time: 40 minutes*

 *Total Time: 1 hour*

DINNER
POULTRY

Ingredients

2 tbsp lard, dripping or goose fat

100g green olives

2 lemons, juice only

2 sprigs fresh thyme

1 pinch sea salt

16 chicken thighs

8 garlic cloves, whole

1 lemon, thickly sliced

100ml water

1 pinch freshly ground black pepper

Preparation

1. Season the chicken thighs with salt and pepper.
2. Heat the fat in a large frying pan. You may need to use two pans.
3. The aim is to fit the chicken in the pan with about an inch between each piece. Overcrowd the pan and it will not brown, but put in too few and it will brown too quickly).
4. Add the chicken pieces to the pan, skin side down and cook until well browned.
5. Turn the chicken over and add the lemon juice, lemon slices, olives, thyme and water.
6. Cover the pan with foil or a lid and cook gently for about 30 minutes until the chicken is tender.
7. Remove the lid or foil and turn up the heat, and allow any residual liquid to cook out. This will leave sticky lemony chicken.
8. Serve half hot with Simple Kale and keep the rest for left over lunches.

PAN FRIED ROSEMARY CHICKEN

 *Servings: 2*

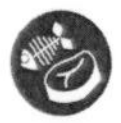 *Preparation Time: 20 minutes*

 *Cooking Time: 30 minutes*

 *Total Time: 50 minutes*

Ingredients

2 tbsp lard, dripping or goose fat
100g green olives
2 lemons, juice only
2 sprigs fresh thyme
1 pinch sea salt
16 chicken thighs
8 garlic cloves, whole
1 lemon, thickly sliced
100ml water
1 pinch freshly ground black pepper

Preparation

1. Prepare the onion and the garlic.
2. Heat the fat in a large frying pan and add the chicken pieces, skin side down.
3. Season with salt and brown on either side.
4. Add the onions, garlic and rosemary.
5. Cook for about 5 minutes until the onion colours.
6. Squeeze over the lemon, cover the pan and turn the heat low.
7. Cook for about 30 minutes, checking the moisture levels every 5 minutes. Top up with a little water if necessary.
8. When the chicken is tender serve hot with the side dishes set out in your weekly meal planner.
9. Keep half to have cold for lunch another day.

PERI-PERI CHICKEN SKEWERS

Peri-Peri sauce is widely available but may contain non-Paleo ingredients. It is a simple enough blend of birds eye chillies, lime juice and salt so can be homemade in no time at all.

You will need metal skewers or wooden/bamboo skewers that have been soaked in water.

 *Servings: 4*

 *Preparation Time: 30 minutes*

 *Cooking Time: 10 minutes*

 *Inactive Time: 45 minutes*

 *Total Time: 1 hour, 25 minutes*

DINNER POULTRY

Ingredients

4 skinless chicken breasts, sliced into long, 2cm wide strips

FOR THE PERI-PERI MARINADE

10 small red birds eye chillies

1 tsp garlic powder

1 tsp sea salt

2 limes, juice only

Preparation

1. Prepare the chicken breasts.
2. Soak the chillies in a little hot water until soft.
3. The liquid will be used so keep the amount of water to a minimum.
4. When the chillies are soft, blitz the marinade ingredients together until smooth.
5. You can use a blender or a mortar and pestle for this.
6. Rub the marinade all over the chicken, using just enough to coat.
7. Keep any remaining marinade that has not been used on the chicken as a dipping sauce (it is great mixed with Paleo Mayonnaise).
8. Thread a strip of chicken loosely onto a skewer; two if small.
9. Set aside to marinate for up to half an hour.
10. Grill the skewers for a few minutes on each side or until tender and cooked through. Be careful not to overcook or they will be dry.
11. Serve hot with the side dishes set out in your weekly meal planner.

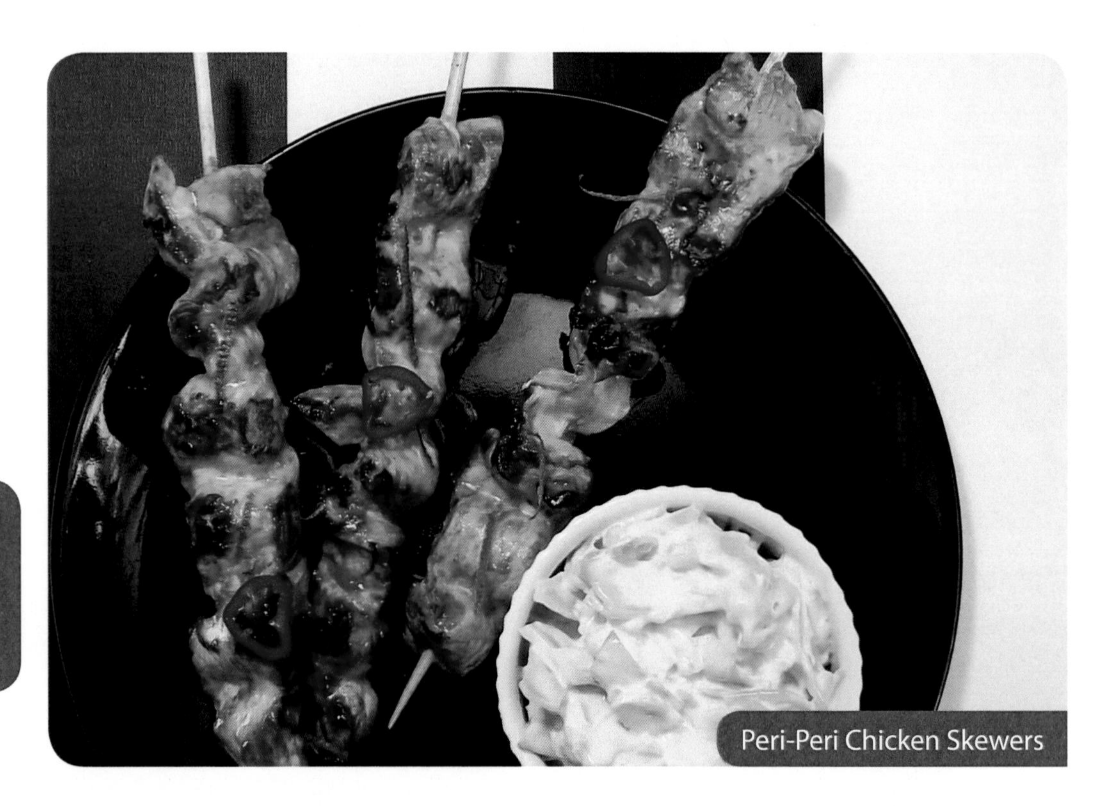

Peri-Peri Chicken Skewers

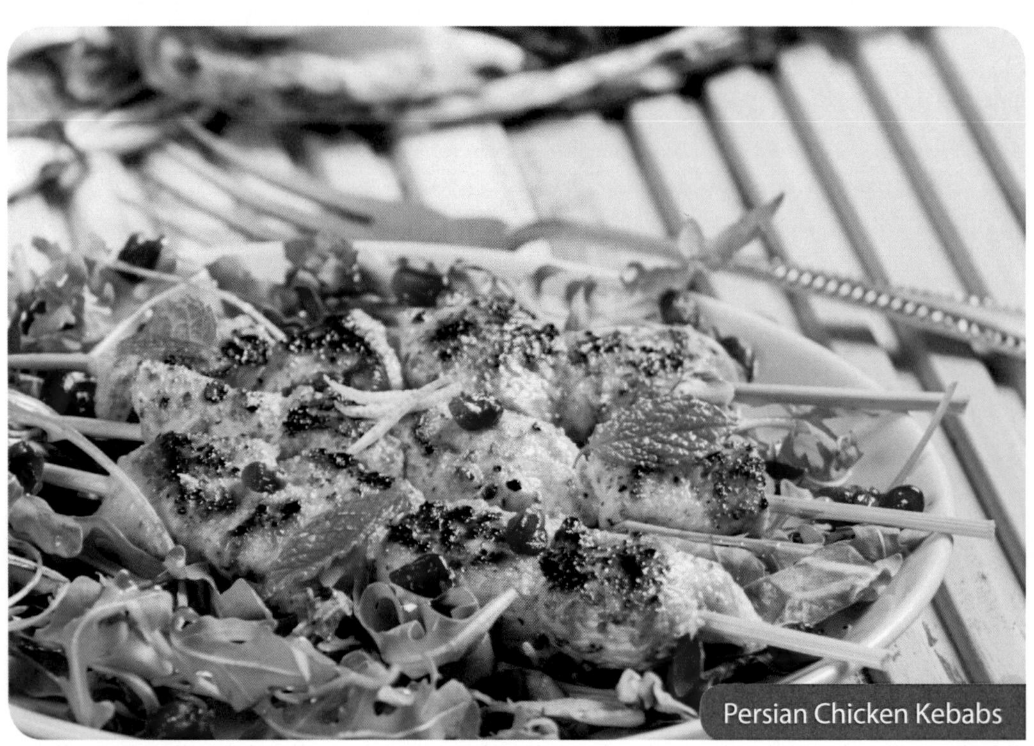

Persian Chicken Kebabs

PERSIAN CHICKEN KEBABS

You will need metal or wooden skewers that have been soaked in water.

 *Servings: 2*

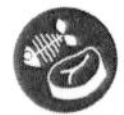 *Preparation Time: 10 minutes*

 *Cooking Time: 10 minutes*

 *Inactive Time: 1 hour*

 *Total Time: 1 hour, 20 minutes*

Ingredients

2 skinless chicken breasts, cut into 1-inch cubes

FOR THE MARINADE

½ tsp garlic powder

½ tsp black pepper

½ tsp ground coriander

½ tsp turmeric

½ tsp ground ginger

1 lemon, juice only

Preparation

1. Combine the marinade ingredients and mix with the chicken.
2. Leave aside for the flavours to develop; the longer the better, but at least 1 hour.
3. Thread onto skewers and grill on each side for about 3 minutes until the chicken is cooked through.
4. Serve hot with Roasted Cauliflower with Mint and Baba Ganoush.

SAGE AND ONION CHICKEN BURGER

A twist on classic flavours to make a healthy Paleo burger. Stack with grilled streaky bacon, tomato and lettuce. A double recipe so there will be leftovers for lunch another day.

 *Servings: 4*

 *Preparation Time: 20 minutes*

 *Cooking Time: 20 minutes*

 *Total Time: 40 minutes*

Ingredients

400g chicken breast

400g chicken thigh meat

1 tsp dried sage

1 red onion

8 rashers streaky bacon

2 large ripe tomatoes, sliced

50g lettuce leaves

Sea salt

Freshly ground black pepper

Preparation

1. Chop the chicken breast and thigh meat into pieces.
2. Chop the red onion into chunky pieces and slice the tomatoes.
3. Blend the onion, sage, salt and pepper into a food processor until finely ground.
4. Add the chicken meat and blend further until a burger mix forms.
5. Create 8 small or 4 large burgers using the mixture.
6. Brush with olive oil and grill or pan fry for about 8 minutes on either side over a moderate heat.
7. Whilst the burgers are cooking grill or fry the bacon.
8. Serve the burgers stacked with bacon, tomato and lettuce and serve with Simple Raw Slaw.
9. Keep half aside for a leftover lunch another day.

ROAST CHICKEN

This chicken not only makes a delicious and satisfying meal but is the basis of several other meals too. We prefer roasting small chickens, and obviously the total time will depend on the size of your chickens. As a general rule of thumb, cook for 20 minutes per pound (45 minutes/kilo), plus 20 minutes, so a 3lb/1.5kg bird will take about 80-90 minutes. Cooking them breast side down keeps the flesh moist; turn over for the last 20 minutes to brown the skin on the breast. Small chickens like this will give you half a bird each for dinner, bones for stock, chicken for a gorgeous salad and cold cuts for the fridge to eat if you get hungry. And the best bit? You get to eat the skin.

Always check your weekly meal planner to see what leftover chicken you will need for lunch recipes.

 *Servings: 4*

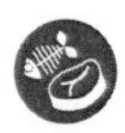 *Preparation Time: 10 minutes*

 *Cooking Time: 1 hr, 30 minutes*
(varies depending on size of bird)

 *Total Time: 1 hr, 40 minutes*

Ingredients

- 2 small roasting chickens
- 2 small onions
- 1 pinch sea salt
- 2 bay leaves
- 1 tbsp olive oil
- Freshly ground black pepper

Preparation

1. Preheat the oven to 180C.
2. Rub the chickens all over with oil, salt and pepper. Place a bay leaf and an onion in each cavity and place upside down in a roasting tray.
3. Roast the chickens for about 70-90 minutes (this is quite a slow temperature for roasting) until the leg pulls away from the rest of the bird with ease and the juices run clear.
4. Turn over for 20 minutes to brown the skin, turning the oven temperature up if need be.
5. Leave the chickens to rest for 15 minutes and then serve with the side dishes set out in your weekly meal planner.
6. Keep plenty aside for other meals during the week.

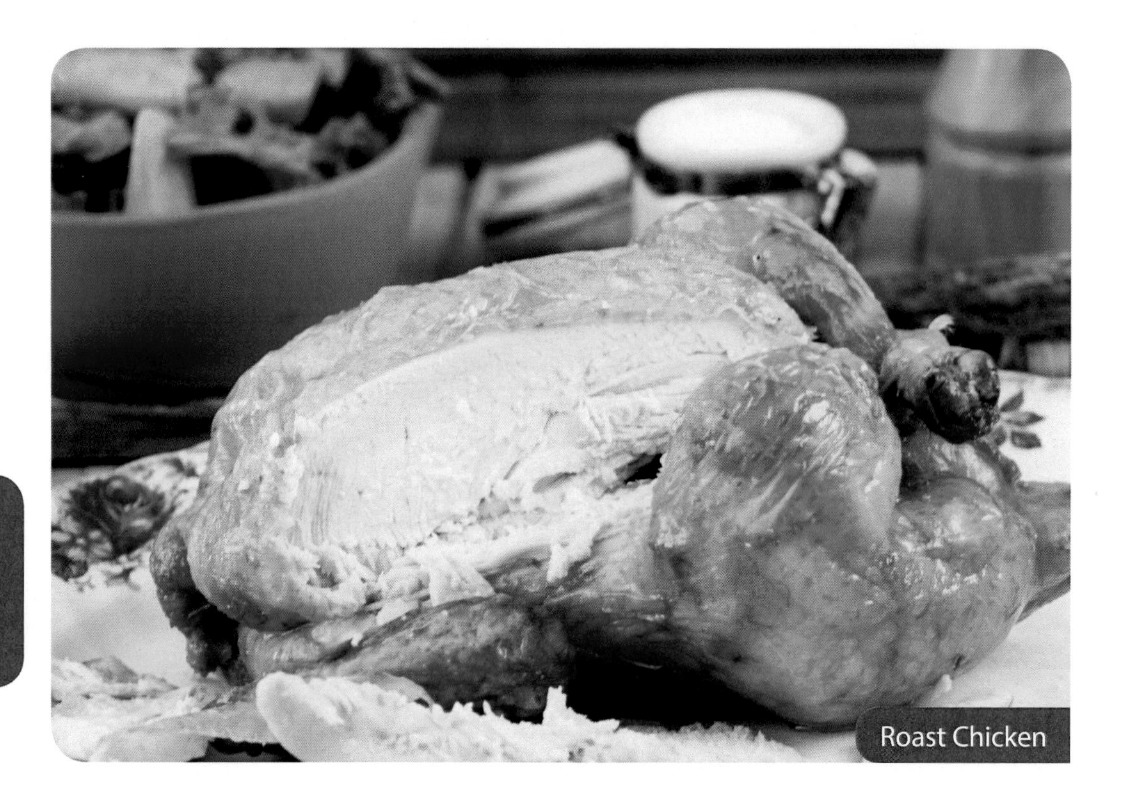

Roast Chicken

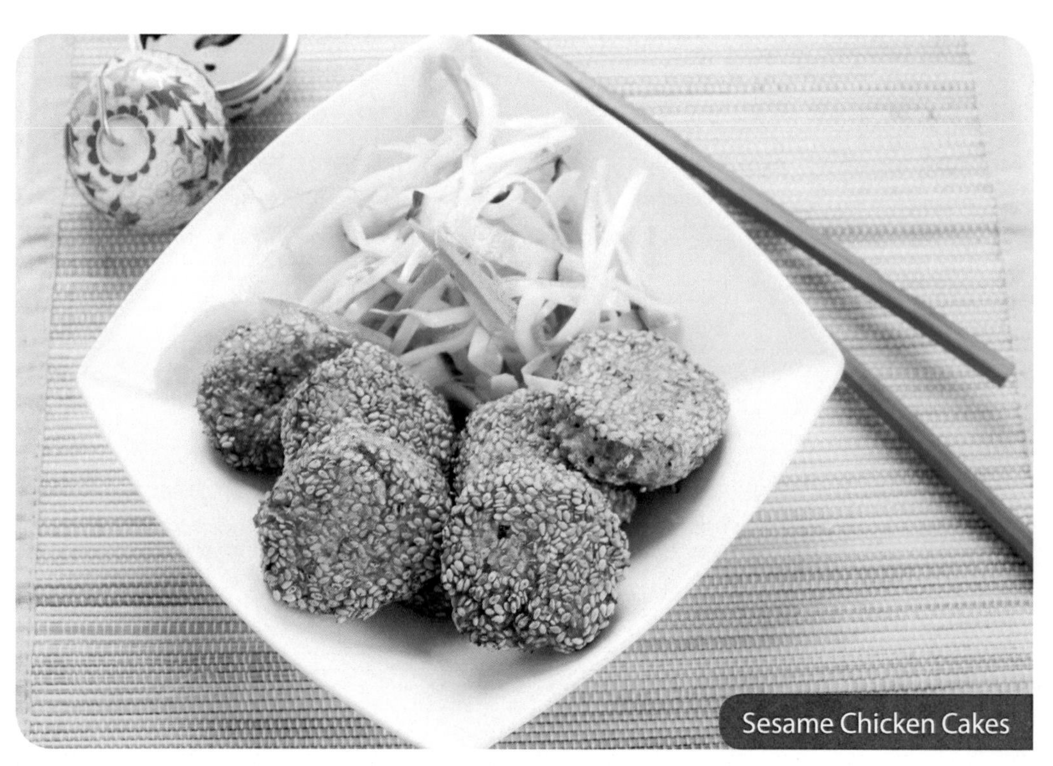

Sesame Chicken Cakes

SESAME CHICKEN CAKES

 *Servings: 2*

 *Preparation Time: 10 minutes*

 *Cooking Time: 15 minutes*

 *Total Time: 25 minutes*

Ingredients

FOR THE BURGERS

400g chicken breast or mince

1 inch ginger, grated

1 garlic clove, crushed

Sea salt

3 tbsp fresh coriander

4 spring onions

2 red chillies, chopped

1 lime, juice only

½ tsp Chinese five spice

Lard, dripping or goose fat for frying

FOR THE COATING

100g sesame seeds

1 egg, beaten

Preparation

1. Place all of the burger ingredients, except the chicken, in a food processor.
2. Mix until you have a medium fine paste.
3. If you have chicken breast then this will need to be chopped.
4. Add the chicken breast pieces or the chicken mince to the food processor.
5. You need to mix the ingredients until you have achieved a burger type consistency.
6. Shape the chicken mixture into small patties of about 1.5 inches diameter.
7. Dip each patty into the beaten egg and roll in the sesame seeds.
8. Heat a little fat in a frying pan until hot and add the patties.
9. Fry for 2 minutes on each side until golden brown and cooked right through.
10. Drain on kitchen paper and serve hot or cold with Sharp Asian Slaw and Asian Dressing to dip.

SMOKY BAKED CHICKEN

 *Servings: 4*

 *Preparation Time: 15 minutes*

 *Cooking Time: 45 minutes*

 *Total Time: 1 hour*

Ingredients

8 bone-in, skin-on, chicken thighs

1 tsp garlic powder

½ tsp dried oregano

1 pinch sea salt

2 tsp smoked paprika

½ tsp ground cayenne

2 tbsp olive oil

1 pinch freshly ground black pepper

Preparation

1. Preheat the oven to 180C.
2. Combine the spices with the oil and rub all over the chicken pieces.
3. Roast for about 45 minutes until the chicken is really tender and the skin crisp.
4. Serve with a Basic Side Salad.

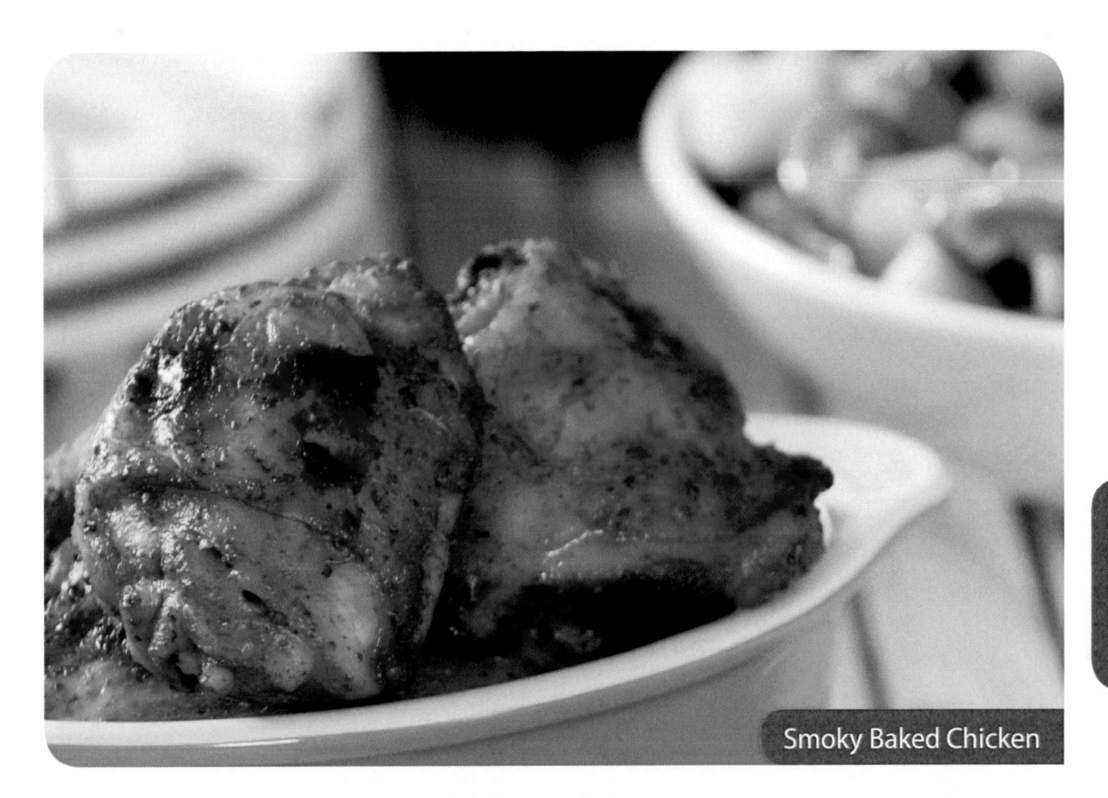
Smoky Baked Chicken

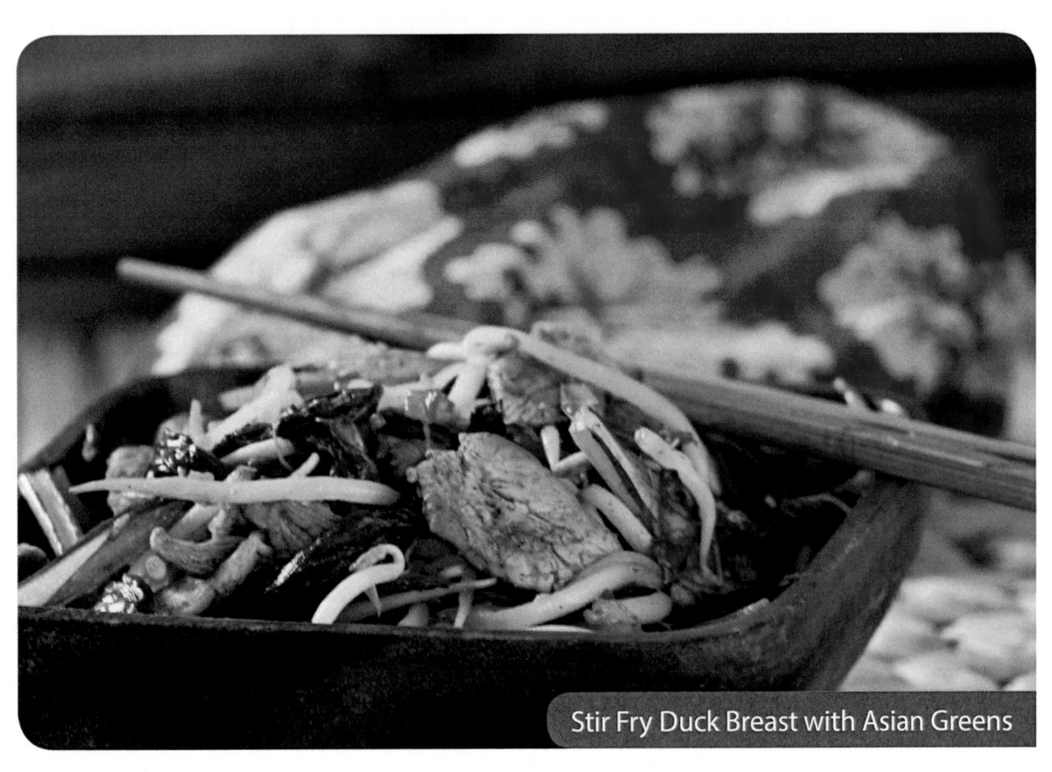
Stir Fry Duck Breast with Asian Greens

TURKEY BURGERS

 *Servings: 4*

 *Preparation Time: 15 minutes*

 *Cooking Time: 15 minutes*

 *Total Time: 30 minutes*

Ingredients

FOR THE BURGER

- 500g turkey mince (or breast)
- 4 rashers streaky bacon, chopped
- 2 tbsp sun dried tomatoes, chopped
- 2 tbsp fresh basil leaves, chopped
- 1 pinch sea salt

FOR THE TOPPINGS

- 1 onion, sliced
- 2 large tomatoes, sliced
- 1 bag rocket
- 1 tbsp extra virgin olive oil
- 1 pinch sea salt
- 1 pinch freshly ground black pepper

Preparation

1. If you have bought turkey breast then this will need to be chopped into pieces.
2. Place all the burger ingredients into a food processor.
3. Mix until it forms a coarse mince.
4. Shape into 4 patties.
5. Heat the oil in a frying pan and add the burgers.
6. Cook for about 5 minutes on each side until cooked through.
7. When cooked served with the toppings and Sweet Potato Fries.

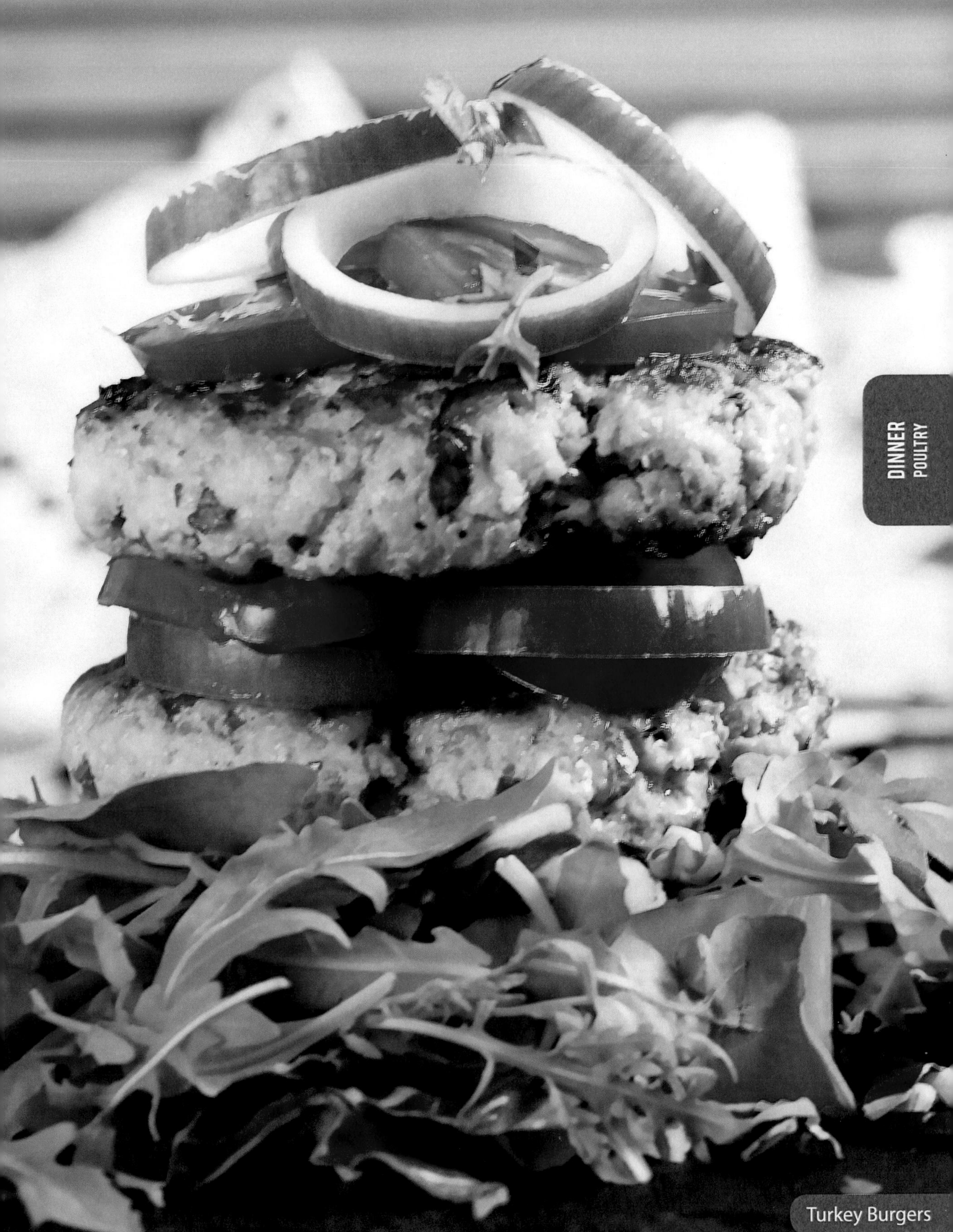

Turkey Burgers

STIR FRY DUCK BREAST WITH ASIAN GREENS

 *Servings: 2*

 *Preparation Time: 15 minutes*

 *Cooking Time: 10 minutes*

 *Total Time: 25 minutes*

Ingredients

2 duck breasts, thinly sliced

1 tsp Chinese five spice

1 red chilli, finely sliced (optional)

100g beansprouts

1 pinch flaked sea salt

1 tsp sesame oil

1 inch ginger, grated

4 bok choi, quartered lengthways

1 large garlic clove, crushed

1 tbsp balsamic vinegar

Preparation

1. Prepare the duck breasts, ginger, chilli, bok choi and garlic.
2. Heat the oil in a wok or large frying pan.
3. When smoking hot add the ginger, chilli, duck and five spice.
4. Stir fry for a few minutes until the duck is cooked.
5. Add the bok choi with the beansprouts and the garlic.
6. Cook until the bok choi wilts.
7. Season with a little salt and balsamic and serve with a Sharp Asian Slaw.

LAMB

BUBBLE AND SQUEAK

 *Servings: 2*

 *Preparation Time: 20 minutes*

 *Cooking Time: 20 minutes*

 *Total Time: 40 minutes*

Ingredients

2 portions leftover lamb

1 portion leftover kale

2 sweet potatoes, chopped into 1cm cubes

2 tbsp lard, dripping or goose fat

2 tbsp fresh mint, chopped

Preparation

1. Chop the sweet potatoes and boil. Drain when tender.
2. Heat the fat in a large frying pan.
3. Add the sweet potatoes, lamb and kale, pressing into the pan and stirring occasionally.
4. Fry until brown and crispy.
5. Season with salt and fresh mint before serving hot.

EASY LAMB CURRY

 *Servings: 2*

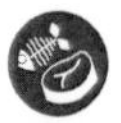 *Preparation Time: 10 minutes*

 *Cooking Time: 1 hour*

 *Total Time: 1 hour, 10 minutes*

Ingredients

1 tbsp coconut oil

1 large onion, chopped

2 garlic cloves, crushed

200g tinned chopped tomatoes

Sea salt

2 tbsp rogan josh spice mix or paste to taste (check label for additives)

400g diced lamb

1 red pepper, chopped

1 inch fresh ginger, grated

200ml water

2 tbsp fresh coriander

Preparation

1. Heat the oil in a large saucepan.
2. Add the onions with the peppers and a pinch of salt.
3. Cook over a low heat until beginning to soften then add the lamb.
4. Stir until the lamb is browned and then add the garlic, ginger and spices.
5. Give it a good stir and add the tomato with the water.
6. Keep over a gentle heat and simmer for about 30-40 minutes until thick and glossy.
7. Garnish with the chopped coriander and serve hot with Cauliflower Rice.

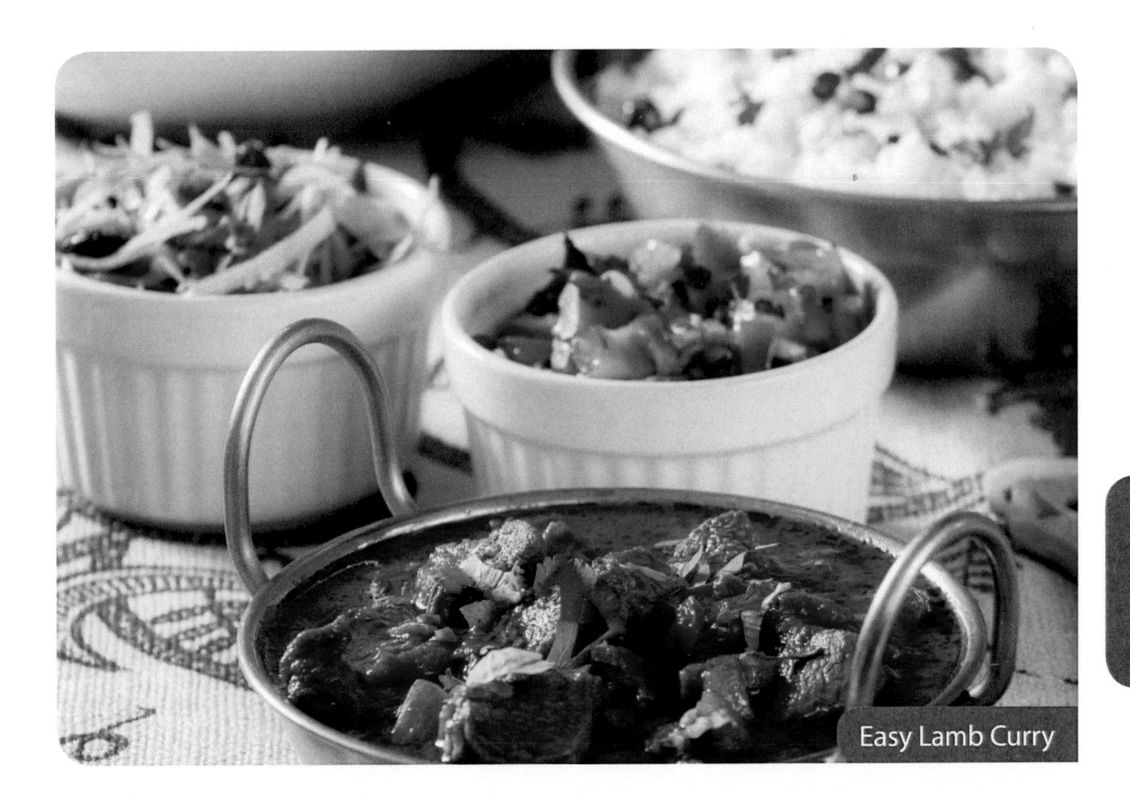

Easy Lamb Curry

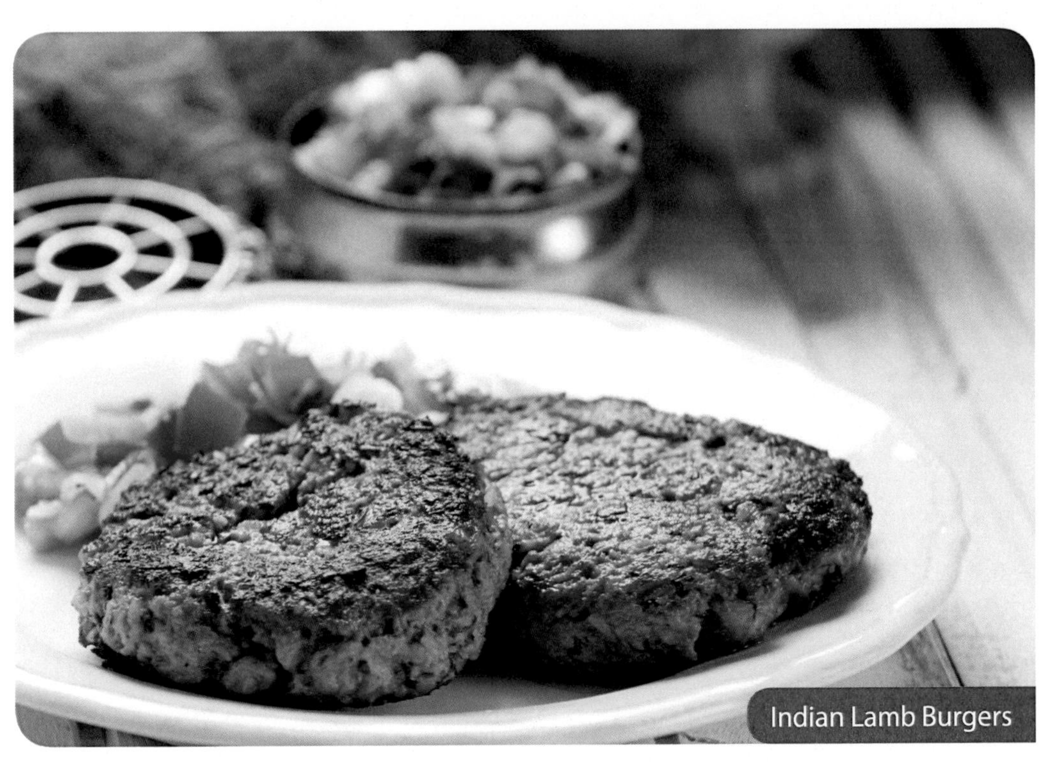

Indian Lamb Burgers

INDIAN LAMB BURGERS

 *Servings: 2*

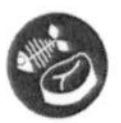 *Preparation Time: 15 minutes*

 *Cooking Time: 20 minutes*

 *Total Time: 35 minutes*

Ingredients

400g lamb mince

1 garlic clove, crushed

1 tbsp fresh mint, chopped

Sea salt

1 finely chopped onion

1 tbsp Madras curry powder

1 tbsp fresh coriander, chopped

Preparation

1. Mix all of the ingredients together and knead to combine thoroughly.
2. Divide the mixture into 2 or 4 depending on the size you want them and grill or fry for roughly 6-8 minutes each side.
3. Serve hot with Tomato and Spring Onion side salad.

KLEFTIKO

A fragrant Greek dish of soft baked lamb with tomato, oregano, onion and garlic. Serve with a chunky Greek style salad. One for the weekend or a late dinner, this dish is best when allowed a long slow bake.

 *Servings: 4*

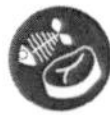 *Preparation Time: 20 minutes*

 *Cooking Time: 2 hours*

 *Total Time: 2 hours, 20 minutes*

Ingredients

2 large onions, sliced

4 tbsp olive oil

1 tsp dried oregano

1 tsp freshly ground black pepper

4 tbsp tomato puree

4 lamb shanks

1 tsp ground coriander

1 tsp sea salt

4 garlic cloves, crushed

500ml water

Preparation

1. Preheat the oven to 160C.
2. Prepare the onion and garlic.
3. Place the sliced onions in the bottom of a deep baking dish.
4. Rub each piece of lamb with the oil and then the herbs, spices and salt.
5. Place, skin side up, on top of the onions.
6. Mix the garlic, tomato puree and water together and then pour over the lamb.
7. Cover the dish tightly with foil, making sure that no steam can escape.
8. Place in the oven for about 2 hours until the sauce is thick.
9. The onions should be soft and the meat falling off the bone.
10. Serve hot with the side dishes set out in your weekly meal planner.

LAMB CHOPS WITH CRACKED CORIANDER

The lemony tang of cracked coriander adds texture and depth to simply grilled lamb chops. You can cook the chops over an outdoor or indoor grill; failing that they pan fry well too. Adding the spice at the end retains the delicate top notes for better contrast with the sweet meat.

 *Servings: 4*

 *Preparation Time: 10 minutes*

 *Cooking Time: 10 minutes*

 *Total Time: 20 minutes*

Ingredients

16 lamb chops

1 tsp coriander seeds

Sea salt

1 tsp olive oil

Preparation

1. Bring the lamb chops to room temperature and rub with the oil.
2. Crack the coriander seeds with the back of a rolling pin or in a pestle and morter.
3. Cook the lamb chops, under the grill or in a hot frying pan, for about three minutes on each side. Sprinkle with salt the minute they go on to the heat.
4. Serve hot, scattered with fragrant cracked coriander seeds and with the side dishes set out in your weekly meal planner.
5. Keep half to eat cold for a lunch.

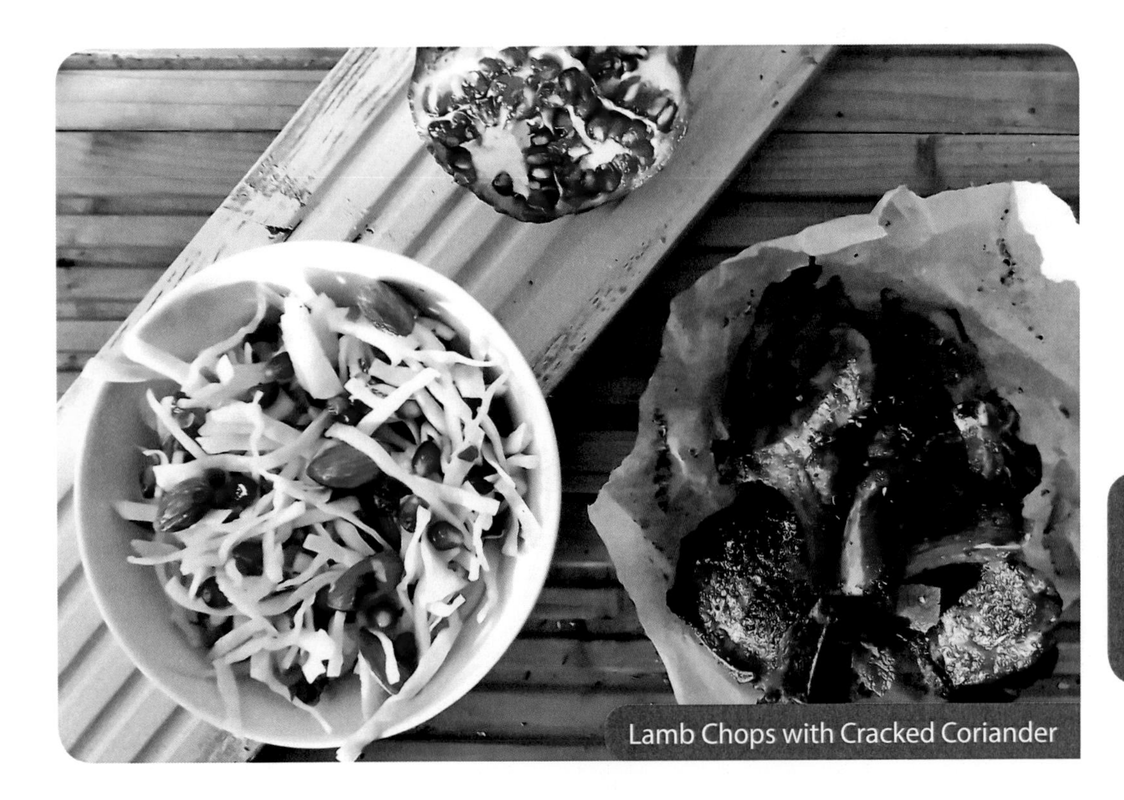
Lamb Chops with Cracked Coriander

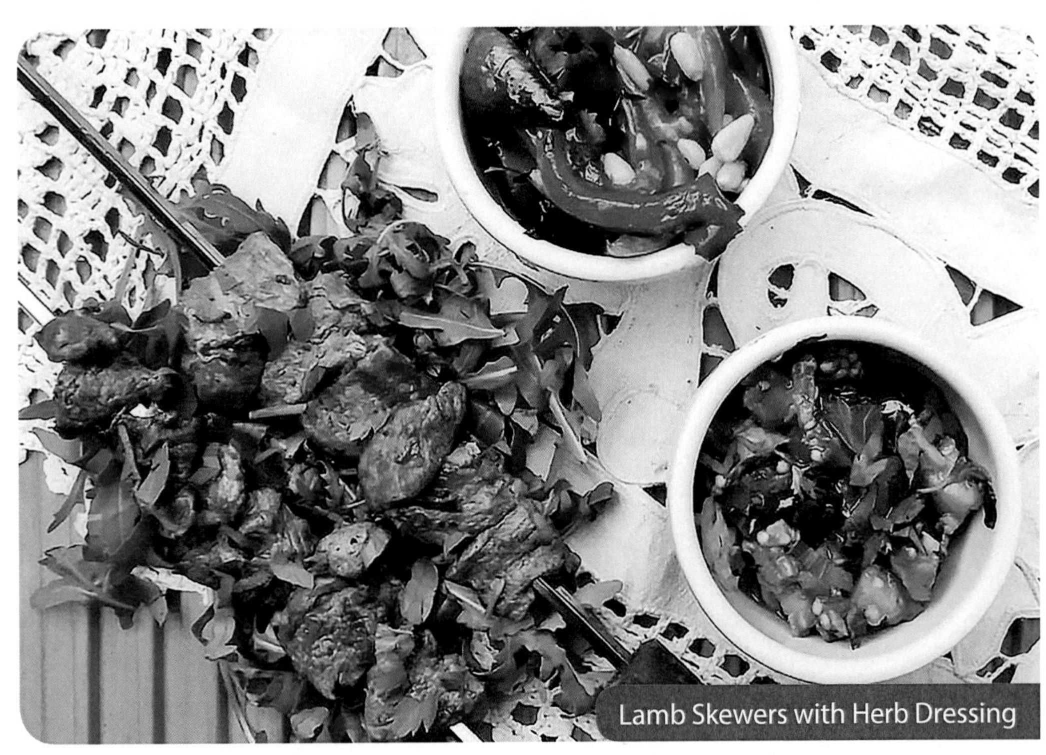
Lamb Skewers with Herb Dressing

LAMB SKEWERS WITH HERB DRESSING

 *Servings: 4*

 *Preparation Time: 15 minutes*

 *Cooking Time: 15 minutes*

 *Inactive Time: 30 minutes*

 *Total Time: 1 hour*

DINNER
LAMB

Ingredients

400g diced lamb, in ½ inch cubes

Bamboo skewers, soaked in water

1 pinch sea salt

FOR THE MARINADE

1 tbsp extra virgin olive oil

1 pinch freshly ground black pepper

½ lemon, juice only

FOR THE DRESSING

1 large garlic clove, chopped

½ bunch fresh parsley, chopped

2 tbsp olive oil

1 red chilli, chopped

½ bunch fresh mint, chopped

1 tbsp white wine vinegar

1 pinch sea salt

Preparation

1. Prepare the lamb and chop the garlic and herbs.
2. Mix together the marinade ingredients.
3. Marinade the lamb for at least half an hour but add no salt until it begins to cook.
4. Either grill the lamb on the barbeque, under an indoor grill or on a skillet.
5. Get the heat as high as you can and cook for only a few minutes on either side.
6. Sprinkle with salt as soon as it goes on the heat.
7. Mix together the dressing ingredients and pour over the lamb.
8. Serve hot with a side dish of Sautéed Courgettes with Lemon.

LAMB MEATBALLS

 *Servings: 2*

 *Preparation Time: 20 minutes*

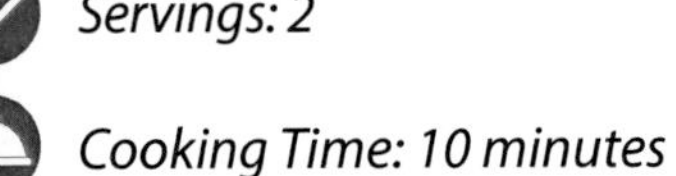 *Cooking Time: 10 minutes*

 *Inactive Time: 15 minutes*

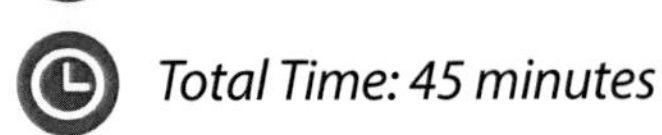 *Total Time: 45 minutes*

Ingredients

400g lamb mince

¼ tsp ground cinnamon

½ tsp fresh grated ginger

1 pinch freshly ground black pepper

¼ tsp ground cumin

¼ tsp ground coriander

1 pinch sea salt

1 tbsp lard, dripping or goose fat

Preparation

1. Mix the lamb mince, cumin, cinnamon, ginger and coriander together in a bowl.
2. Add salt and pepper to taste.
3. Place the lamb mixture in the fridge for 15 minutes.
4. Remove from the fridge and heat the fat in a frying pan over a medium heat.
5. Use your hands to create small meatballs, about a teaspoon in size.
6. Fry the meatballs for about 6-8 minutes, turning occasionally until cooked through.
7. Remove from the heat and serve, hot or cold with Greek Style Salad.

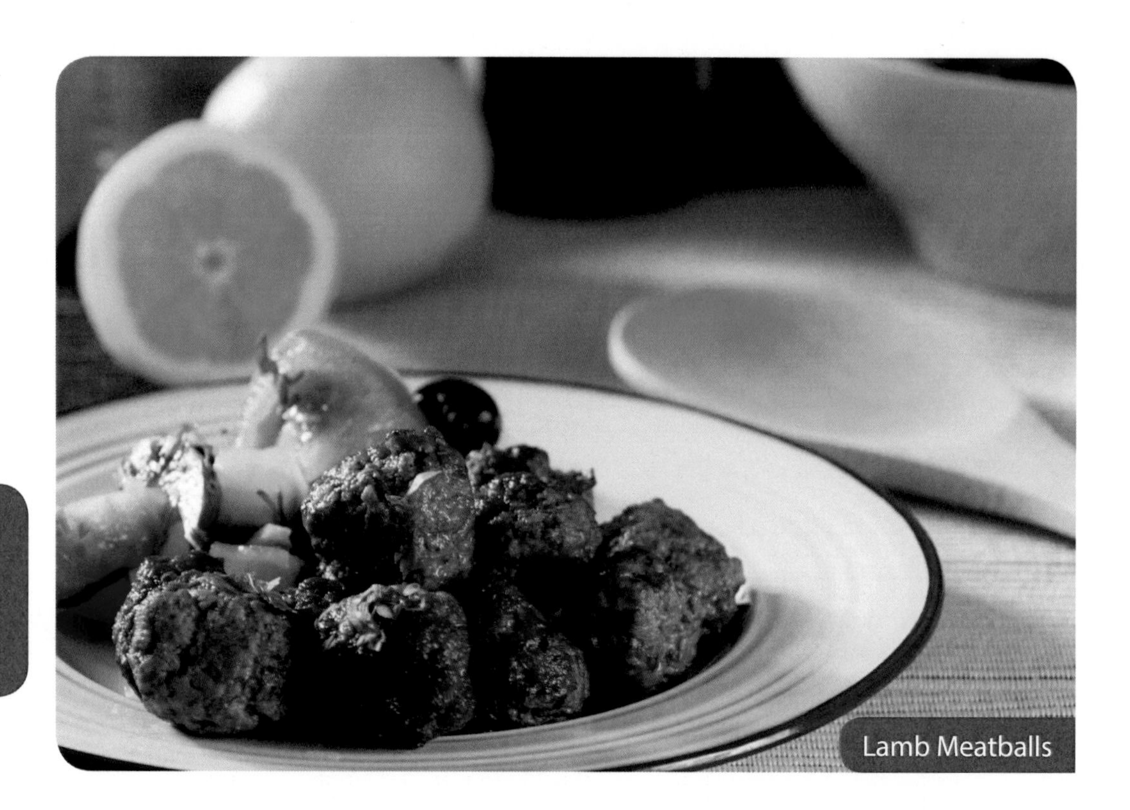

Lamb Meatballs

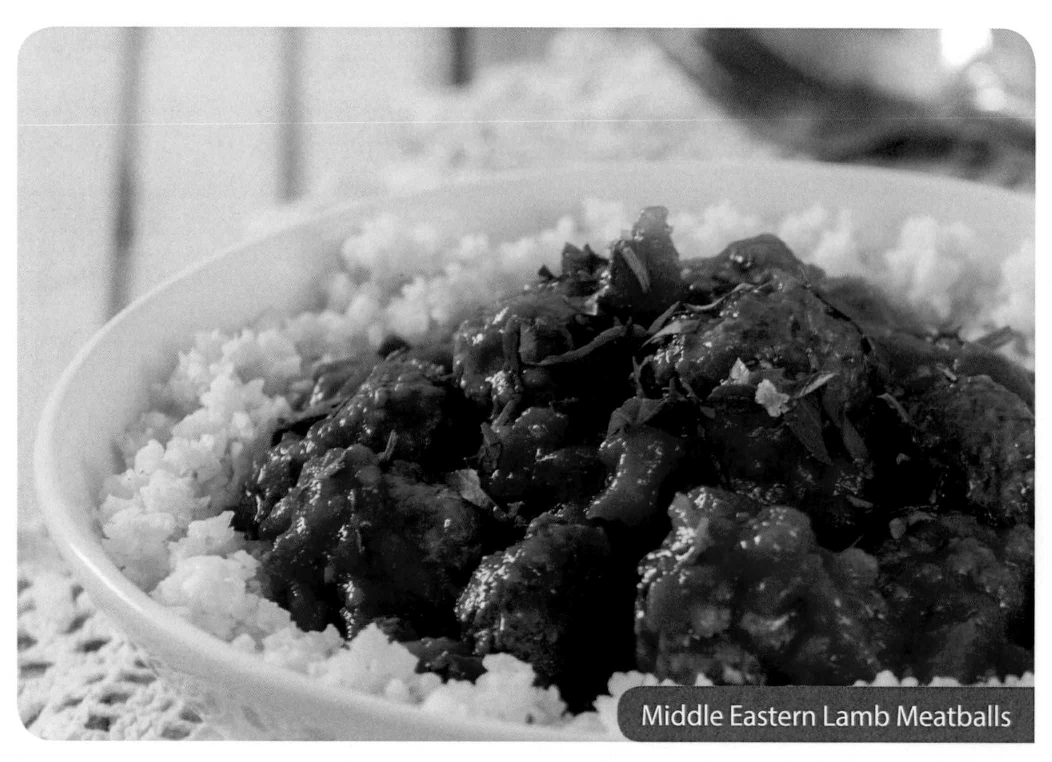

Middle Eastern Lamb Meatballs

MIDDLE EASTERN LAMB MEATBALLS

 *Servings: 4*

 *Preparation Time: 15 minutes*

 *Cooking Time: 30 minutes*

 *Total Time: 45 minutes*

Ingredients

FOR THE MEATBALLS

500g minced lamb

1 tsp ground cumin

1 pinch sea salt

1 onion, finely chopped

1 tsp ground coriander

2 tbsp fresh parsley, finely chopped

FOR THE SAUCE

400g tin chopped tomatoes

125ml olive oil

1 small bunch fresh coriander, chopped

1 tbsp olive oil, for frying

2 tbsp tomato puree

2 garlic cloves, crushed

1 pinch sea salt

Preparation

1. Chop the onion and the parsley and place in a bowl.
2. Add the remainder of the meatball ingredients and mix together.
3. Roll the meatballs into teaspoon sized balls; use wet hands to stop it sticking.
4. Pour all of the sauce ingredients into a large pan, except the coriander.
5. Place over a medium heat. Simmer gently for about 20 minutes.
6. Heat the oil in a large frying pan and add the meatballs to brown.
7. Once browned place them into the pan with the sauce.
8. Continue to cook the sauce and meatballs for a further 10 minutes.
9. Stir in the coriander and serve hot with Cauliflower Rice.

SHEPHERDS PIE

 *Servings: 2*

 *Preparation Time: 20 minutes*

 *Cooking Time: 1 hr, 20 minutes*

 *Total Time: 1 hr, 40 minutes*

Ingredients

FOR THE TOPPING

1 celeriac, chopped into 1cm cubes
2 tbsp ground almonds
Sea salt

FOR THE FILLING

600g lamb mince
1 onion, chopped
1 large carrot, sliced
1 bay leaf
Freshly ground black pepper
1 tbsp lard, dripping, goose fat
1 garlic clove, crushed
1 tbsp tomato paste
Sea salt

Preparation

1. Preheat the oven to 180C.
2. Prepare the celeriac, onion and garlic.
3. Cook the celeriac until soft in a large pan of boiling salted water.
4. Drain and lay kitchen paper over the surface to soak up moisture whilst it cools.
5. Heat the fat in a saucepan and add onions, garlic, mince, bay leaf and a pinch of salt.
6. Cook for about 10 minutes, stirring regularly to ensure an even cook.
7. Stir in the tomato puree and the carrots.
8. Pour in some water, just enough to cover, and bring to the boil.
9. Once boiling, turn down and simmer for 30 minutes or until the water has reduced by half.
10. Place the cooked filling in the bottom of an oven proof dish.
11. Mash the celeriac and stir in the ground almonds to stiffen it up.
12. Spread the celeriac over the filling and bake in the oven for 30 minutes when it should be brown and bubbling.
13. Serve with a side dish of Sautéed Carrots with Fresh Herbs.

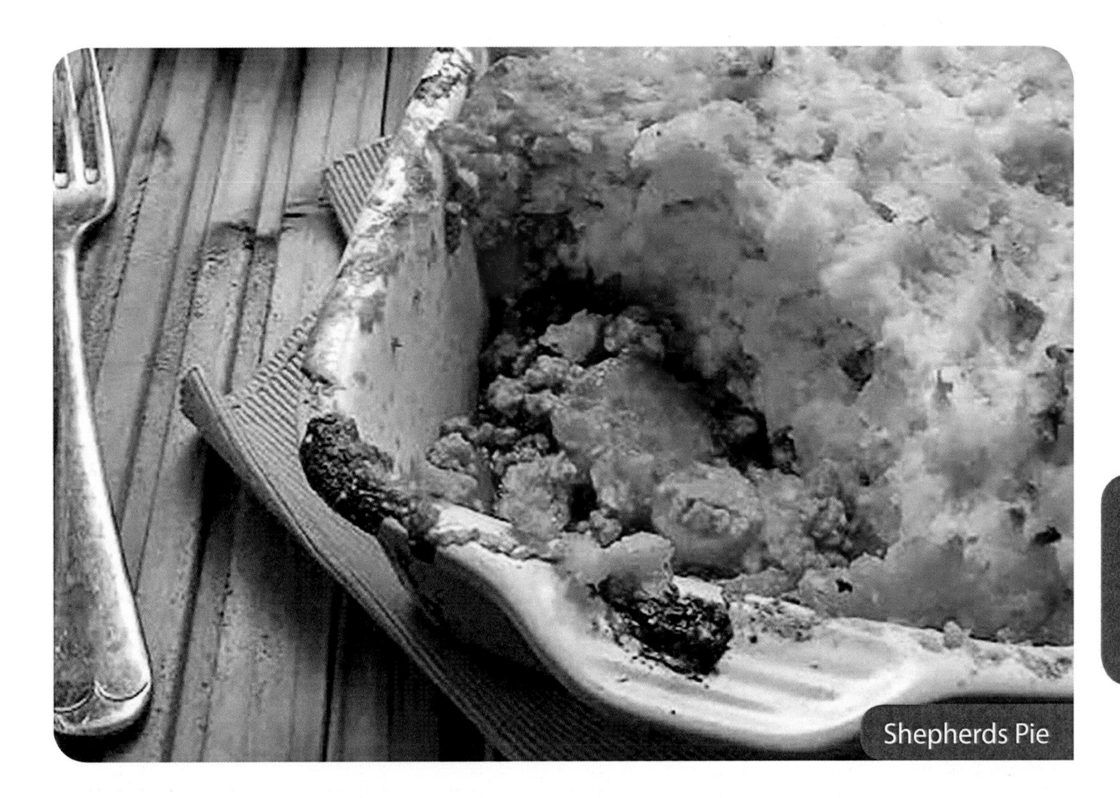
Shepherds Pie

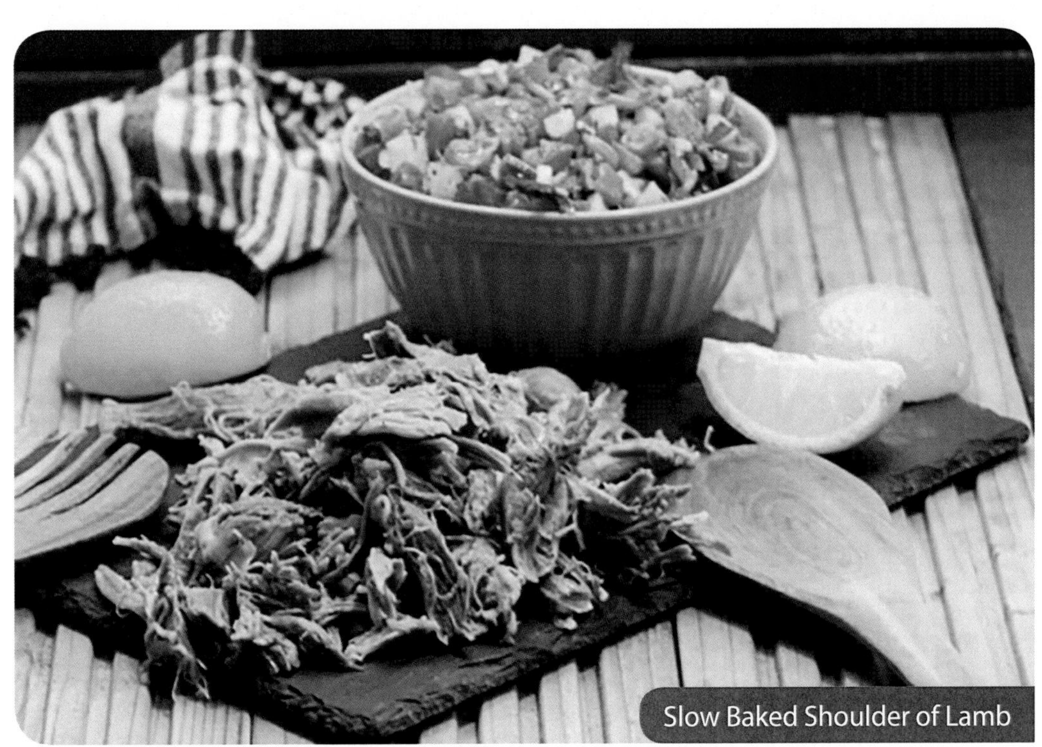
Slow Baked Shoulder of Lamb

SLOW BAKED SHOULDER OF LAMB

Get a full shoulder for a really long slow and tender roast. The leftovers can be used for lunch during the week.

 *Servings: 6*

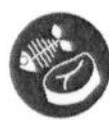 *Preparation Time: 10 minutes*

 *Cooking Time: 4 hours*

 *Total Time: 4 hours, 10 minutes*

Ingredients

1 small shoulder of lamb
2 sprigs fresh rosemary
2 bay leaves
Sea salt
6 garlic cloves, whole
1 lemon, quartered
2 tbsp olive oil
Freshly ground black pepper

Preparation

1. Preheat the oven to 170C.
2. Season the lamb, and place in a roasting tin with the oil, herbs, garlic and lemon.
3. Cover with tin foil and cook for about 4 hours until the meat falls of the bone.
4. Bring from the oven (no need to rest) and shred the meat with two forks.
5. Serve hot with the side dishes set out in your weekly meal planner.

PORK

AWESOME PULLED PORK

When making pulled pork you really need a large piece of meat, otherwise it can dry out and become tough during the cooking process. Feel free to use a larger piece of meat if you like and maybe invite friends over for a Paleo lunch and/or keep some leftovers for another meal.

 *Servings: 8*

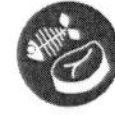 *Preparation Time: 15 minutes*

 *Cooking Time: 4 hours*

 *Total Time: 4 hours, 15 minutes*

Ingredients

2kg pork shoulder

2 onions, sliced

FOR THE DRY RUB

3 tbsp paprika

2 tsp ground cumin

1 tsp chipotle powder or flakes

1 tsp ground coriander

1 tsp garlic powder

2 tsp sea salt

Preparation

1. Preheat the oven to 150C.
2. Mix the dry rub ingredients and massage into the pork.
3. Lay in a deep roasting dish with the sliced onions and cover tightly with foil.
4. Cook for about 4 hours until the pork shreds easily with two forks.
5. Serve hot with the side dishes set out in your weekly meal planner.
6. Don't forget to use the pan juices as a dip.

BBQ PORK BURGER

 *Servings: 2*

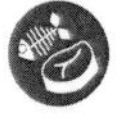 *Preparation Time: 10 minutes*

 *Cooking Time: 25 minutes*

 *Total Time: 35 minutes*

Ingredients

400g pork mince

1 tsp sweet paprika

1 pinch celery seed

1 bag mixed salad leaf

1 pinch freshly ground black pepper

¼ tsp garlic powder

1 tbsp lard, melted

FOR THE SAUCE

½ small onion, finely chopped

1 tbsp Dijon mustard

1 pinch sea salt

1 tbsp raw honey

2 tbsp apple cider vinegar

Preparation

1. Prepare the onion.
2. Place the lard in a saucepan over a medium heat.
3. Place the onions into the saucepan and cook until translucent.
4. Add the honey, mustard, and vinegar and stir to combine.
5. Reduce the heat and simmer for about 5 minutes to reduce the mixture.
6. Add a pinch of salt and set aside.
7. Mix the pork mince with the spices and form into 4 small burgers.
8. Grill or fry for about 5 minutes on each side or until just cooked through.
9. Serve the burgers, drizzled with sauce, on a bed of crisp salad leaf with Sweet Potato Fries.

GAMMON STEAKS

Cook all four gammon steaks and keep two for a leftover lunch later in the week.

 *Servings: 4*

 *Cooking Time: 10 minutes*

Ingredients

4 thick gammon steaks

Preparation

1. Make slits along the rind of the gammon to prevent it curling up on the grill.
2. Grill under a hot grill for about 2 minutes each side.
3. You want it to be cooked through, yet juicy and moist.
4. Serve hot with our Roast Cinnamon Apples and Squash.
5. Don't forget to keep two for leftover lunch.

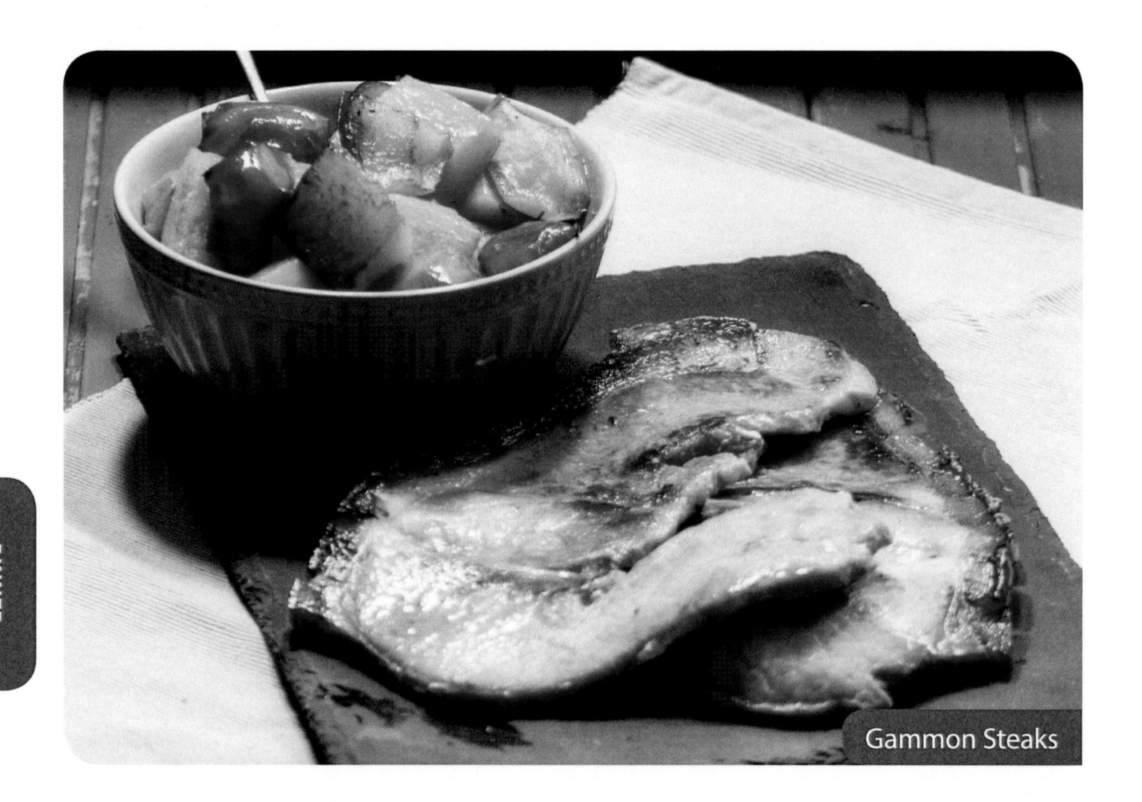
Gammon Steaks

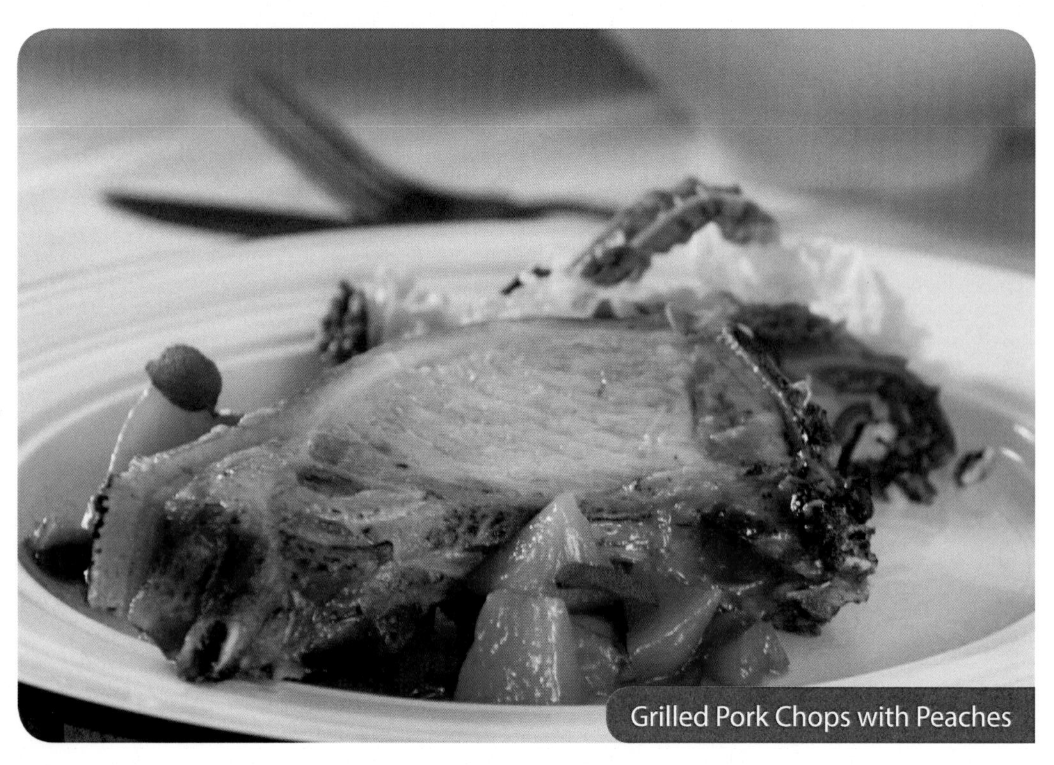
Grilled Pork Chops with Peaches

GRILLED PORK CHOPS WITH PEACHES

 *Servings: 2*

 *Preparation Time: 10 minutes*

 *Cooking Time: 30 minutes*

 *Total Time: 40 minutes*

Ingredients

2 pork chops, bone-in

FOR THE SAUCE

½ red onion, sliced

½ large garlic clove, crushed

1 tbsp water

1 tsp sage leaves, chopped

Freshly ground black pepper

1 tbsp extra virgin olive oil

1 large peach or nectarine, chopped

1 tbsp apple cider vinegar

Sea salt

Preparation

1. Prepare the onions, garlic, peach/nectarine and sage.
2. Heat the olive oil in a pan over a medium heat and add the onions.
3. Fry until soft and slightly brown.
4. Rub the chops with a little seasoning and cook under a hot grill or in a skillet/frying pan turning occasionally.
5. Timing will vary depending on thickness but they need at least 20 minutes.
6. Add the rest of the sauce ingredients to the onions.
7. Cook for about 5 minutes until the peach has softened.
8. When the chops are cooked, serve hot with the sauce and the side dishes set out in your weekly meal planner.

PORK TENDERLOIN WITH SAGE AND TOMATO

 *Servings: 2*

 *Preparation Time: 20 minutes*

 *Cooking Time: 40 minutes*

 *Total Time: 1 hour*

Ingredients

500g whole pork tenderloin

1 tsp fresh sage, finely chopped

2 tbsp olive oil

Freshly ground black pepper

6 sun-dried tomatoes, chopped

1 garlic clove, minced

Sea salt

Ingredients

1. Preheat the oven to 180C.
2. Chop the tomatoes and sage.
3. Place a piece of foil, large enough to loosely wrap the tenderloin, over a baking dish.
4. Add the tenderloin, oil, tomatoes, sage, garlic and seasoning.
5. Wrap the meat loosely and bake for about 30 minutes or until the pork is tender.
6. Allow to rest for 10 minutes before slicing to serve.
7. Serve with our Beetroot and Peach Salad.

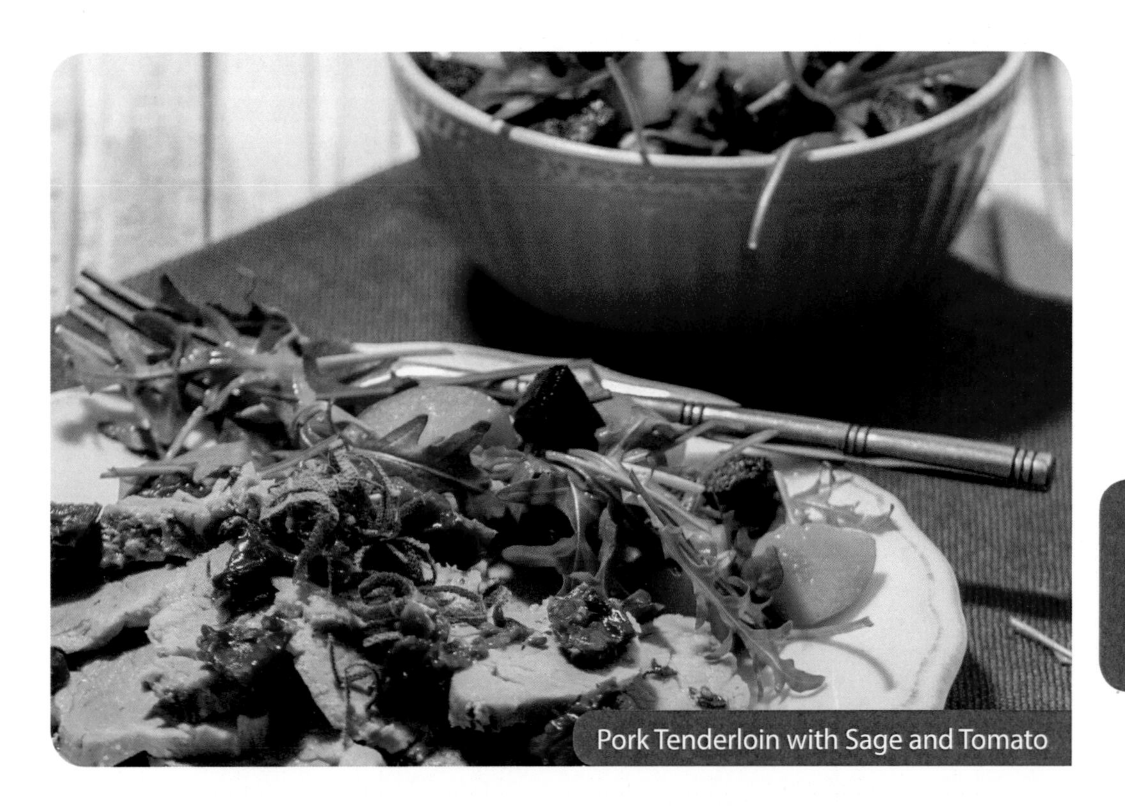
Pork Tenderloin with Sage and Tomato

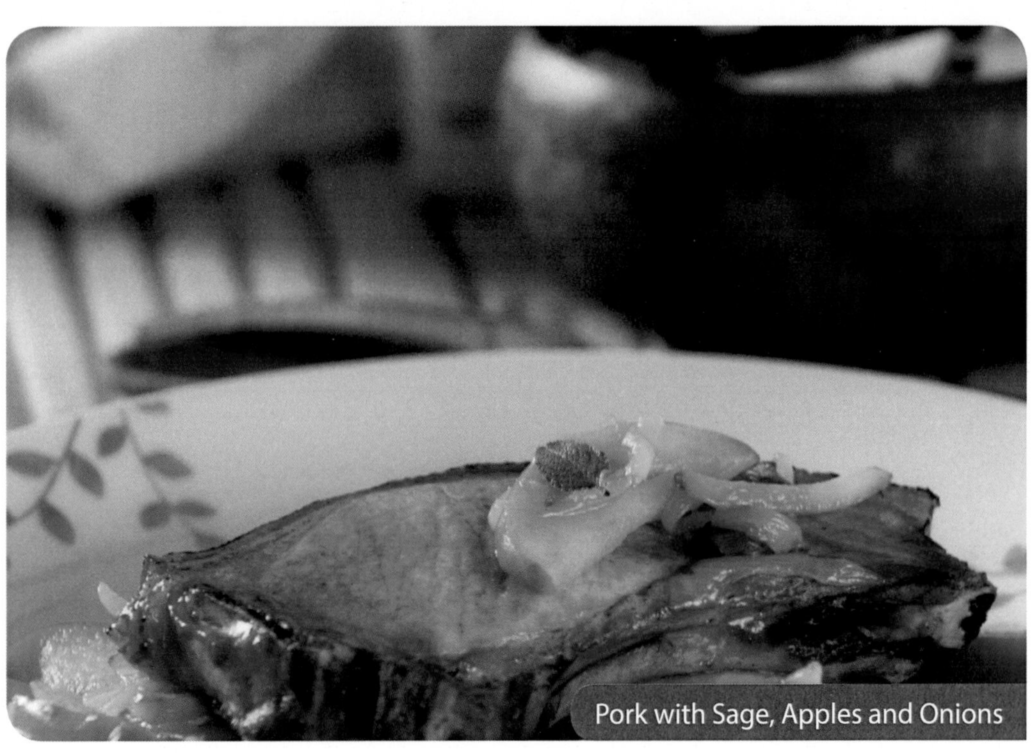
Pork with Sage, Apples and Onions

PORK WITH SAGE, APPLES AND ONIONS

 *Servings: 2*

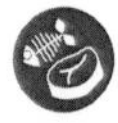 *Preparation Time: 10 minutes*

 *Cooking Time: 20 minutes*

 *Total Time: 30 minutes*

Ingredients

2 bone-in pork chops

1 large onion, sliced

4 fresh sage leaves, chopped

1 tbsp lard

2 apples, sliced

Sea salt

Preparation

1. Prepare the onion and the apples.
2. Heat the lard in a frying pan and add the pork chops.
3. Season with salt and pepper and cook for about 5 minutes on each side.
4. Add the onions, sage and apples to the pan.
5. Add a few drops of water if needed to keep the pan moist.
6. Cook gently for a further 10 minutes.
7. The apples and sage should be soft and the pork cooked through.
8. Serve hot with a side dish of Wilted Spinach.

SAUSAGES WITH CARAWAY CABBAGE

You can choose a few interesting varieties of good quality sausages to make this dish more interesting. Something German or Polish suits the caraway cabbage. If you don't like caraway then just season your choice of cabbage well.

 *Servings: 2*

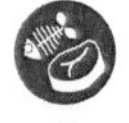 *Preparation Time: 5 minutes*

 *Cooking Time: 40 minutes*

 *Total Time: 45 minutes*

DINNER
PORK

Ingredients

400g pork sausages
(or any sausage of your choice)
½ tsp caraway seeds
1 pinch sea salt
½ head Savoy cabbage, shredded
½ tbsp lard
1 tsp lemon juice, freshly squeezed
1 pinch freshly ground black pepper

Preparation

1. Preheat the oven to 180C.
2. Toast the caraway seeds in a small hot dry pan and set aside to cool.
3. Place the sausages on a baking tray and cook in the oven for 40 minutes (or according to the individual instructions provided).
4. Whilst the sausages are cooking, heat the lard or oil in a frying pan.
5. Add the cabbage and a pinch of salt.
6. Cook slowly over a gentle heat so that the cabbage browns slightly yet softens too.
7. Remove the cabbage from the heat and add the caraway seeds with plenty of black pepper and a drop of lemon juice.
8. Serve the sausages hot with the cabbage.

SAUSAGE AND PEPPER CASSEROLE

 *Servings: 2*

 *Preparation Time: 10 minutes*

 *Cooking Time: 30 minutes*

 *Total Time: 40 minutes*

Ingredients

6 pork sausages, cut into chunks

1 red onion, peeled and sliced

3 garlic cloves, finely chopped

4 sprigs fresh thyme

1 pinch sea salt

1 red pepper, sliced

400g tinned chopped tomatoes

2 tbsp lard, dripping or goose fat

2 bay leaves

1 pinch freshly ground black pepper

Preparation

1. Prepare the peppers, onion, garlic and the sausages.
2. Heat the fat in a large frying pan over a medium heat.
3. Add all of the ingredients except the tomato and sauté for about 20 minutes.
4. Stir in the chopped tomatoes, turn down the heat and cover the pan.
5. Simmer for a further 10 minutes or until the sauce is thick and the sausages are cooked through.
6. Once the sausage is cooked you can remove the lid and reduce the sauce if it needs it.
7. Serve hot with a side dish of Greens with Chilli and Walnut.

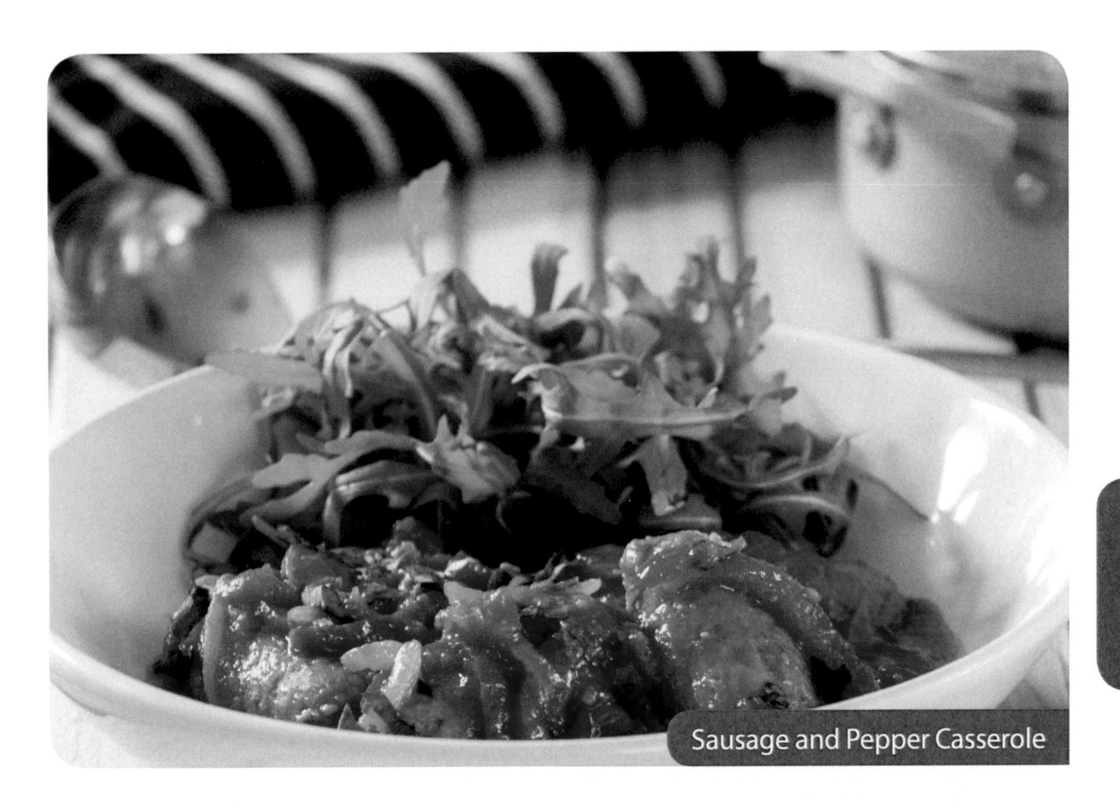
Sausage and Pepper Casserole

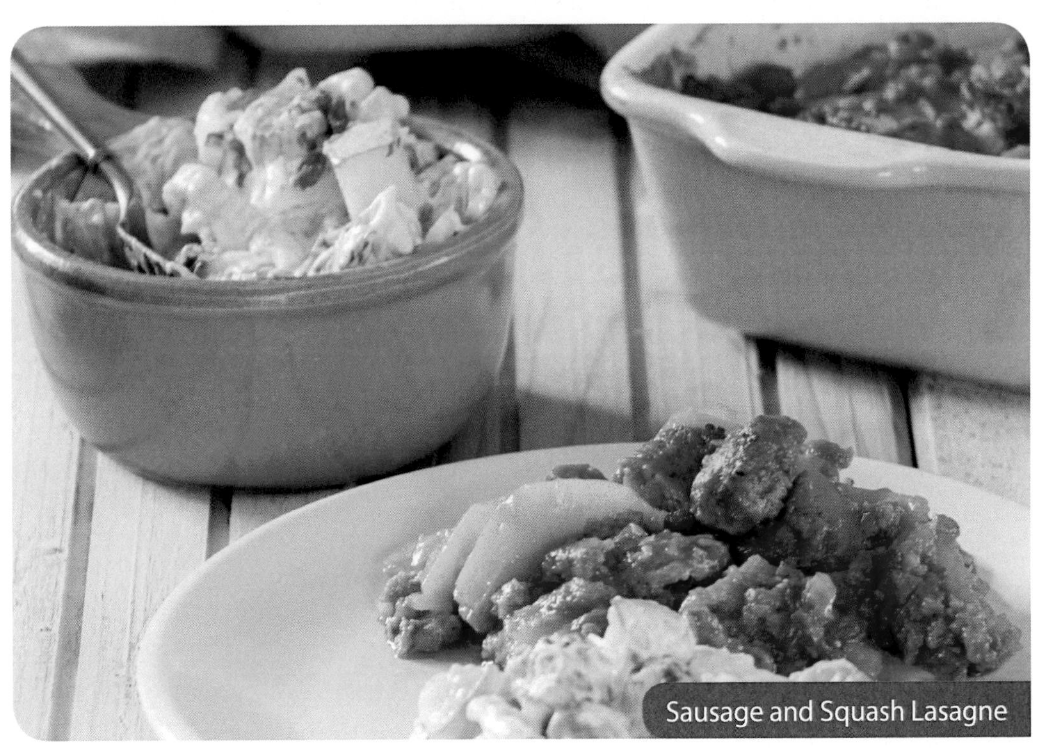
Sausage and Squash Lasagne

SAUSAGE AND SQUASH LASAGNE

 *Servings: 2*

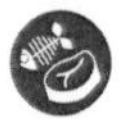 *Preparation Time: 15 minutes*

 *Cooking Time: 60 minutes*

 *Total Time: 1 hour, 15 minutes*

Ingredients

300g cumberland sausage, chopped

½ recipe Basic Tomato Sauce

1 onion, chopped

1 small butternut squash

Preparation

1. Preheat the oven to 180C.
2. Prepare the onion and sausage.
3. Peel the butternut squash and slice as thinly as you can manage.
4. Heat a pan and when hot add the chopped sausage. There should be enough fat in the sausage to release into the pan, so there is no need for additional oil.
5. Add the onion and fry gently, stirring occasionally.
6. When the onions are soft, pour in the tomato sauce and simmer for about 10 minutes.
7. In a medium sized casserole dish, alternate layers of sauce with layers of squash, ending with a layer of sauce.
8. Cover with foil and bake in the oven for about 40 minutes or until the squash is soft.
9. Allow to stand and cool slightly before serving with Pear and Walnut Waldorf Salad and Simple Leaf Salad.

SWEET AND SOUR PORK

 *Servings: 2*

 *Preparation Time: 30 minutes*

 *Cooking Time: 20 minutes*

 *Total Time:50 minutes*

Ingredients

FOR THE SAUCE

½ mango, chopped

1 onion, sliced

4 tbsp white wine vinegar

¼ pineapple, chopped

1 garlic clove, crushed

FOR THE PORK

400g pork loin, cubed

1 tsp Chinese 5-spice powder

1 red pepper, chopped

1 tsp ginger, crushed

2 tbsp lard, dripping or goose fat

1 onion, sliced

1 garlic clove, minced

Preparation

1. Prepare all of the ingredients and cut up the pork loin.
2. Put all of the sauce ingredients in a pan and simmer gently for about 10 minutes.
3. Heat the fat in a frying pan and add the onions, peppers, garlic, ginger and pork.
4. Stir fry for about 5 minutes or until the pork is cooked through.
5. Add the spice to the pork and stir through before pouring on the sauce.
6. Serve hot with Cauliflower Rice.

FISH

AROMATIC FISH PARCELS

 *Servings: 2*

 *Preparation Time: 15 minutes*

 *Cooking Time: 15 minutes*

 *Total Time: 30 minutes*

Ingredients

2 chunky white fish fillets

2 garlic cloves, whole

2 red chilli peppers, chopped

200ml coconut milk

2 lemongrass, chopped

2 inches ginger, chopped

2 limes, juice only

Fresh coriander for garnish

Preparation

1. Preheat the oven to 200C.
2. Prepare the lemongrass, garlic, ginger and chilli and place into a bowl.
3. Add the coconut milk and the lime juice and mix well.
4. Prepare 2 squares of greaseproof paper large enough to fit a piece of fish.
5. Srumple the paper squares at the edges to form a shallow dish.
6. Place a piece of fish onto each piece of greaseproof paper.
7. Divide the topping between each parcel and then wrap the paper up into a parcel.
8. Place in the oven and cook for about 15 minutes until the fish is cooked through.
9. Serve in the parcels and cut open at the table to release fragrant steam.
10. Sprinkle with coriander and serve with a side of Broccoli with Mustard Seeds.

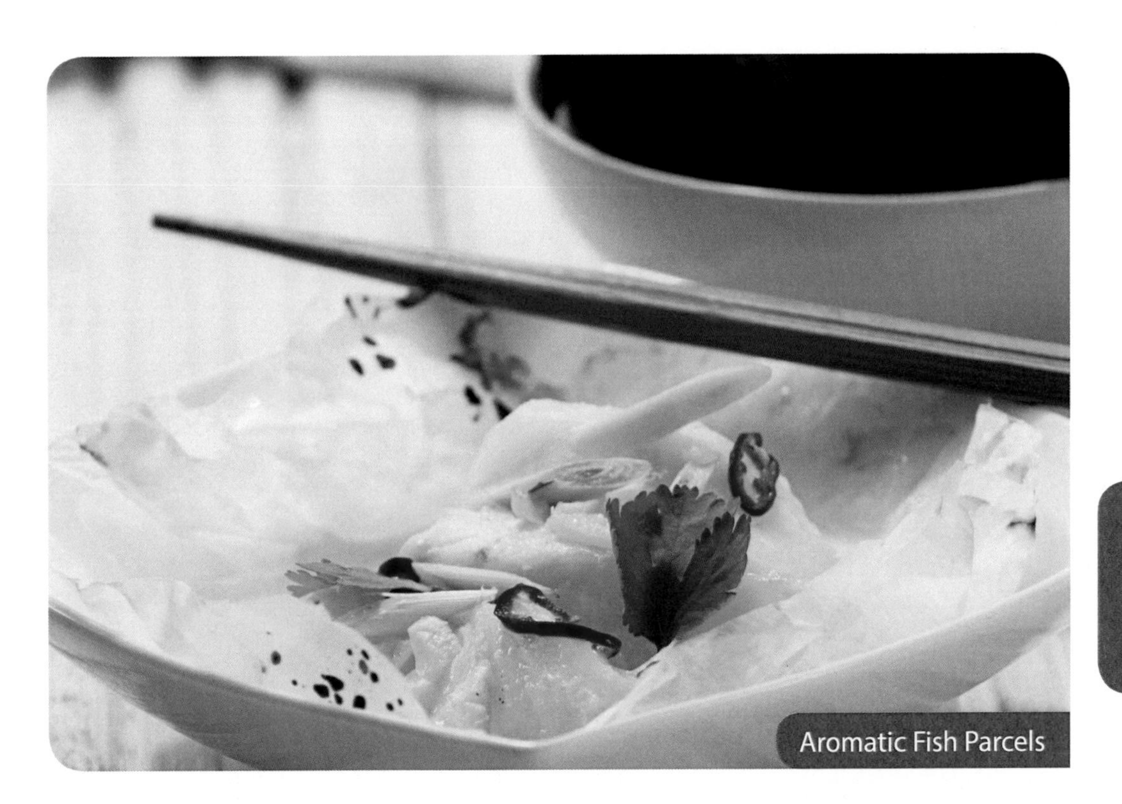

Aromatic Fish Parcels

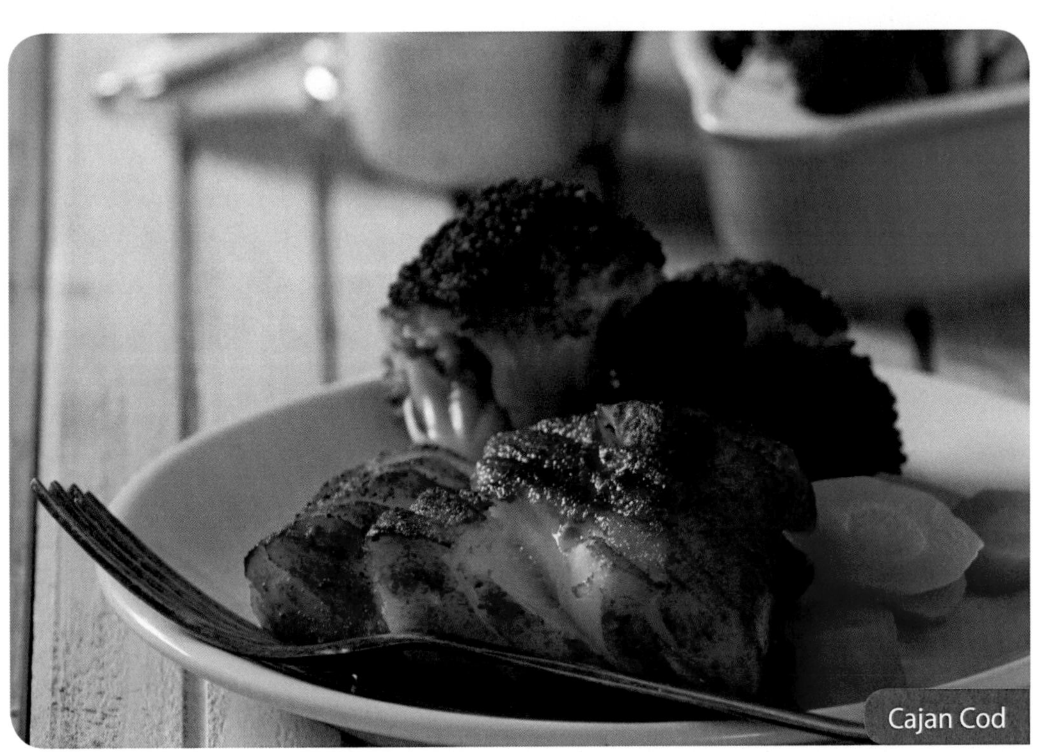

Cajan Cod

CAJUN COD

 *Servings: 2*

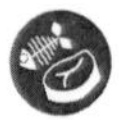 *Preparation Time: 5 minutes*

 *Cooking Time: 20 minutes*

 *Total Time: 25 minutes*

Ingredients

2 chunky cod fillets

1 tbsp smoked paprika

1 tsp ground coriander

1 tsp garlic powder

1 tbsp lard, dripping or goose fat

1 tsp chilli powder

1 tsp oregano

Sea salt

Preparation

1. Preheat oven to 200C.
2. Mix spices together and rub all over the fish.
3. Heat the fat in a frying pan or skillet and cook the fish for a few minutes on each side to colour the spices.
4. Transfer to a shallow pan and finish cooking in oven for 5 - 10 minutes or until the fish flakes easily with a fork.
5. Serve with side dishes of Pan Steamed Broccoli and Pan Steamed Carrots.

GRILLED FRESH TROUT WITH LEMON AND PARSLEY

 *Servings: 2*

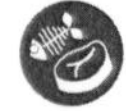 *Preparation Time: 20 minutes*

 *Cooking Time: 20 minutes*

 *Total Time: 40 minutes*

Ingredients

2 fresh trout, gutted with heads on

Sea salt

1 lemon, sliced

2 tbsp olive oil

Freshly ground black pepper

4 sprigs fresh parsley

Preparation

1. Preheat the oven to 200C.
2. Slash the trout diagonally and rub all over with oil, salt and pepper.
3. Lay the trout on a baking tray and stuff the cavity with lemon slices and parsley sprigs.
4. Bake in the hot oven for about 20 minutes until the flesh flakes away from the bone. There is no need to turn over.
5. Transfer the trout carefully to warm plates and serve with Peas with Onions and Bacon.

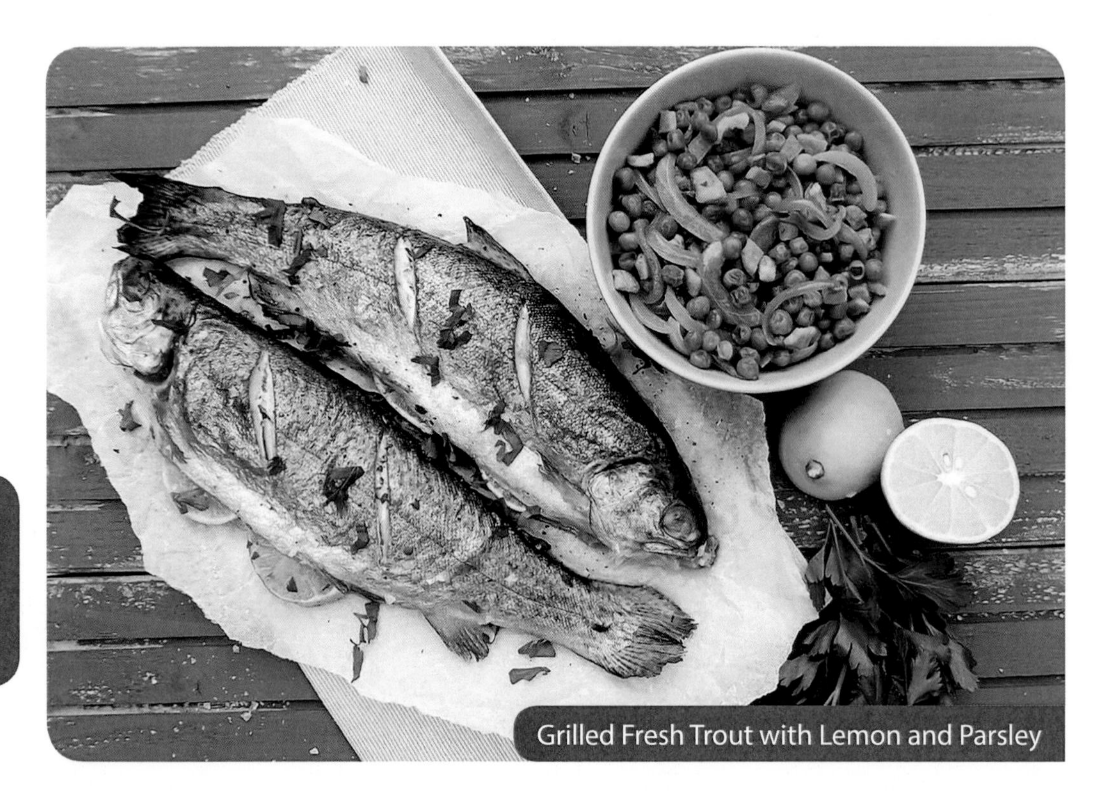
Grilled Fresh Trout with Lemon and Parsley

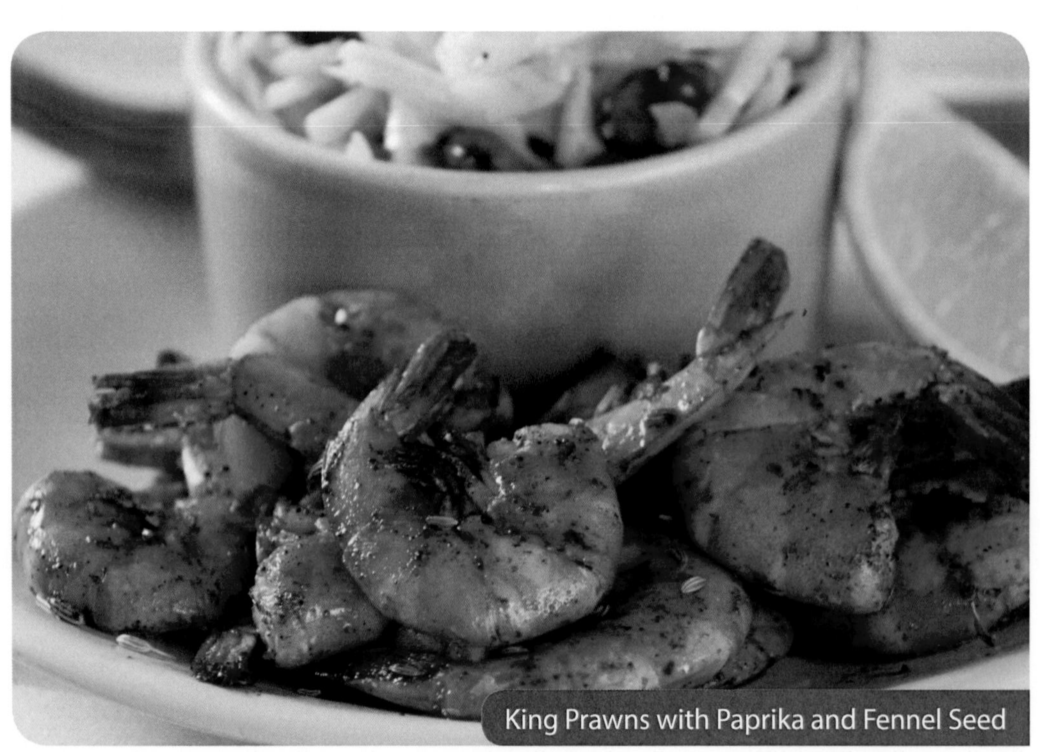
King Prawns with Paprika and Fennel Seed

KING PRAWNS WITH PAPRIKA AND FENNEL SEED

 *Servings: 2*

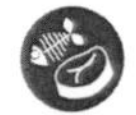 *Preparation Time: 5 minutes*

 *Cooking Time: 10 minutes*

 *Total Time: 15 minutes*

Ingredients

16 shell on king prawns

1 tbsp paprika

1 lemon, juice only

2 tbsp lard, dripping or goose fat

1 tsp fennel seed

Sea salt

Preparation

1. Heat the fat in a frying pan and add the prawns.
2. Toss for a few minutes until they turn pink and opaque.
3. Add the spices and salt.
4. Cook for a further few minutes and squeeze over the lemon juice to serve.
5. Serve with a side dish of Simple Raw Slaw.

LEMON AND GARLIC SCALLOPS

 *Servings: 2*

 *Preparation Time: 10 minutes*

 *Cooking Time: 5 minutes*

 *Total Time: 15 minutes*

Ingredients

400g scallops, white only

1 garlic clove, crushed

1 tbsp fresh parsley, chopped

1 pinch freshly-ground black pepper

1 tbsp lard, dripping or goose fat

1 tbsp lemon juice

1 pinch sea salt

Preparation

1. Heat a pan over a high heat and add the fat.
2. Add the scallops and sear for a minute on each side. They need to be cooked through, but can overcook very easily. The scallops will be slightly firm to the touch, and opaque when done.
3. Turn off the heat, add the garlic, parsley and lemon then season with salt and pepper.
4. Serve the scallops whilst hot with a side dish of Green Beans and Lemon.

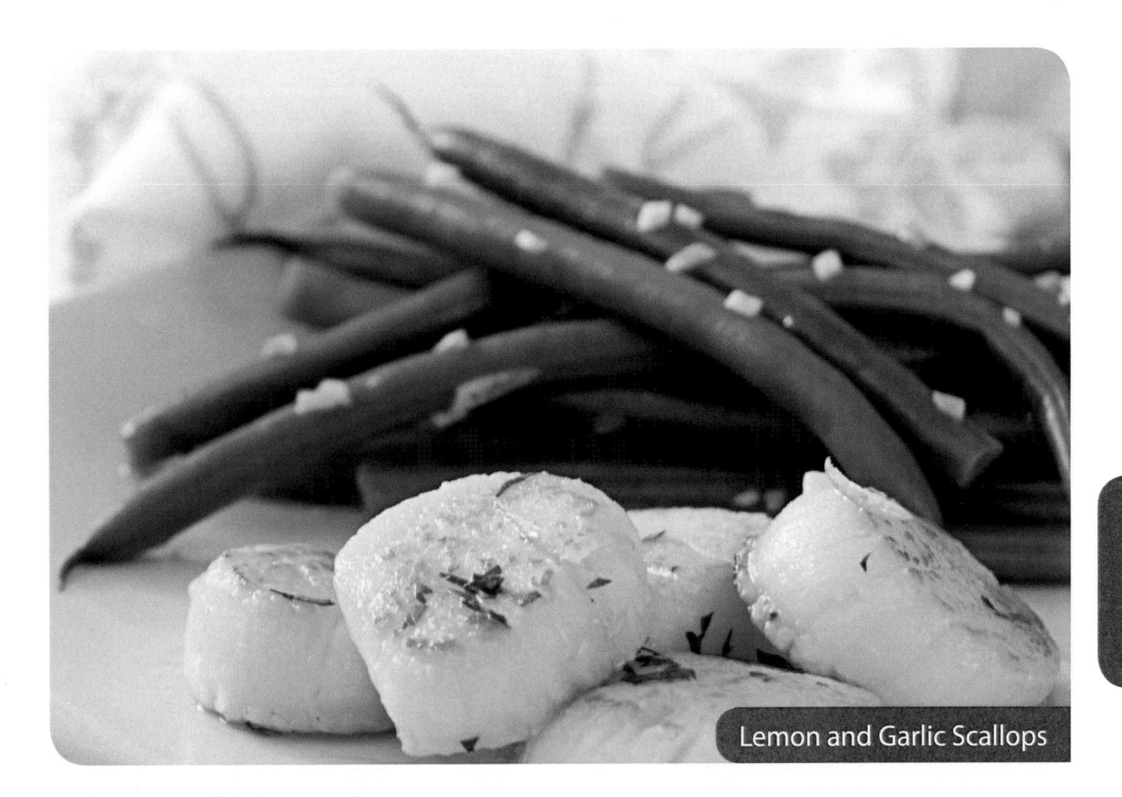
Lemon and Garlic Scallops

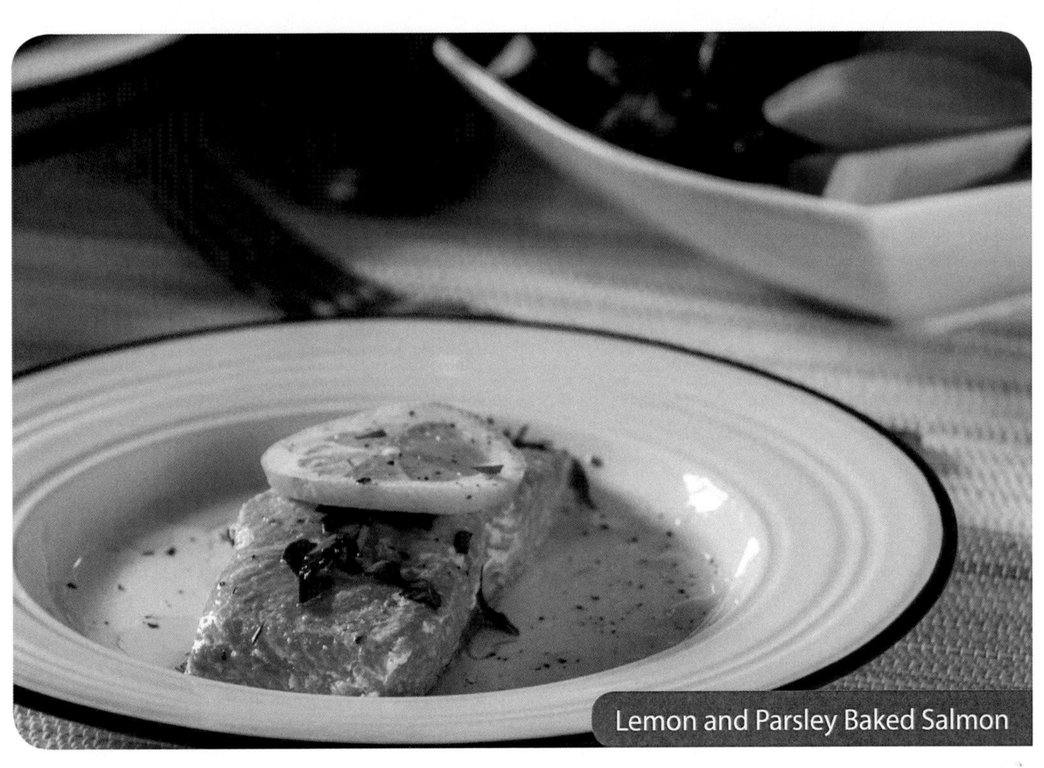
Lemon and Parsley Baked Salmon

LEMON AND PARSLEY BAKED SALMON

 *Servings: 2*

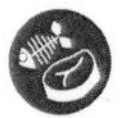 *Preparation Time: 10 minutes*

 *Cooking Time: 20 minutes*

 *Total Time: 30 minutes*

Ingredients

2 salmon fillets

2 lemons, juice and zest

Sea salt

Freshly ground black pepper

4 tbsp parsley

1 tbsp olive oil

1 tsp paprika

Preparation

1. Preheat the oven to 180C.
2. Place the salmon fillets in a baking dish and top with parsley, garlic and lemon zest.
3. Drizzle with oil and lemon juice, season with salt, pepper and paprika.
4. Bake in the oven for roughly 20 minutes.
5. Serve hot with Pan Steamed Broccoli and Pan Steamed Carrots.

MARINATED TUNA STEAKS

 *Servings: 2*

 *Preparation Time: 15 minutes*

 *Cooking Time: 5 minutes*

 *Inactive Time: 1 hour*

 *Total Time: 1 hour, 20 minutes*

Ingredients

2 tuna steaks

1 tbsp olive oil

FOR THE MARINADE

2 tbsp vinegar (white wine vinegar works well)

2 tbsp water

2 red chillies, chopped

2 garlic cloves, finely chopped

1 bay leaf

Sea salt

Freshly ground black pepper

Preparation

1. Mix all of the ingredients for the marinade and pour over the tuna steaks.
2. Cover and set aside for an hour (or a minimum of 20 minutes if pushed for time).
3. Heat the oil in a frying pan to a high heat.
4. Cook the tuna steaks. For a rare steak a minute either side will suffice. Be careful not to overcook as tuna gets dry and tough very quickly.
5. Serve hot with a side dish of Avocado, Red Onion and Green Pepper Salsa.

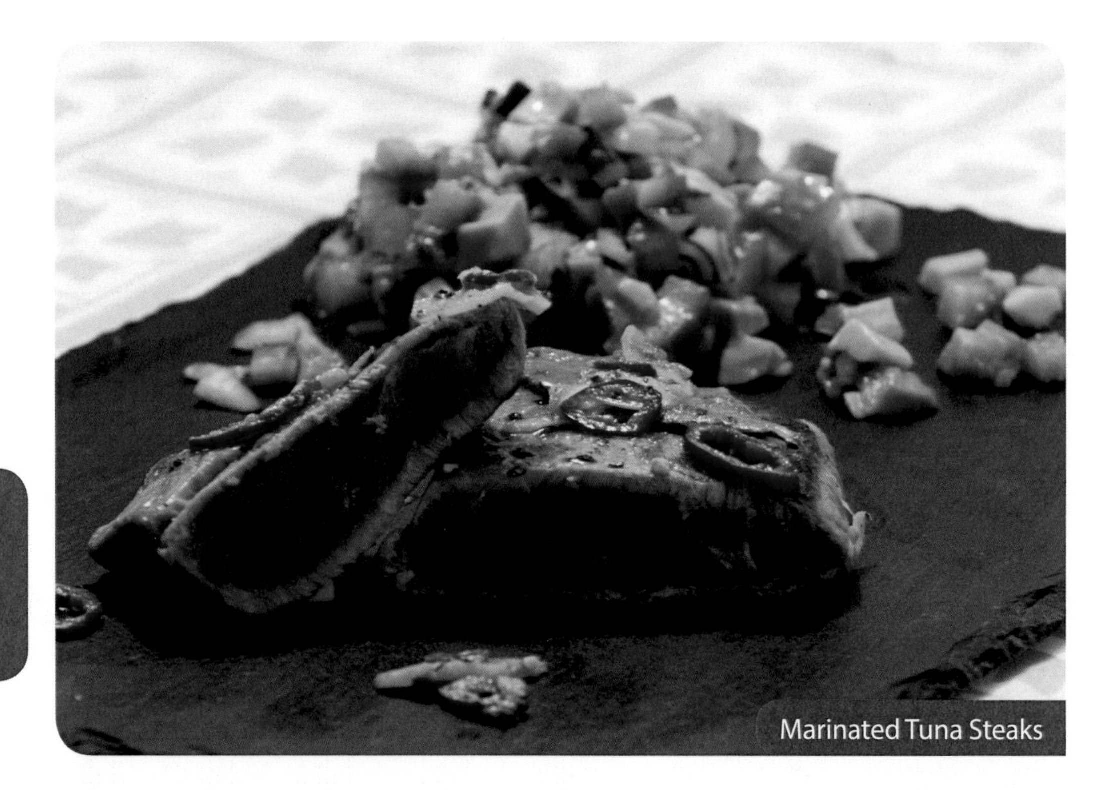
Marinated Tuna Steaks

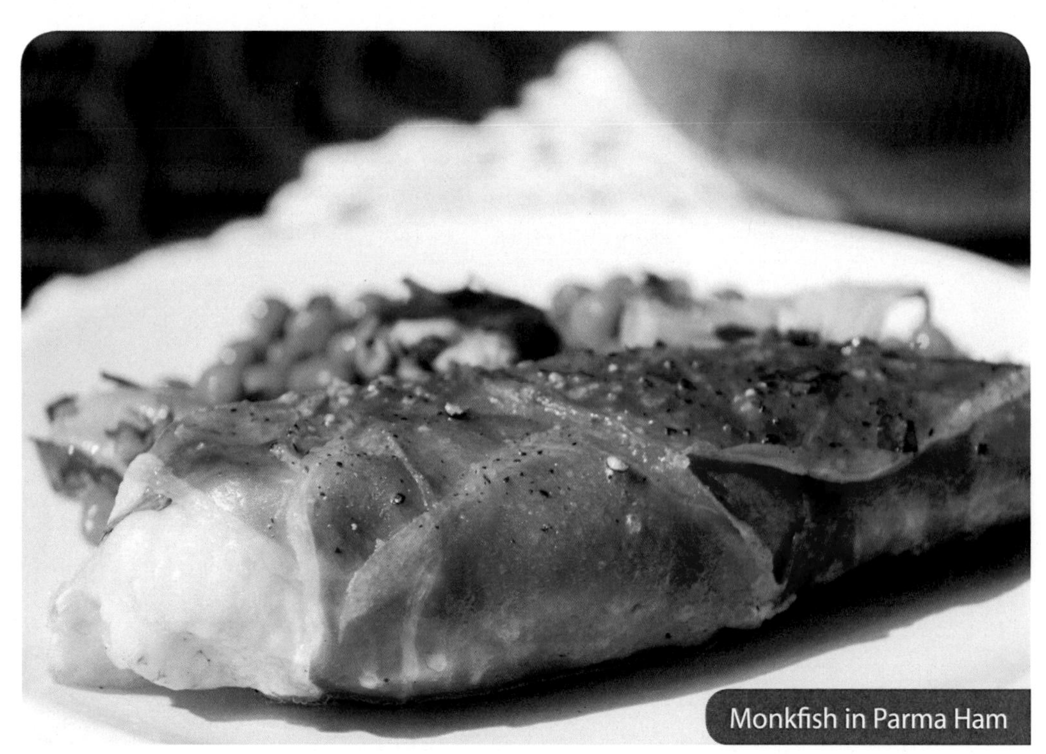
Monkfish in Parma Ham

MONKFISH IN PARMA HAM

 *Servings: 2*

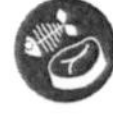 *Preparation Time: 10 minutes*

 *Cooking Time: 20 minutes*

 *Total Time: 30 minutes*

Ingredients

2 monkfish fillets

2 slices parma ham

1 tbsp lard, dripping or goose fat

1 tbsp water

Freshly ground black pepper

Preparation

1. Preheat the oven to 200C.
2. Wrap the parma ham around the monkfish. You may need to secure with a toothpick.
3. Place the monkfish in an oven proof dish with a tbsp of water.
4. Add the fat or oil to the dish, season with black pepper.
5. Roast for about 20 minutes or until the monkfish is cooked through.
6. Serve with a side dish of Peas with Artichokes.

PRAWN CURRY

 *Servings: 2*

 *Preparation Time: 10 minutes*

 *Cooking Time: 30 minutes*

 *Total Time: 40 minutes*

Ingredients

400g king prawns, shelled and deveined
1 onion, coarsely chopped
2 garlic cloves, crushed
2 tbsp tomato puree
1 pinch sea salt
2 tbsp coconut oil
1 tbsp fresh ginger, grated
1 tbsp Madras curry powder or paste
200ml coconut milk
1 tbsp fresh coriander, chopped

Preparation

1. Prepare the onion, ginger, garlic and prawns.
2. Heat the oil in a pan. Add the onion and cook over medium heat.
3. Stir occasionally, until softened and just beginning to brown.
4. Reduce the heat, add the ginger, garlic, curry powder, and tomato puree.
5. Stir for about 2 minutes.
6. Then add the coconut milk and simmer until thickened; about 10 minutes.
7. Throw in the prawns and season with salt. Remove from the heat and cover.
8. After 5 minutes the prawns will have cooked through.
9. Add the coriander and add seasoning to taste.
10. Serve hot with Cauliflower Rice.

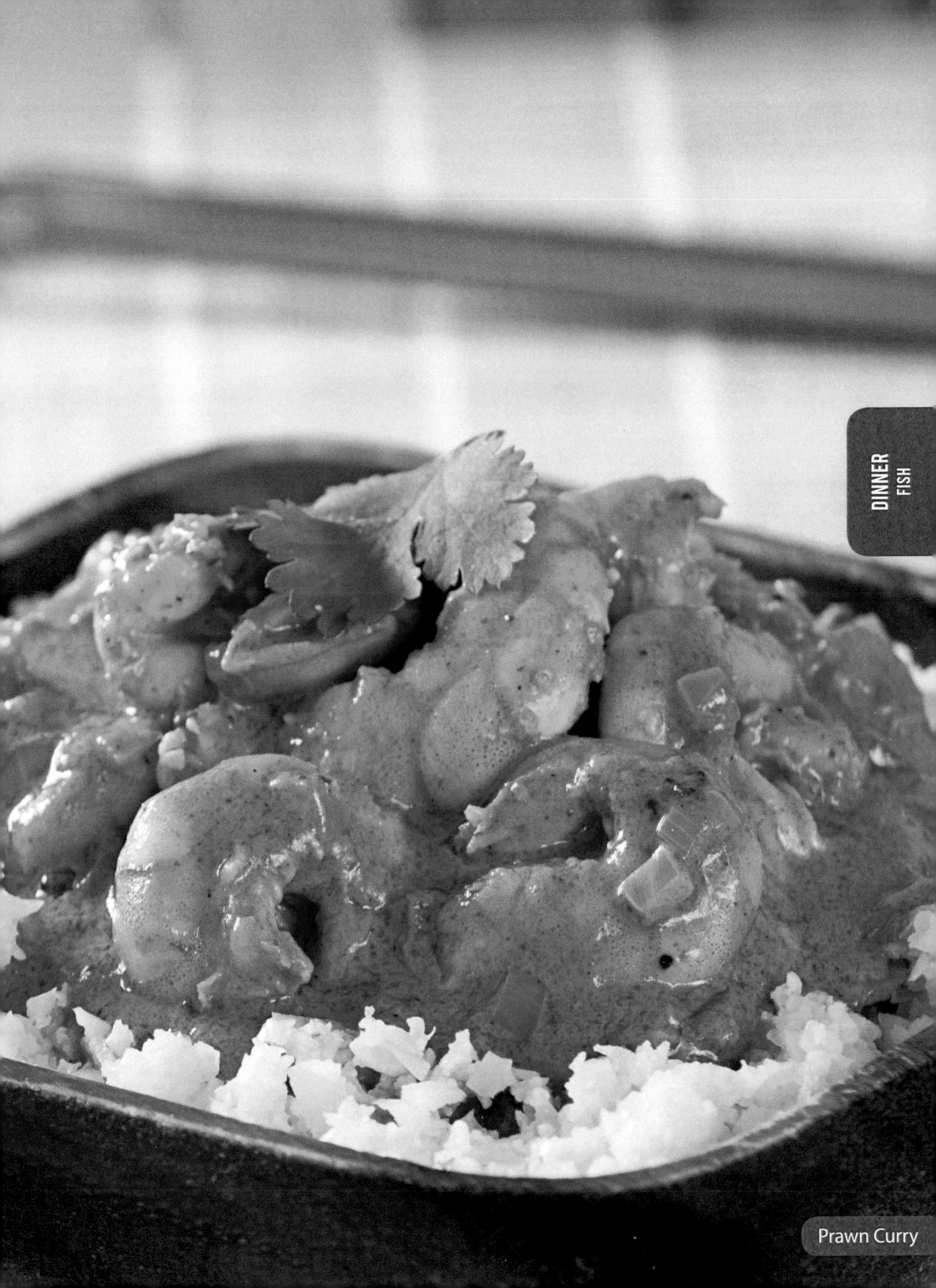

Prawn Curry

SALMON WITH AVOCADO SALSA

When you are cooking the salmon fillets, as a general rule a 1 inch deep fillet will take about 8-10 minutes. If you give the sides a squeeze, the flakes will separate easily and be opaque all the way through. If the outsides are cooking more quickly than you want them to, add a splash of water to create steam or transfer to a hot oven for 10 minutes to finish off.

 *Servings: 2*

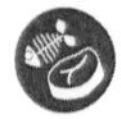 *Preparation Time: 20 minutes*

 *Cooking Time: 20 minutes*

 *Total Time: 40 minutes*

Ingredients

2 wild salmon fillets

1 tbsp lard, dripping or goose fat

FOR THE SALSA

2 ripe avocados, cut into 1inch chunks

1 lime, juice only

½ garlic clove, crushed

1 pinch sea salt

1 tsp extra virgin olive oil

½ punnet cherry tomatoes, quartered

½ red onion, finely sliced

1 tbsp fresh coriander, chopped

1 pinch freshly ground black pepper

FOR THE BLACKENING SPICES

1 tbsp smoked paprika

½ tsp ground cumin

½ tsp oregano

1 tsp chilli powder

½ tsp sea salt

½ tsp garlic powder

Preparation

1. Prepare the avocado, onions, tomatoes and garlic.
2. Mix with the other ingredients for the salsa and set aside.
3. Mix all the blackening spices together and rub into the top side of the salmon fillets.

4 Heat the fat in a large frying pan over medium heat.

5 Add the salmon, spice side down.

6 Cook the salmon for as long as you can on this side without actually burning it. The spices will blacken which is fine. Just watch that the flesh itself does not catch.

7 Turn the salmon over and finish cooking on the other side.

8 Serve the hot salmon with the salsa and a Basic Side Salad.

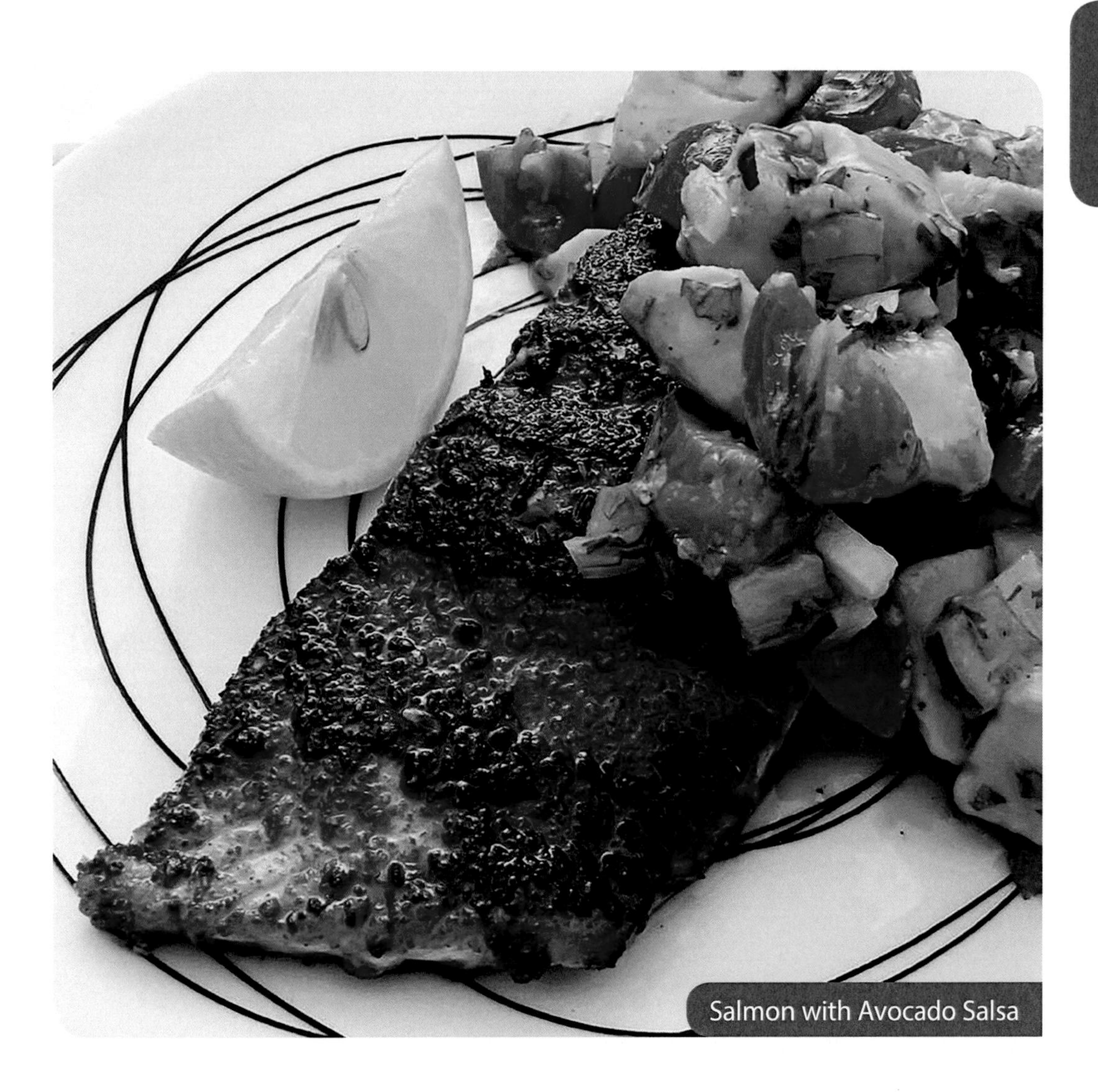

Salmon with Avocado Salsa

SALMON WITH TOMATO AND CAPER DRESSING

 *Servings: 2*

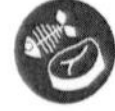 *Preparation Time: 10 minutes*

 *Cooking Time: 15 minutes*

 *Total Time: 25 minutes*

Ingredients

FOR THE SALMON

2 salmon fillets, skin on

1 pinch sea salt

1 tbsp coconut oil

1 squeeze lemon juice

FOR THE TOMATO DRESSING

1 small red onion, finely chopped

2 tbsp capers, finely chopped

2 tbsp fresh parsley, chopped

2 medium tomatoes, finely chopped

2 tbsp extra virgin olive oil

Preparation

1. Prepare the red onion, tomatoes and capers and place into a bowl.
2. Add the olive oil and parsley to the dressing ingredients and mix well.
3. Heat the coconut oil in a frying pan and place the salmon, skin down, into the pan.
4. Cook for about 8 minutes and then turn over and cook for a further 2 minutes.
5. The salmon is cooked when you can squeeze the side of the fish and it flakes apart easily.
6. Top the salmon with the dressing and serve with a side dish of Green Beans with Lemon.

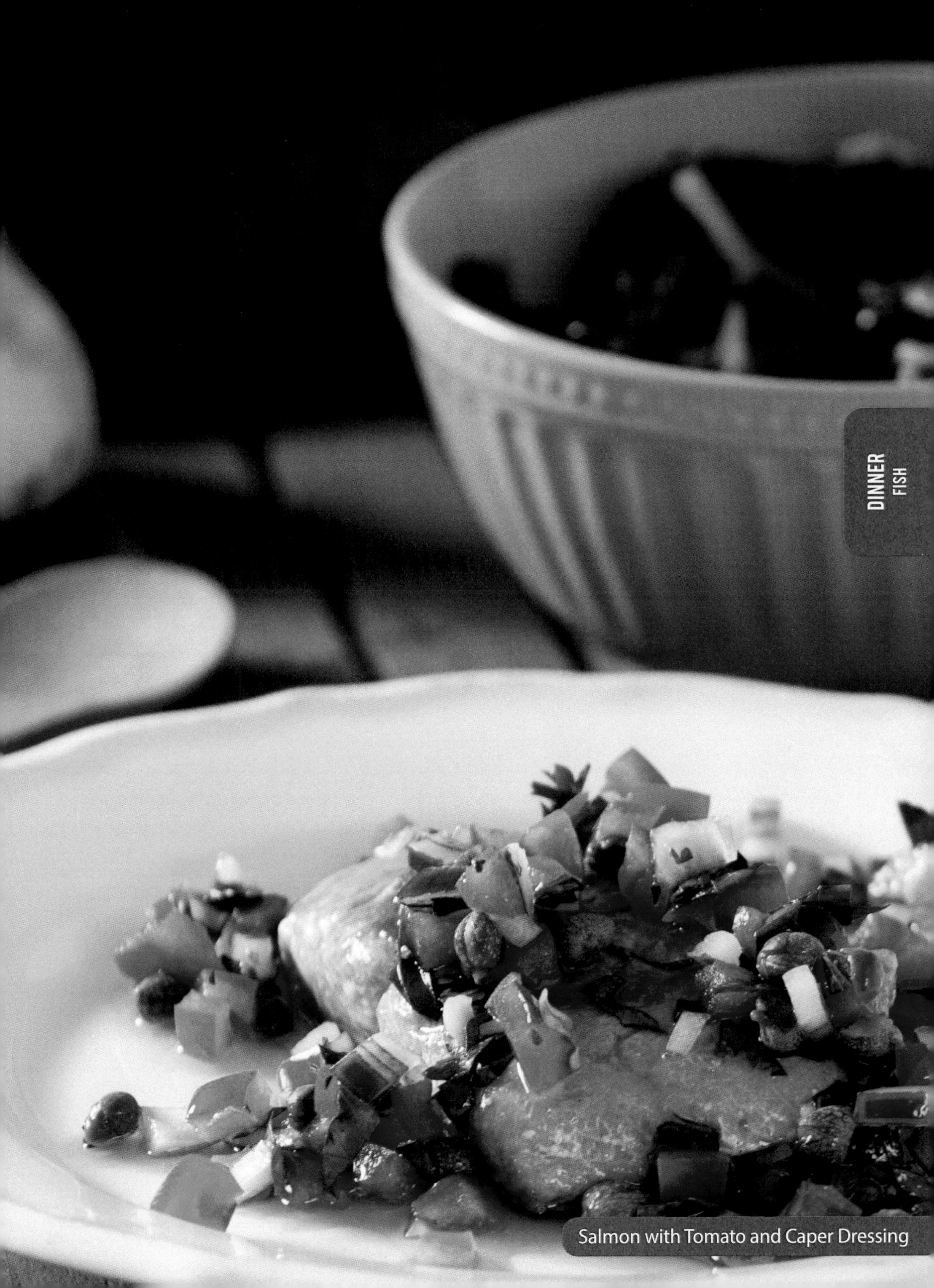

Salmon with Tomato and Caper Dressing

WHITE WINE AND GARLIC MUSSELS

Mussels are a delicious shellfish and take just moments to cook, however they do require some preparation/cleaning prior to use. The 'beards' need to be taken off and the shells should be given a quick scrub under cold running water to ensure they are clean. Ask you local fishmonger to help you with this if you can.

Also important with mussels is freshness. If a mussel is open before cooking, tap it lightly on a hard surface. If it closes it is fine, if not discard. Once cooked, it is the closed mussels you need to be wary of. Any which remain closed after cooking should also be discarded. There will always be one or two in a batch which need discarding so don't be concerned if you do find the odd one.

 *Servings: 2*

 *Preparation Time: 20 minutes*

 *Cooking Time: 15 minutes*

 *Total Time: 35 minutes*

Ingredients

1kg fresh mussels

200ml white wine

1 onion, chopped

3 garlic cloves, finely chopped

2 tbsp parsley, chopped

Preparation

1. To prepare the mussels, wash and remove the beards.
2. Make sure you discard any of the opened mussels prior to cooking.
3. In a saucepan, combine the wine, onions and garlic.
4. Bring to a boil and simmer for about 5 minutes.
5. Add the mussels to the saucepan, cover and increase the heat to medium-high.
6. As soon as all the mussels have opened add the herbs.
7. Remove from the heat and ladle into bowls.

8

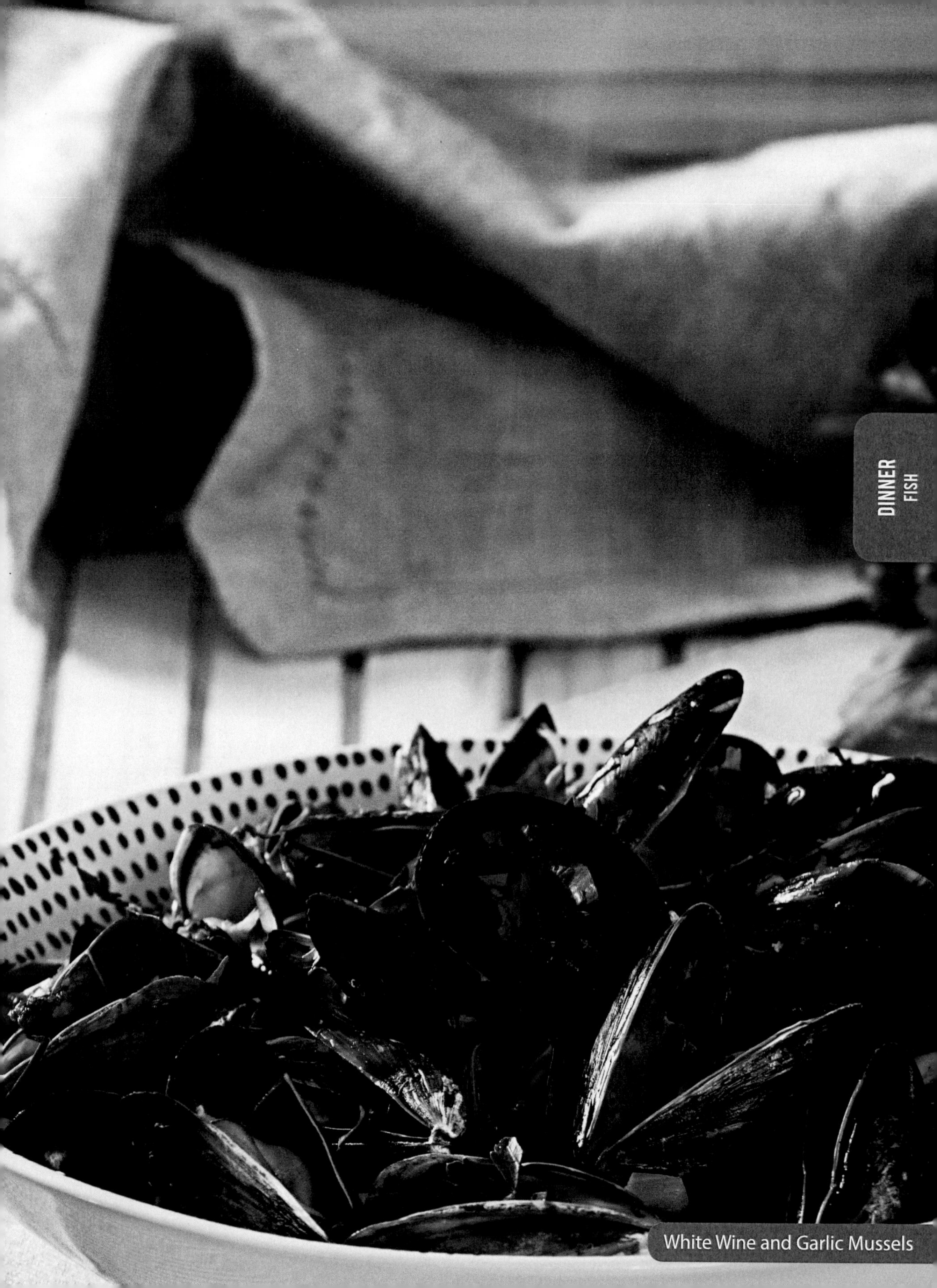

White Wine and Garlic Mussels

SOLE WITH LEMON AND THYME

 *Servings: 2*

 *Preparation Time: 10 minutes*

 *Cooking Time: 10 minutes*

 *Total Time: 20 minutes*

Ingredients

2 sole fillets

2 sprigs thyme

1 squeeze lemon juice

1 tbsp lard, dripping or goose fat

Sea salt

Preparation

1. Heat the fat in a frying pan and lay in the fish fillets.
2. Sprinkle with salt and add the thyme sprigs.
3. Cook for 2 minutes on either side.
4. Remove from the pan and squeeze over lemon to taste.
5. Serve with Pan Steamed Broccoli and Pan Steamed Carrots.

SIDES

If any of you think that vegetables are boring and tasteless then you are in for a surprise. We have prepared over 50 salad, vegetable, dressing and dip recipes for you to use. They are quick and easy to prepare and add a great variety of tastes to any meal.

We will be giving you suggestions in the weekly meal plans of which sides to use with each meal but you can swap these around if you wish. We would encourage you to try all of these recipes – you will see vegetables in a whole new light!

You will also find useful recipes for Chicken stock and Basic Tomato Sauce in this section. Both are tasty and easy to prepare and are included in lots of the recipes.

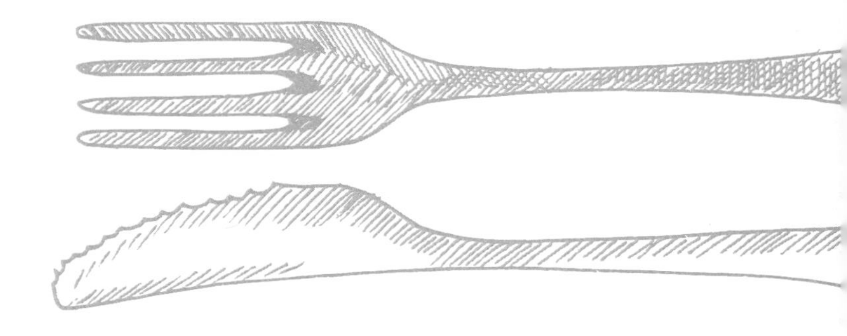

DRESSINGS & DIPS

ASIAN DRESSING

 *Servings: 2*

 *Preparation Time: 10 minutes*

Ingredients

2 limes, juice only

1 red chilli, finely sliced

1 tbsp sesame oil

1 tbsp fresh mint, chopped

Preparation

1. Mix all the ingredients together in a bowl. A good way to do this is to pop the ingredients into a clean jar, screw on the top and shake vigorously.

AVOCADO, RED ONION AND GREEN PEPPER SALSA

 *Servings: 2*

 *Preparation Time: 10 minutes*

Ingredients

½ green pepper, finely chopped

2 avocado, sliced into small cubes

Sea salt

½ red onion, sliced thin

2 tbsp olive oil

Freshly ground black pepper

Preparation

1. Prepare the pepper, onion and avocado.
2. Place ingredients into a bowl, season to taste and drizzle with good olive oil.

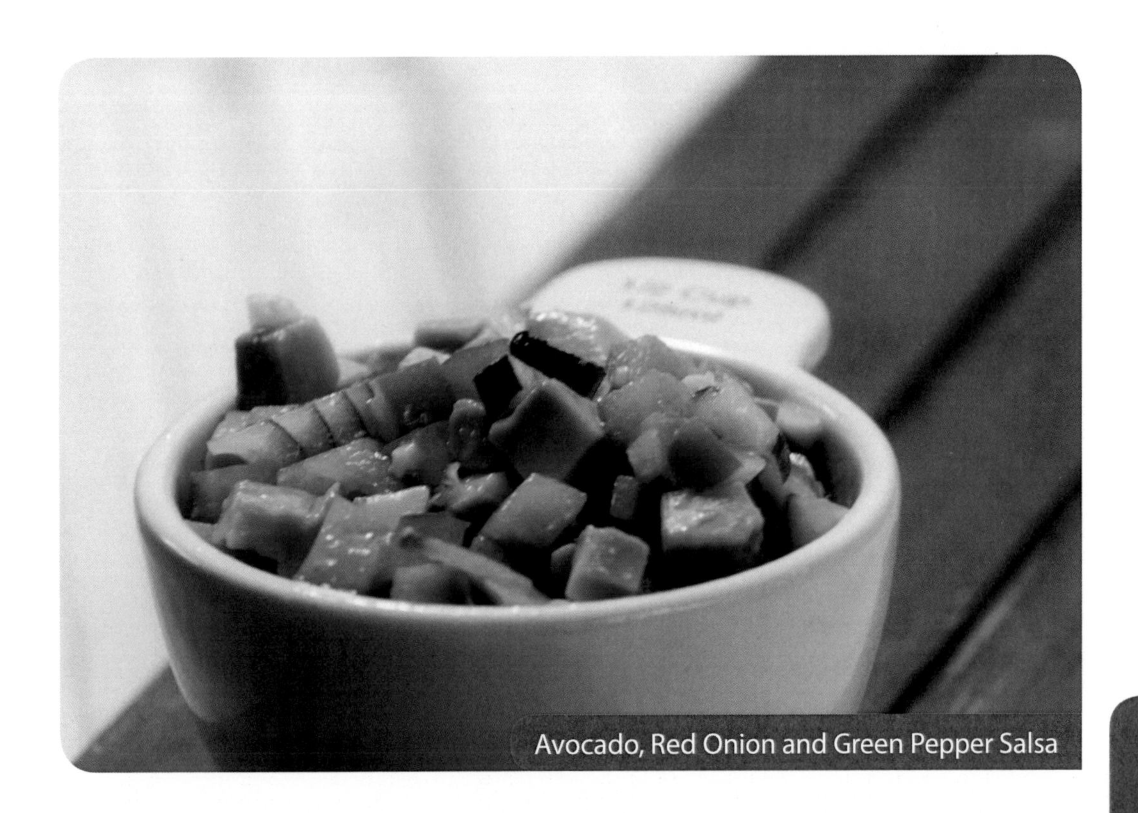
Avocado, Red Onion and Green Pepper Salsa

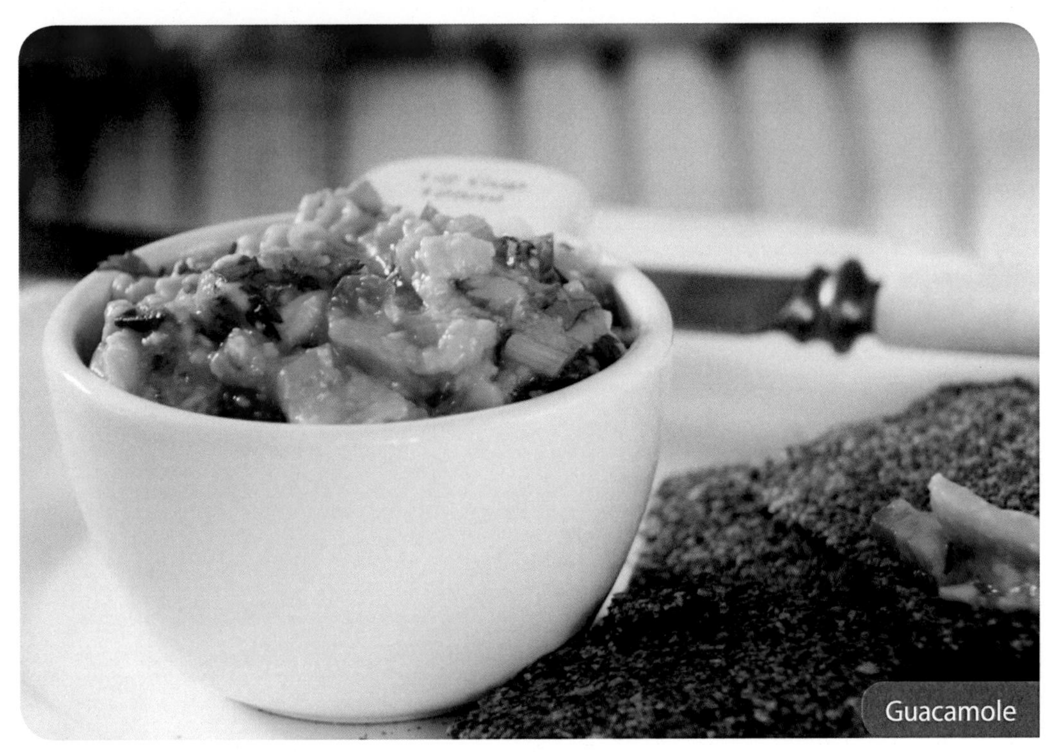
Guacamole

GUACAMOLE

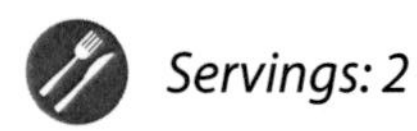 *Servings: 2*

 *Preparation Time: 10 minutes*

Ingredients

2 ripe avocado

2 spring onions, finely chopped

2 tbsp lime juice

1 red chilli, finely chopped

1 tomato, finely diced and deseeded

2 tbsp fresh coriander, chopped

2 tbsp extra virgin olive oil

1 pinch sea salt

Preparation

1 Mash the guacamole ingredients together to form a coarse, chunky dip.

2 Eat immediately to prevent browning.

FIERY AUBERGINE DIP

 *Servings: 2*

 *Preparation Time: 10 minutes*

 *Cooking Time: 30 minutes*

 *Total Time: 40 minutes*

Ingredients

1 aubergine, chopped to 1 inch slices
1 pinch flaked sea salt
1 tbsp harissa paste
1 tbsp fresh parsley, chopped
4 tbsp olive oil
Freshly ground black pepper
1 tbsp fresh mint, chopped

Preparation

1. Prepare the aubergine and chop the herbs.
2. Heat the oil in a large frying pan over a medium low heat.
3. Fry the aubergine slices until golden brown on the outside and soft through the middle; use more oil if needed.
4. Drain the slices on kitchen paper and leave to cool slightly.
5. Once cooled, remove the skin and mash with the harissa and herbs until smooth.
6. Season to taste and serve at room temperature.

MAYONNAISE

This can be made by hand or in a food mixer if you have one available.

 *Servings: 4*

 *Preparation Time: 20 minutes*

Ingredients

1 egg yolk

½ tsp Dijon mustard

½ tbsp white wine vinegar

150ml groundnut or extra virgin olive oil

1 pinch salt

Preparation

1. In a bowl, beat the yolk with the salt, mustard and the vinegar.
2. Beating continuously, drizzle the oil into the bowl very slowly until you have used almost all the oil.
3. Taste and decide if you want it to be sharper or not. If so, add a little vinegar. If not, then continue with oil or stop if you are happy with it.
4. Season with salt and pepper.
5. Please note that oil will make the mayonnaise thicker and vinegar will thin it down.

MUSTARD VINAIGRETTE

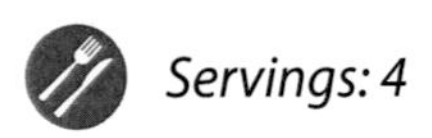
Servings: 4

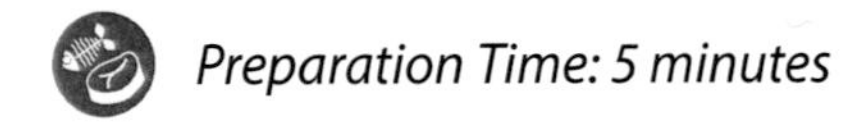
Preparation Time: 5 minutes

Ingredients

4 tbsp extra virgin olive oil

1 tbsp balsamic vinegar

1 tbsp Dijon mustard

1 pinch sea salt

1 pinch fresh ground black pepper

Preparation

1. Mix all of the ingredients together. We recommend using a clean, empty jar with a secure lid. Shake well and serve.

SALADS

APPLE SALAD

This recipe can be bulked out by adding to a bag of mixed salad leaves for a great lunch. We would recommend keeping the nuts separate until ready to eat though to prevent from going soft.

 *Servings: 2*

 *Preparation Time: 10 minutes*

Ingredients

3 apples, cored and chopped

2 oranges, chopped segments and juice

25g pecan halves

25g walnut pieces

Preparation324

1. Segment the oranges, ensuring any juice is also kept from the leftovers. Slice the apples, pecans and walnuts.
2. Mix together well and eat.

AVOCADO AND APPLE SALAD

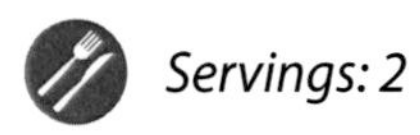 *Servings: 2*

 *Preparation Time: 15 minutes*

Ingredients

1 bag mixed leaves

4 spring onion, chopped

2 avocado, chopped

2 green apples, cored and chopped

2 tbsp fresh parsley, chopped

FOR THE DRESSING

2 tbsp walnut oil

1 lemon, juice only

Sea salt

Preparation

1. Prepare and chop the salad ingredients
2. Toss all of the salad ingredients together in a bowl.
3. Mix the ingredients for the dressing together and drizzle over the salad.
4. Season to taste.

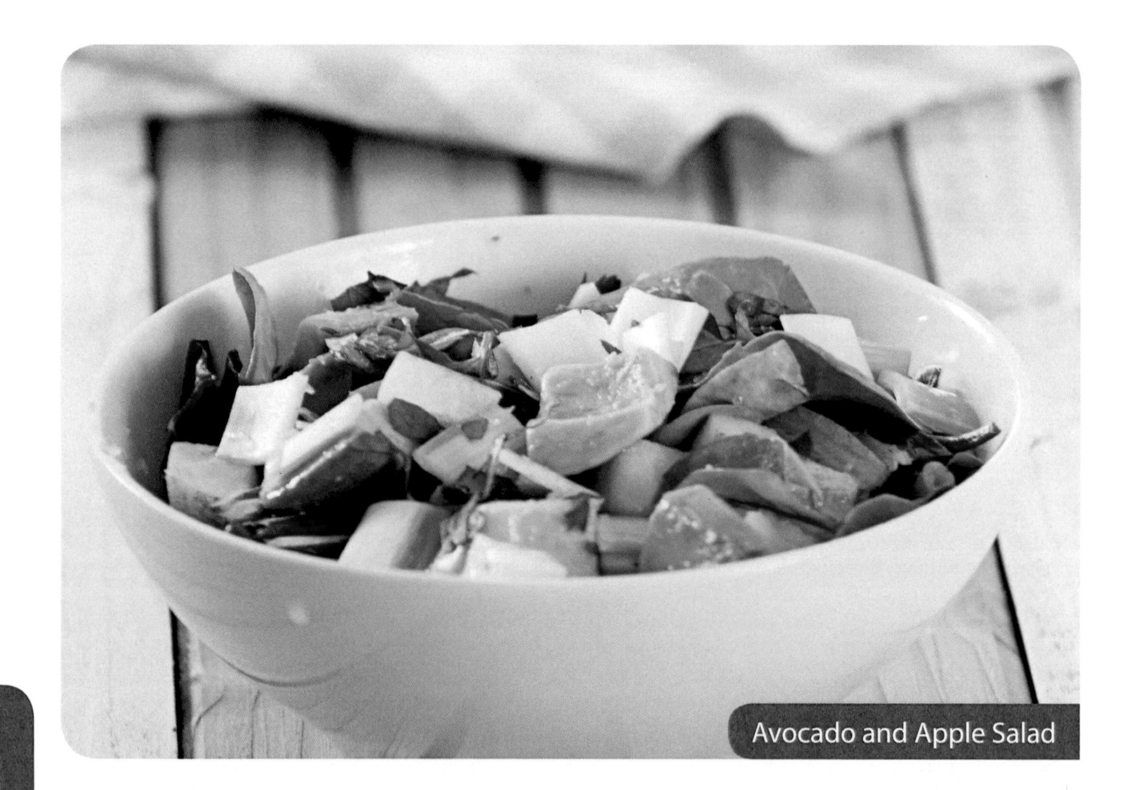
Avocado and Apple Salad

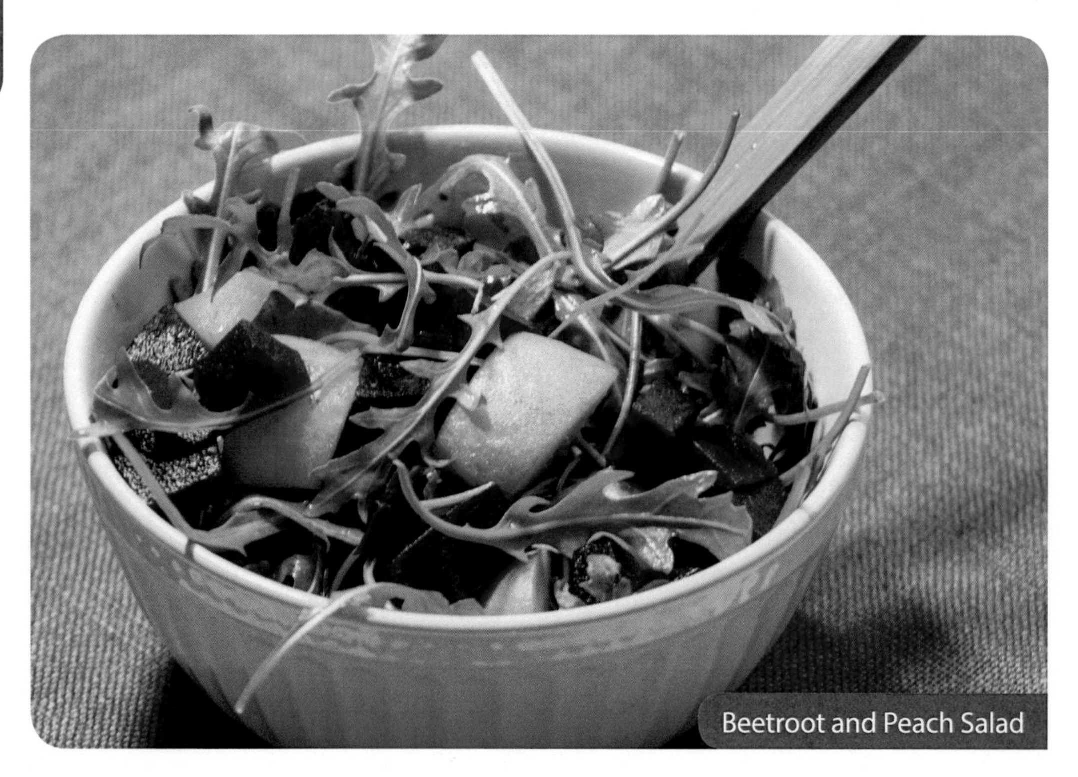
Beetroot and Peach Salad

BEETROOT AND PEACH SALAD

Servings: 2

Preparation Time: 10 minutes

Cooking Time: 50 minutes

Inactive Time: 20 minutes

Total Time: 1 hour, 20 minutes

Ingredients

100g raw beetroot

2 peaches, chopped

1 bag rocket

FOR THE DRESSING

1 tbsp good quality balsamic vinegar

1 tbsp extra virgin olive oil

1 pinch sea salt

1 pinch freshly ground black pepper

SIDES
SALADS

Preparation

1. Preheat the oven to 200C.
2. Top and tail the beetroot and place on a lined baking tray.
3. Place in the oven for 40 – 50 minutes or until the flesh is tender.
4. Once soft and tender remove from the oven and allow to cool.
5. Remove the skin and chop into pieces.
6. Place the beetroot into a bowl with the rocket and add the chopped peaches.
7. Mix the dressing together and toss with the rocket, beetroot and peaches.
8. Season to taste and serve immediately.

BASIC SIDE SALAD

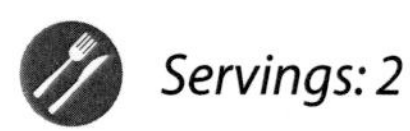
Servings: 2

Preparation Time: 10 minutes

Ingredients

½ bag salad leaf

½ cucumber, diced

1 apple, cored and diced

10 cherry tomatoes, halved

1 carrot, grated

1 red onion, diced

FOR THE DRESSING

1 tbsp extra virgin olive oil

1 pinch sea salt

1 tbsp balsamic vinegar

1 pinch freshly ground black pepper

Preparation

SIDES
SALADS

1. Prepare all the salad vegetables and place into a bowl.
2. Mix together the ingredients for the dressing and season to taste.
3. Pour the dressing over the salad, mix thoroughly and enjoy.

CARROT AND CORIANDER SALAD

 *Servings: 2*

 *Preparation Time: 10 minutes*

 *Standing Time: 10 minutes*

 *Total Time: 20 minutes*

Ingredients

2 large carrots, grated
1 tbsp fresh coriander, chopped
2 tbsp raisins
1 red onion, sliced thinly
2 tbsp white wine vinegar
Sea salt

Preparation

1. Prepare the carrots, onion and coriander and place in a bowl.
2. Add the remainder of the ingredients (except the salt) and mix together well.
3. Season to taste.
4. Leave to stand for 10 minutes before serving to allow flavours to fully develop.

COLESLAW

We recommend making to order when needed as water from the vegetables can leach into the mayonnaise and make it runny if kept for over 24 hours.

 *Servings: 2*

 *Preparation Time: 20 minutes*

Ingredients

¼ white cabbage, shredded
1 carrot, grated or finely shredded
½ onion, finely shredded
4 tbsp Paleo Mayonnaise

Preparation

1. Prepare the cabbage, onion and carrot.
2. Toss all of the shredded vegetable together and then stir in the mayonnaise, ensuring a consistent covering.

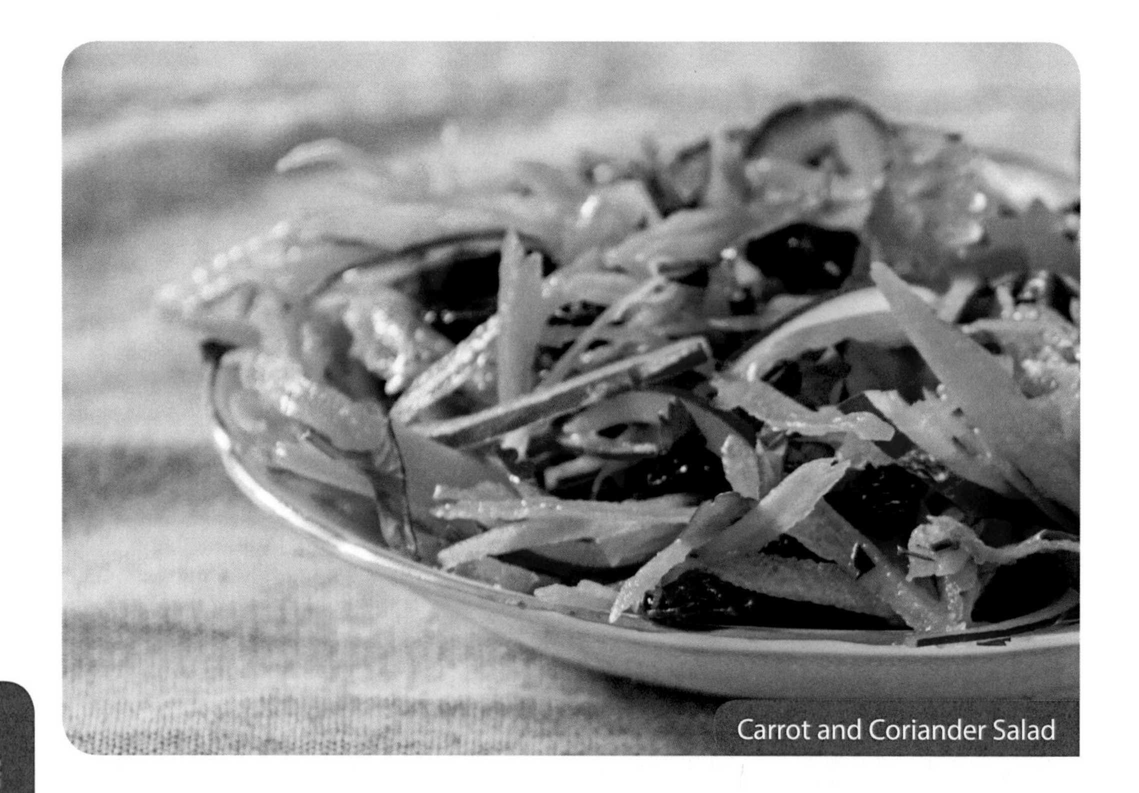
Carrot and Coriander Salad

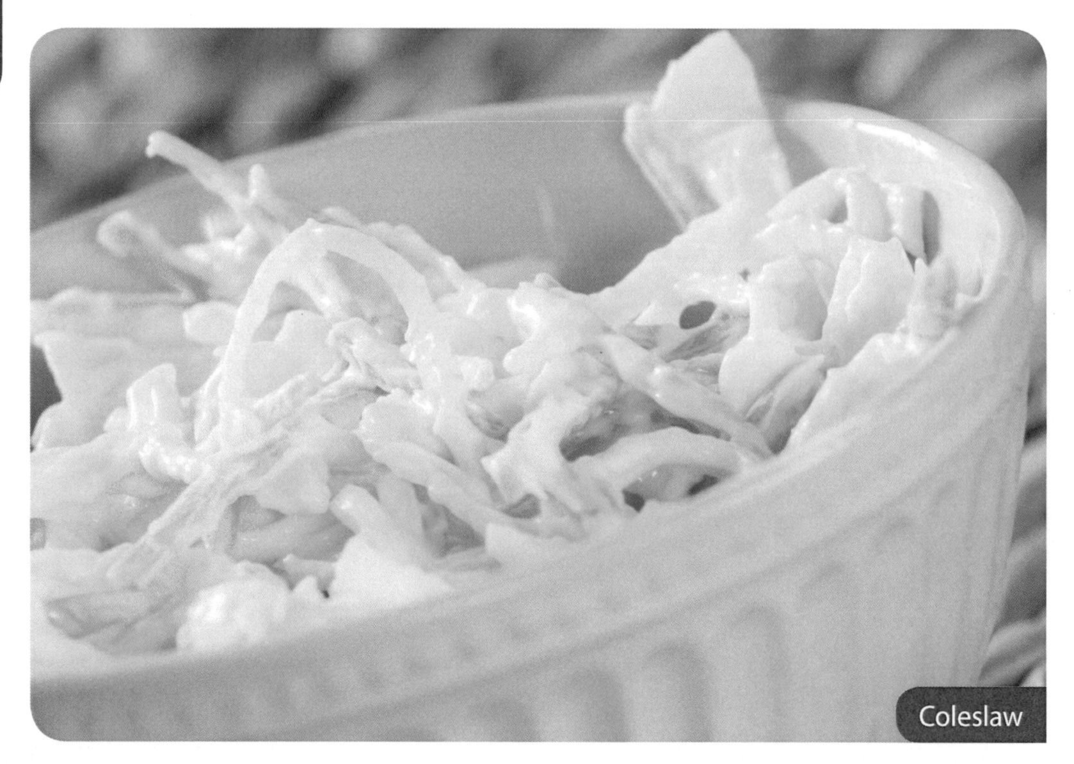
Coleslaw

FENNEL, ALMOND AND POMEGRANATE SALAD

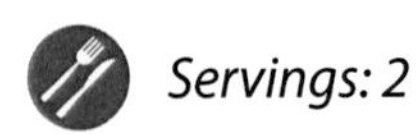

Servings: 2 *Preparation Time: 20 minutes*

Ingredients

1 bulb young fennel, finely shredded

1 pomegranate, seeds only

2 tbsp fresh mint, chopped

2 tbsp extra virgin olive oil

¼ white cabbage, finely shredded

20 whole almonds

½ lemon, juice only

Sea salt

Preparation

1. Prepare the fennel, cabbage and mint.
2. Place all of the ingredients into a bowl and mix together.
3. Season to taste.
4. Serve immediately as almonds go soft if left to stand amongst vegetables. If making for later in the day, keep the nuts separate and add when ready to eat.

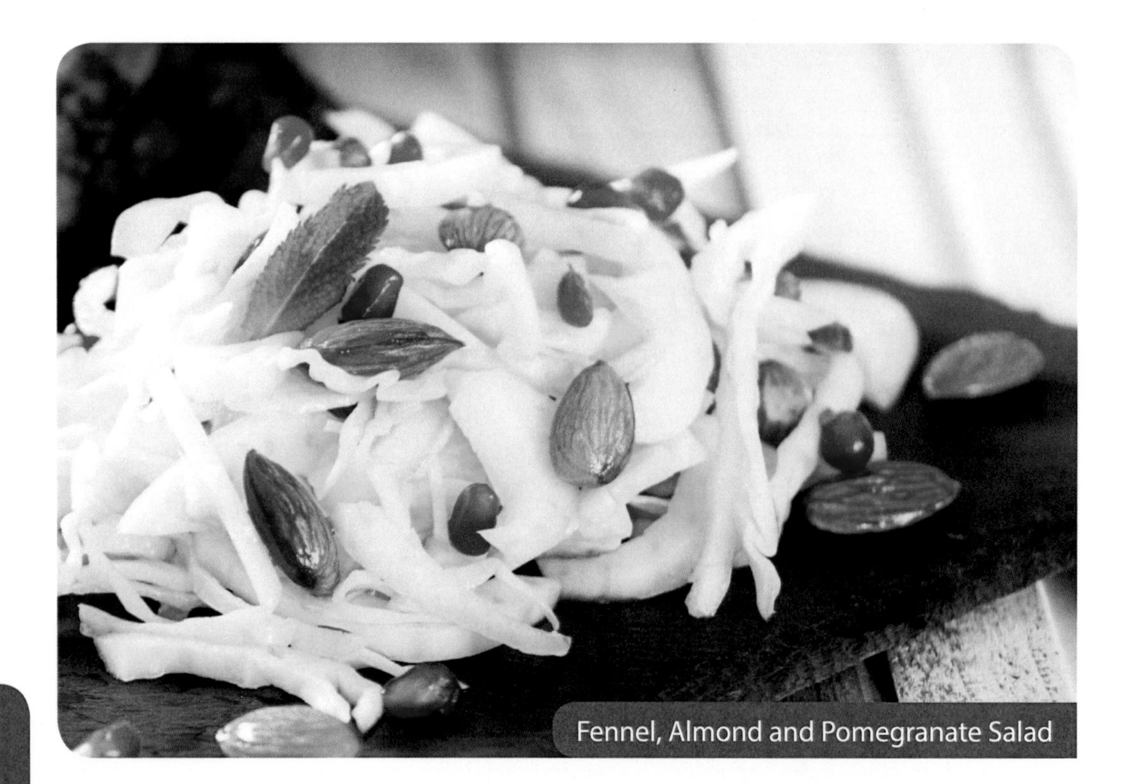
Fennel, Almond and Pomegranate Salad

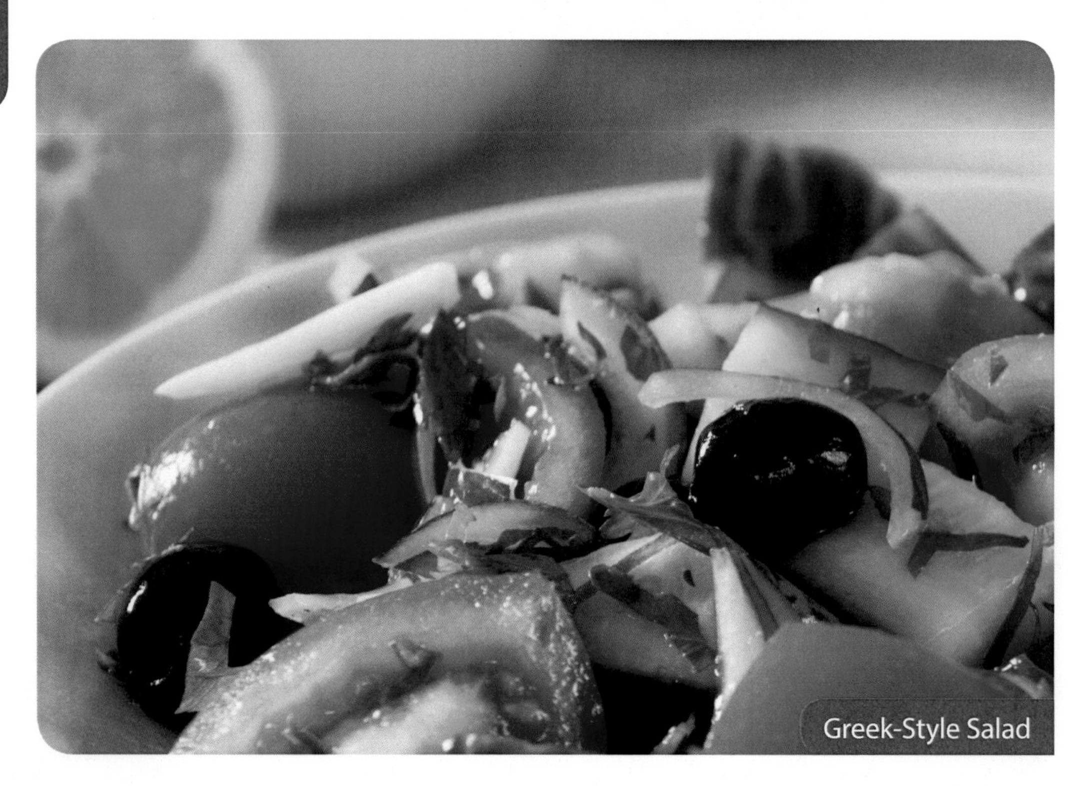
Greek-Style Salad

GREEK-STYLE SALAD

This salad will keep for several hours with the dressing on so makes an ideal packed lunch.

 *Servings: 2*

 *Preparation Time: 10 minutes*

Ingredients

½ cucumber, chopped

½ red onion, chopped

2 tbsp fresh parsley, chopped

1 large tomato, chopped

16 black olives

1 garlic clove, minced

FOR THE DRESSING

1 tbsp lemon juice

1 pinch sea salt

1 tbsp extra virgin olive oil

1 pinch freshly ground black pepper

Preparation

1. Prepare all the salad ingredients and place into a bowl and mix together.
2. Prepare the dressing and pour over the salad. Toss thoroughly to ensure all ingredients are coated with the dressing.
3. Season to taste.

MIDDLE EASTERN HERB SALAD

 *Servings: 2*

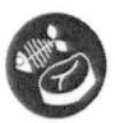 *Preparation Time: 10 minutes*

 *Standing Time: 30 minutes*

 *Total Time: 40 minutes*

Ingredients

1 large cucumber, finely diced

6 medium tomatoes, finely diced

1 bunch spring onion, very finely chopped

1 bunch parsley, finely chopped

1 bunch mint, finely chopped

FOR THE DRESSING

4 tbsp olive oil

1 lemon, juice only

Sea salt

Preparation

1. Prepare the cucumber, tomato, spring onion, parsley and mint and place in a bowl.
2. Mix together the dressing and toss with the salad.
3. Add seasoning to taste.
4. Leave to stand for 30 minutes before serving at room temperature.

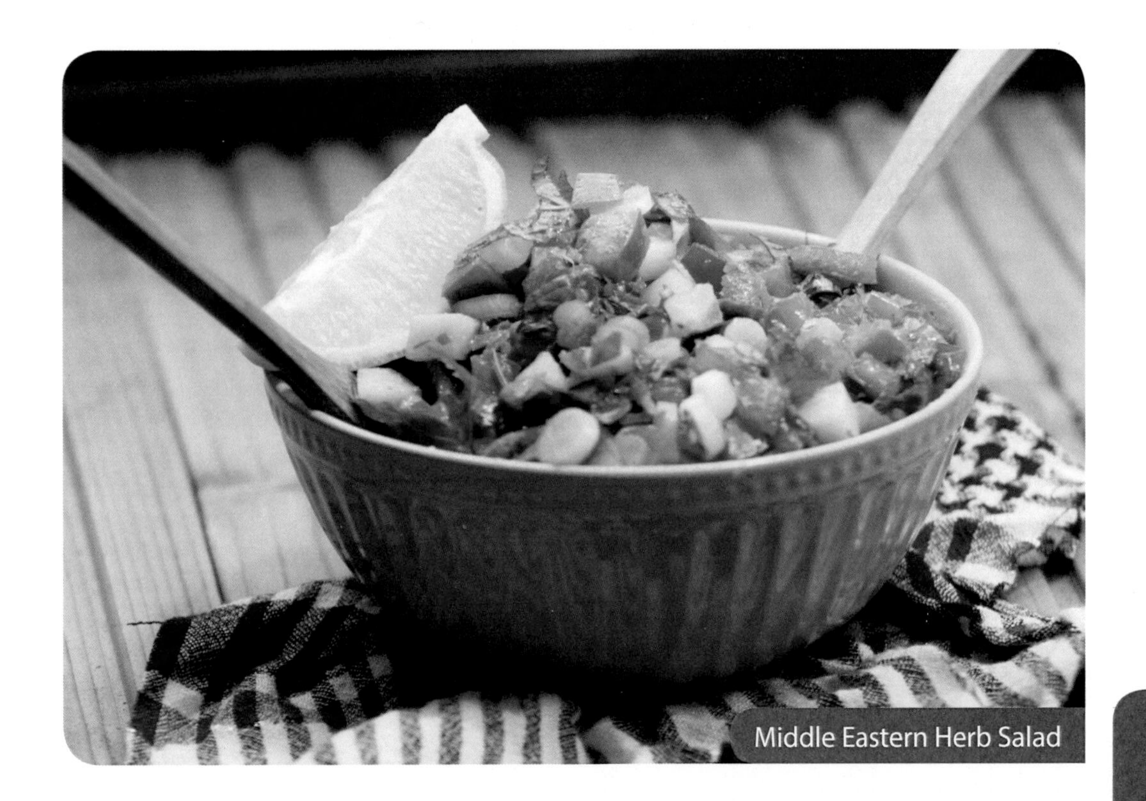

Middle Eastern Herb Salad

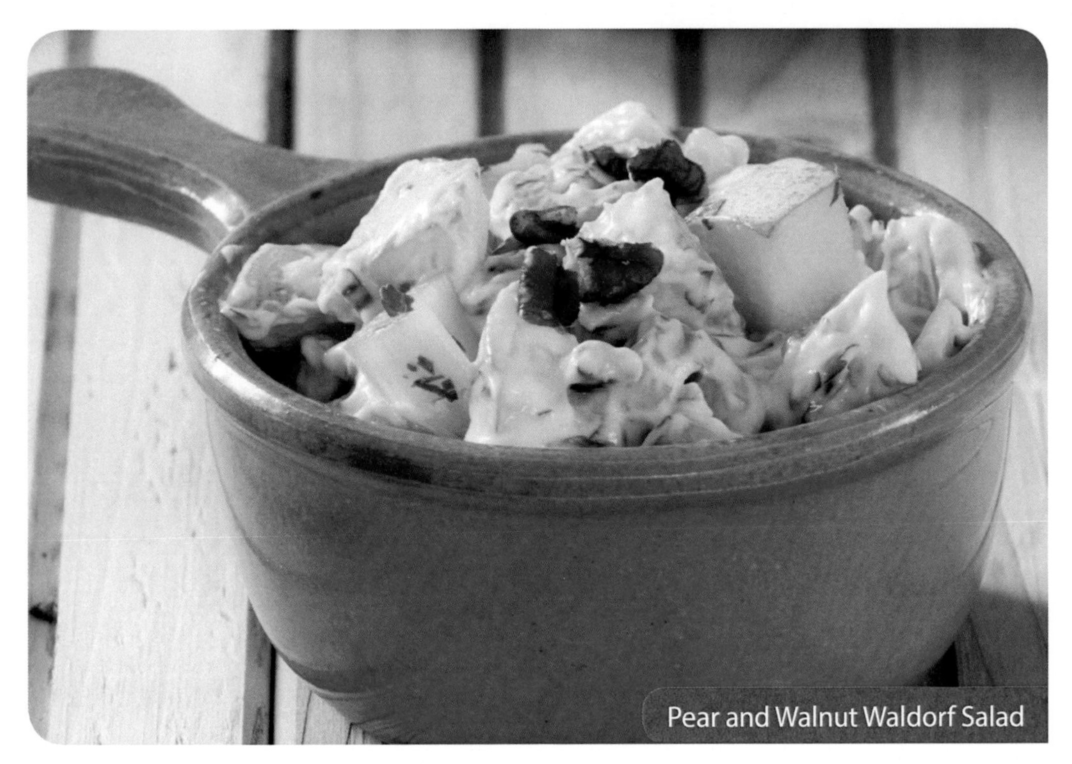

Pear and Walnut Waldorf Salad

PEAR AND WALNUT WALDORF SALAD

 *Servings: 2*

 *Preparation Time: 15 minutes*

Ingredients

3 sticks celery, chopped

8 walnuts, chopped

4 tbsp Paleo Mayonnaise

2 pears, chopped

2 tbsp fresh parsley, chopped

Preparation

1. Prepare the celery, pears, walnuts and parsley.
2. Place into a bowl and mix with the mayonnaise.
3. Serve as an unusual yet refreshing side dish.

RADICCHIO AND ORANGE SALAD

 *Servings: 2*

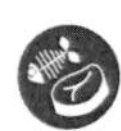 *Preparation Time: 10 minutes*

Ingredients

1 head radicchio, torn into pieces

1 large orange, peeled and segmented

1 pinch sea salt

1 tbsp balsamic vinegar

2 tbsp raisins

Preparation

1. Prepare the radicchio and orange.
2. Mix all of the ingredients together and serve.

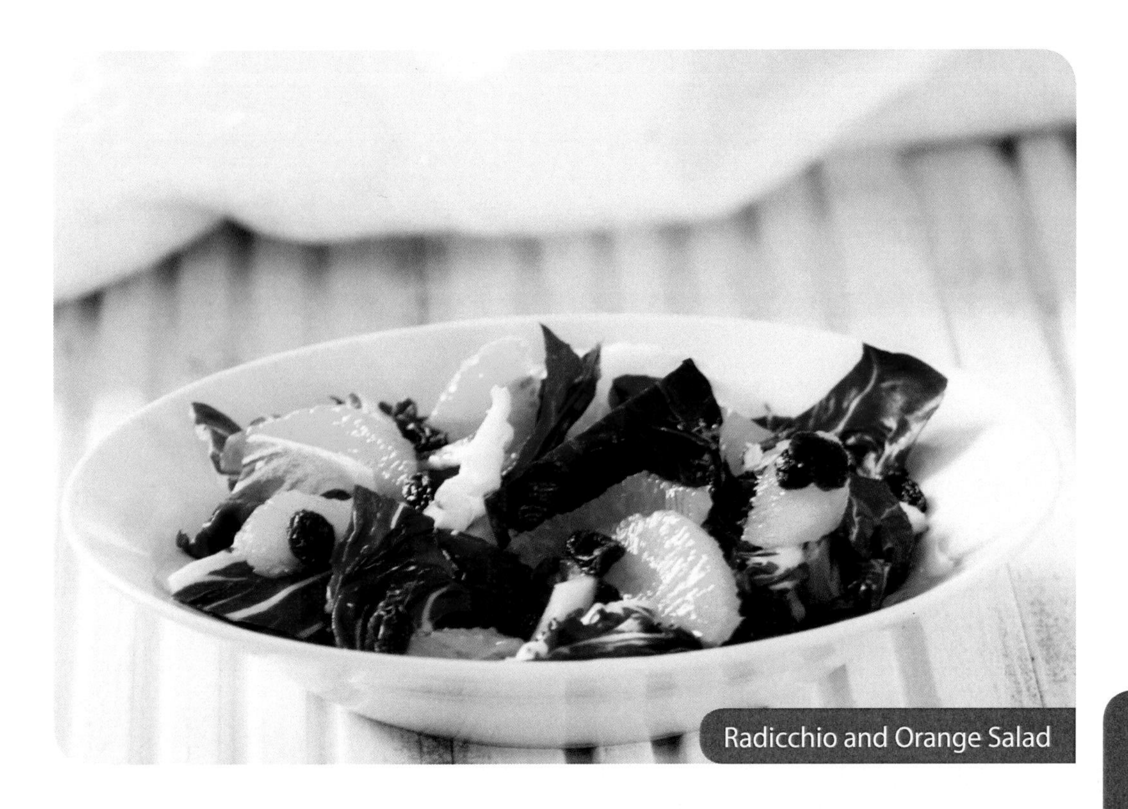

Radicchio and Orange Salad

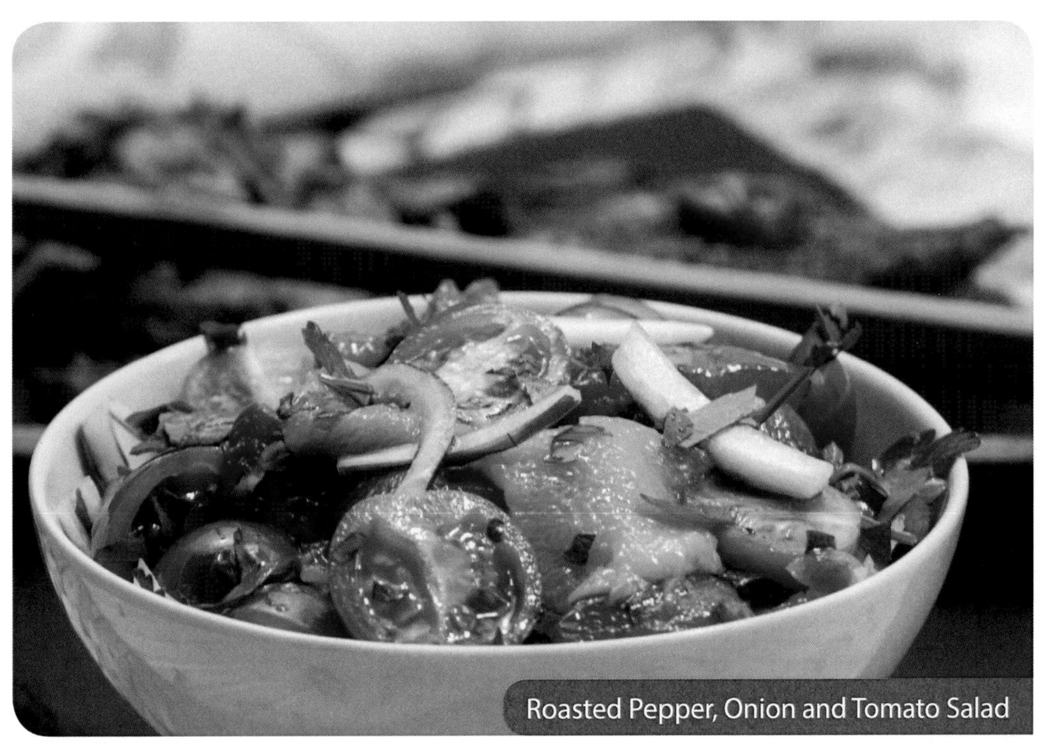

Roasted Pepper, Onion and Tomato Salad

ROASTED PEPPER, ONION AND TOMATO SALAD

This dish will happily stand for a few days so feel free to make extra if you wish. Use deli style peppers for this dish; it isn't always practical to make absolutely everything from scratch. The recipe makes enough for two meals.

 *Servings: 2*

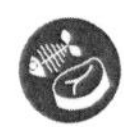 *Preparation Time: 10 minutes*

Ingredients

200g roasted red peppers, sliced
2 red onion, chopped
4 tbsp fresh parsley, chopped
3 tbsp extra virgin olive oil
4 tomatoes, chopped
2 garlic cloves, crushed
Sea salt

Preparation

1 Prepare the tomatoes, onion, peppers, garlic and parsley.
2 Mix all the ingredients together
3 Season to taste and serve.

RED SALAD

To cook the beetroot, roast in a preheated oven at 200C for 40-50 minutes. Once cooked, cool to room temperature before peeling and chopping. We recommend covering your countertop/chopping board with a layer of cling film to stop the beetroot staining surfaces.

 *Servings: 2*

 *Preparation Time: 15 minutes*

Ingredients

¼ red cabbage, shredded

2 cooked beetroot, chopped

2 spring onions, sliced

1 red apple, sliced

1 tbsp parsley chopped

Preparation

1. Prepare the cabbage, spring onions, beetroot, apple and the parsley.
2. Place all the ingredients into a bowl and mix together.
3. Season to taste and dress with Mustard Vinaigrette.

ROCKET, CUCUMBER, PISTACHIO AND POMEGRANATE SALAD

 *Servings: 2*

 *Preparation Time: 15 minutes*

Ingredients

100g rocket
1 pomegranate, seeds only
1 tbsp white wine vinegar
30g shelled pistachios
½ cucumber, thinly sliced
2 tbsp fresh coriander leaves

Preparation

1. Prepare the cucumber and pomegranate and shell the pistachios.
2. Toss all of the ingredients together in a bowl and serve immediately.

SHARP ASIAN SLAW

 *Servings: 2*

 *Preparation Time: 10 minutes*

Ingredients

¼ red cabbage, shredded
4 spring onions, chopped diagonally
50g beansprouts
1 inch ginger, grated
½ garlic clove, crushed
1 large leek, shredded
1 large carrot, shredded
1 lime, juice only
1 red chilli, finely chopped
2 tbsp fresh coriander, chopped

Preparation

1. Prepare the cabbage, leek, spring onion, carrot, ginger, chilli and garlic.
2. Place into a bowl with the beansprouts and mix well.
3. Pour over the lime juice and sprinkle the coriander before serving.
4. Add more chilli or lime if required; it is best when lip puckeringly sharp.

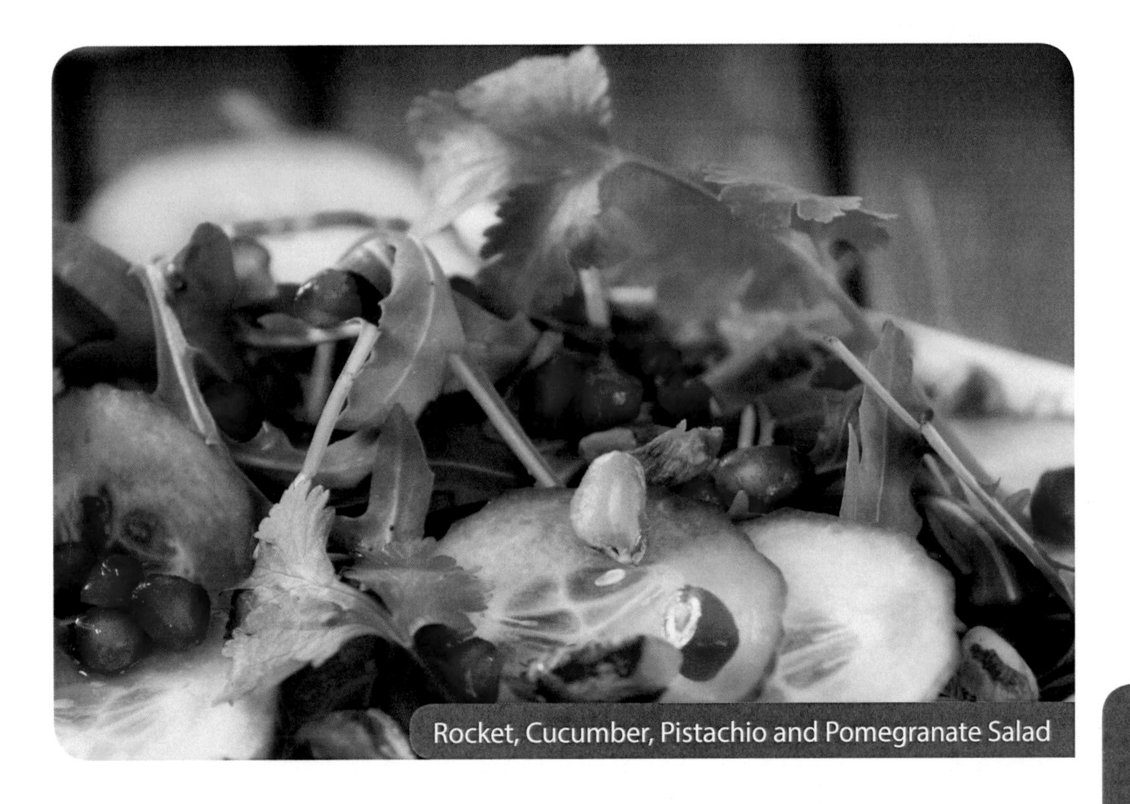

Rocket, Cucumber, Pistachio and Pomegranate Salad

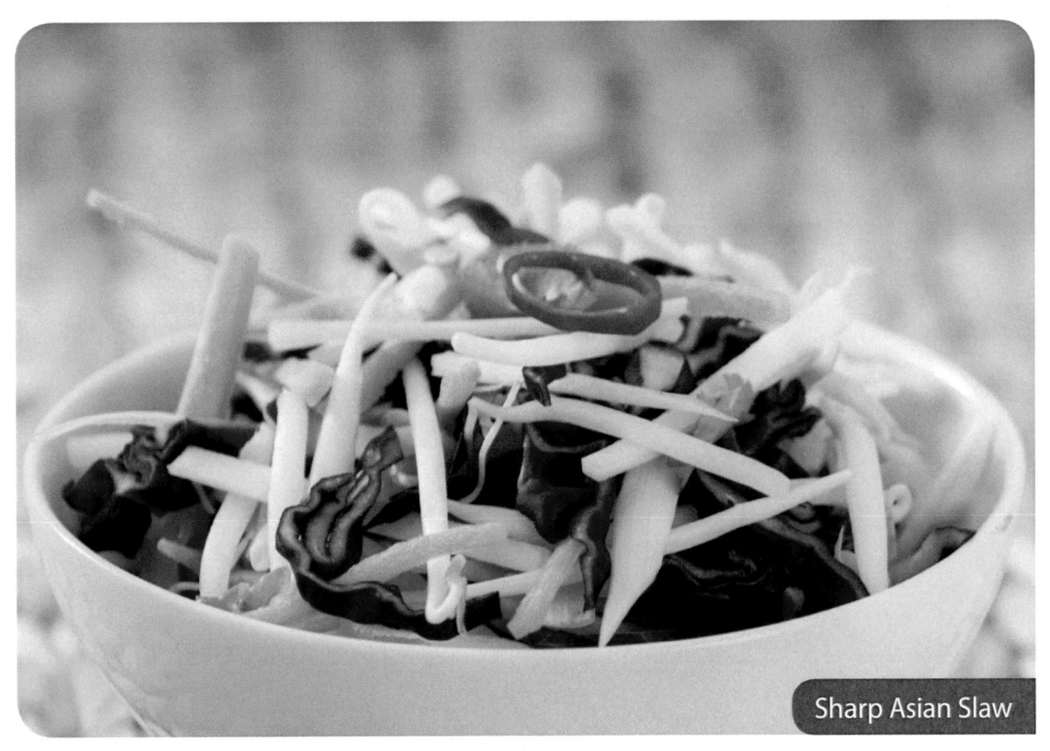

Sharp Asian Slaw

ROASTED ROOT SALAD WITH ORANGE AND THYME

If you cannot get baby vegetables (you are looking for long skinny ones rather than tiny fat ones) use full sized vegetables and cut into thin wedges.

 *Servings: 2*

 *Preparation Time: 15 minutes*

 *Cooking Time: 45 minutes*

 *Total Time: 1 hour*

Ingredients

2 tbsp lard, dripping or goose fat

150g baby parsnips

6 garlic cloves, smashed

4 sprigs fresh thyme

100g rocket

150g baby carrots

4 small beetroots, quartered

8 shallots, peeled and halved

Sea salt

FOR THE DRESSING

2 tbsp walnut oil

1 orange, juice only

Preparation

1. Preheat the oven to 200C.
2. Prepare the vegetables.
3. Arrange all of the roots on a baking tray, with the shallots, thyme, fat and garlic.
4. Season with salt and place in the oven.
5. Bake for about 30-40 minutes, turning occasionally until everything is soft and caramelised.
6. Toss the rocket with the oil and orange juice, then top with the roasted roots.
7. Eat whilst still warm.

SIMPLE RAW SLAW

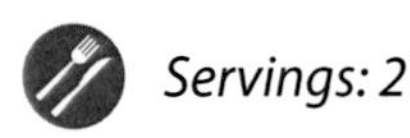
Servings: 2

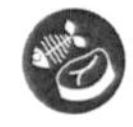
Preparation Time: 10 minutes

Ingredients

¼ white cabbage, shredded
¼ red cabbage, shredded
50g beansprouts
2 tbsp fresh parsley, chopped
1 red onion, finely sliced
2 carrots, grated
1 lemon, juice only

Preparation

1 Prepare the cabbage, red onion and carrots and place into a bowl.
2 Add the beansprouts and the lemon juice and mix well.
3 Sprinkle the fresh parsley over the top.
4 Do not salt or it will become waterlogged.

SIMPLE LEAF SALAD

Servings: 2

Preparation Time: 10 minutes

Ingredients

1 bag mixed salad greens
2 tbsp whole almonds
3 spring onions, chopped

FOR THE DRESSING

1 tbsp extra virgin olive oil
Sea salt
2 tbsp fresh parsley, chopped
1 tbsp balsamic vinegar
Freshly ground black pepper

Preparation

1 Prepare the spring onions and place in a bowl with the mixed salad and the almonds.
2 Mix together the olive oil and the balsamic vinegar and toss into the salad.
3 Season to taste and sprinkle with the fresh parsley.

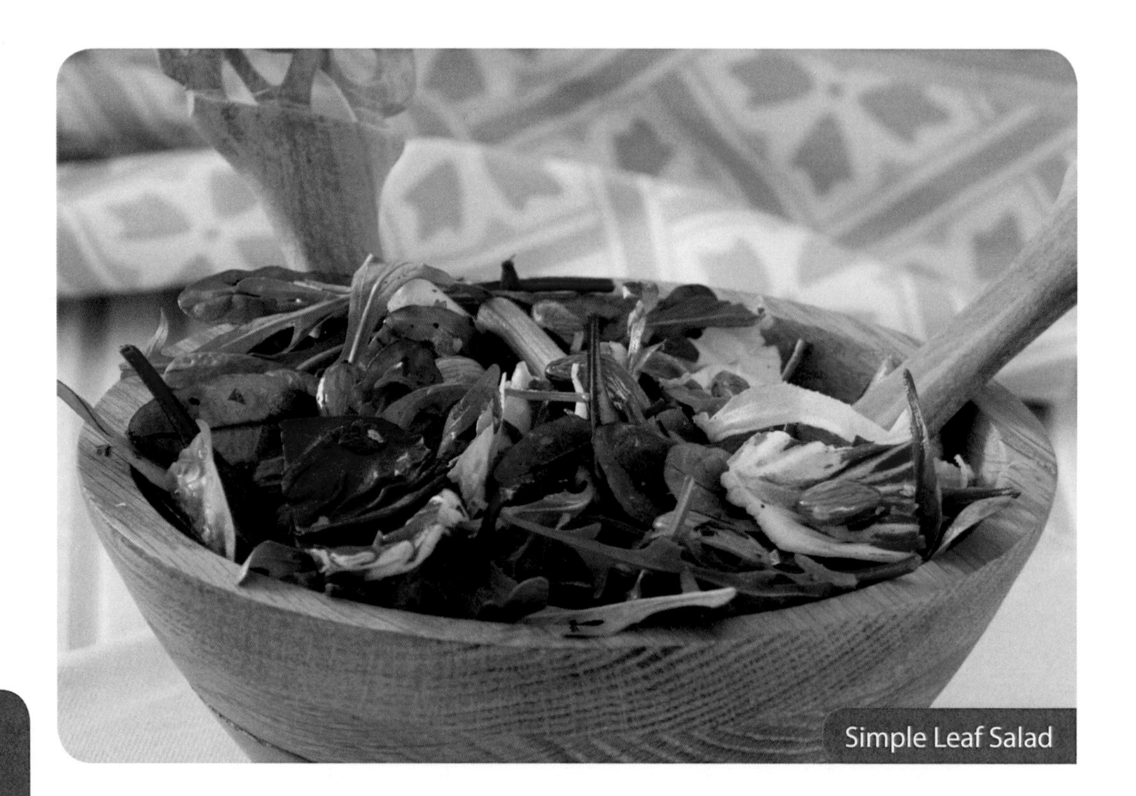

Simple Leaf Salad

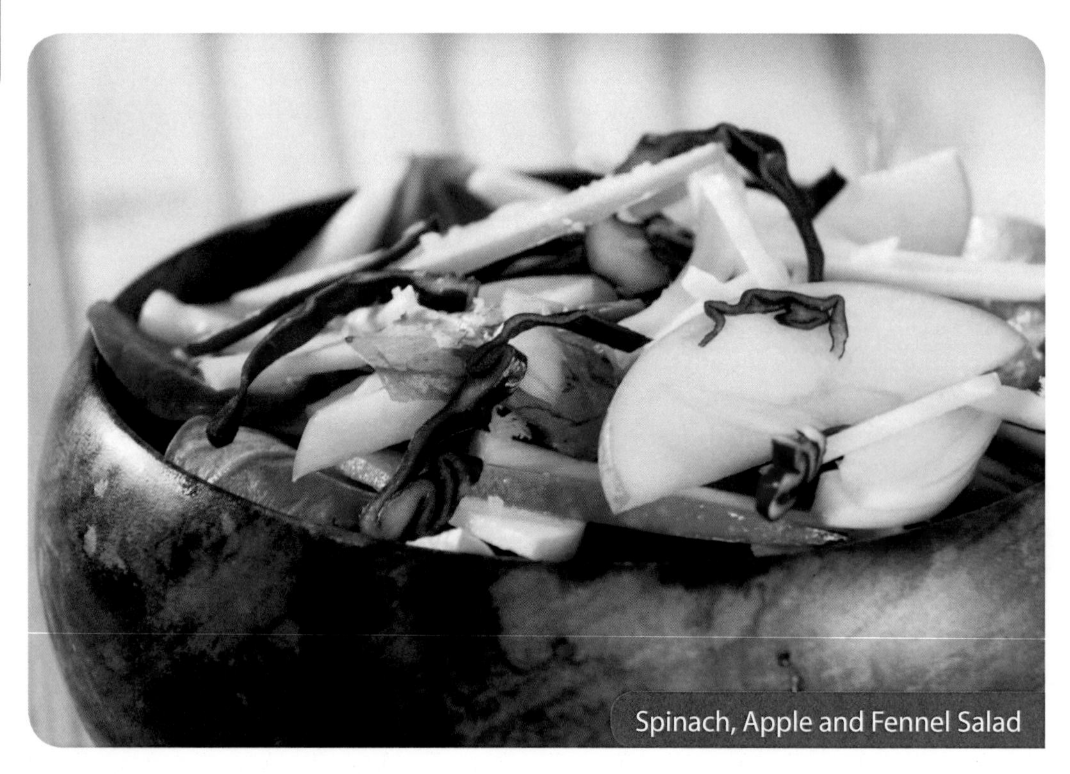

Spinach, Apple and Fennel Salad

SPINACH, APPLE AND FENNEL SALAD

This lovely crunchy salad pairs the robust green flavour of baby spinach and sweetens it with crunchy fresh apple. Red cabbage brings extra crunch and the anise tones of fennel elevate it into something special.

This salad is a masterclass in using a few simple ingredients rather than throwing the whole salad compartment at the bowl.

 *Servings: 2*

 *Preparation Time: 15 minutes*

Ingredients

75g baby spinach leaves

¼ red cabbage, shredded

1 bulb young fennel, shredded

2 crisp green apples, cored and finely sliced

FOR THE DRESSING

1 tbsp walnut oil

2 tsp balsamic vinegar

1 pinch sea salt

Preparation

1. Prepare the cabbage, fennel and apple and place into a bowl with the spinach.
2. Mix the dressing and then toss with the salad.
3. Season to taste and serve.

TOMATO AND AVOCADO SALAD

 *Servings: 2*

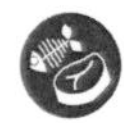 *Preparation Time: 15 minutes*

Ingredients

2 ripe avocado, chopped

½ red onion, finely sliced

1 tbsp red wine vinegar

Sea salt

1 punnet cherry tomatoes, halved

2 tbsp olive oil

1 garlic clove, crushed

3 tbsp fresh parsley, chopped

Preparation

1. Prepare the avocado, onion, tomatoes, garlic and parsley and place in a bowl.
2. Mix gently but thoroughly.
3. Season to taste and serve at room temperature.

TOMATO AND SPRING ONION SALAD

 *Servings: 2*

 *Preparation Time: 10 minutes*

Ingredients

4 ripe tomatoes, chopped

2 tbsp fresh parsley, chopped

2 tbsp olive oil

1 pinch ground pepper

4 spring onions, chopped

1 lemon, juice only

1 pinch sea salt

Preparation

1. Combine all the ingredients and serve at room temperature.

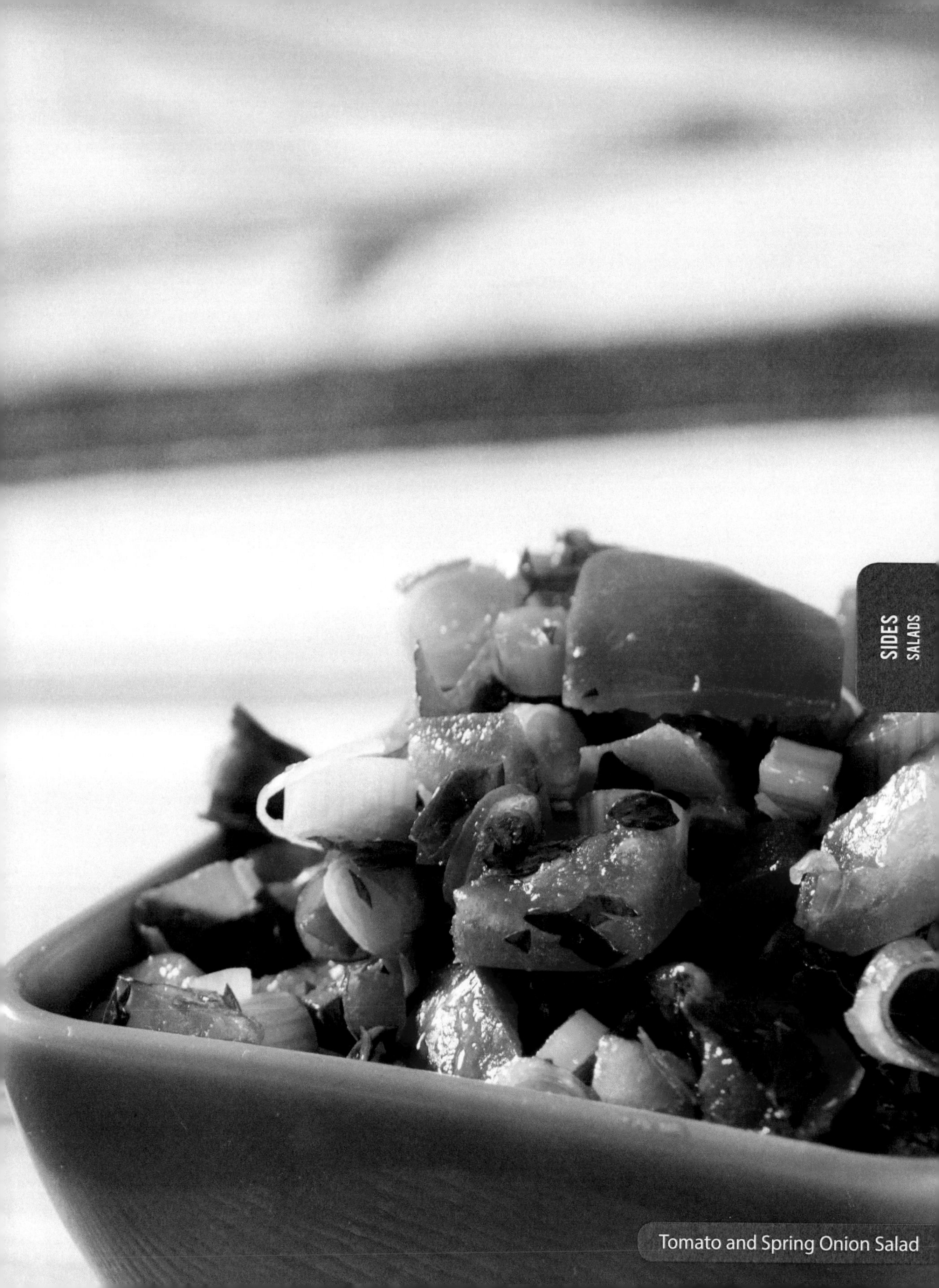

Tomato and Spring Onion Salad

BABA GANOUSH

This recipe makes a delicious accompaniment for our Paleo Flax Crackers. Ideal for a snack or when you are entertaining.

 *Servings: 2*

 *Preparation Time: 15 minutes*

 *Cooking Time: 35 minutes*

 *Total Time: 50 minutes*

Ingredients

1 aubergine

1 tbsp fresh lemon juice

2 tbsp extra virgin olive oil

1 pinch sea salt

2 garlic cloves, crushed

1 tbsp tahini

1 tsp ground cumin

1 tbsp fresh parsley, chopped

Preparation

1. Preheat the oven to 200C
2. Prick the skin of the aubergine with a fork and roast whole for about 35 minutes.
3. Remove and once cool enough to handle, peel off the skin.
4. Blend all the ingredients to a rough paste and serve warm or cold.

BALSAMIC GREEN BEANS

 *Servings: 2*

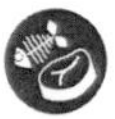 *Preparation Time: 10 minutes*

 *Cooking Time: 10 minutes*

 *Total Time: 20 minutes*

Ingredients

200g green beans, topped and tailed

1 sprig thyme

1 tbsp balsamic vinegar

Freshly ground black pepper

4 shallots, quartered

1 tbsp olive oil

Sea salt

Preparation

1. Place a large pan of water on to boil and blanch the green beans for about 5 minutes, or until tender crisp. Drain, and unless you are using immediately, refresh under cold water.
2. Heat the oil in a frying pan and cook the shallots, with a pinch of salt and the sprig of thyme, over a low heat until they are soft and browned around the edges.
3. Tip in the beans, cook for a few more minutes and add the balsamic.
4. Check your seasoning and serve.

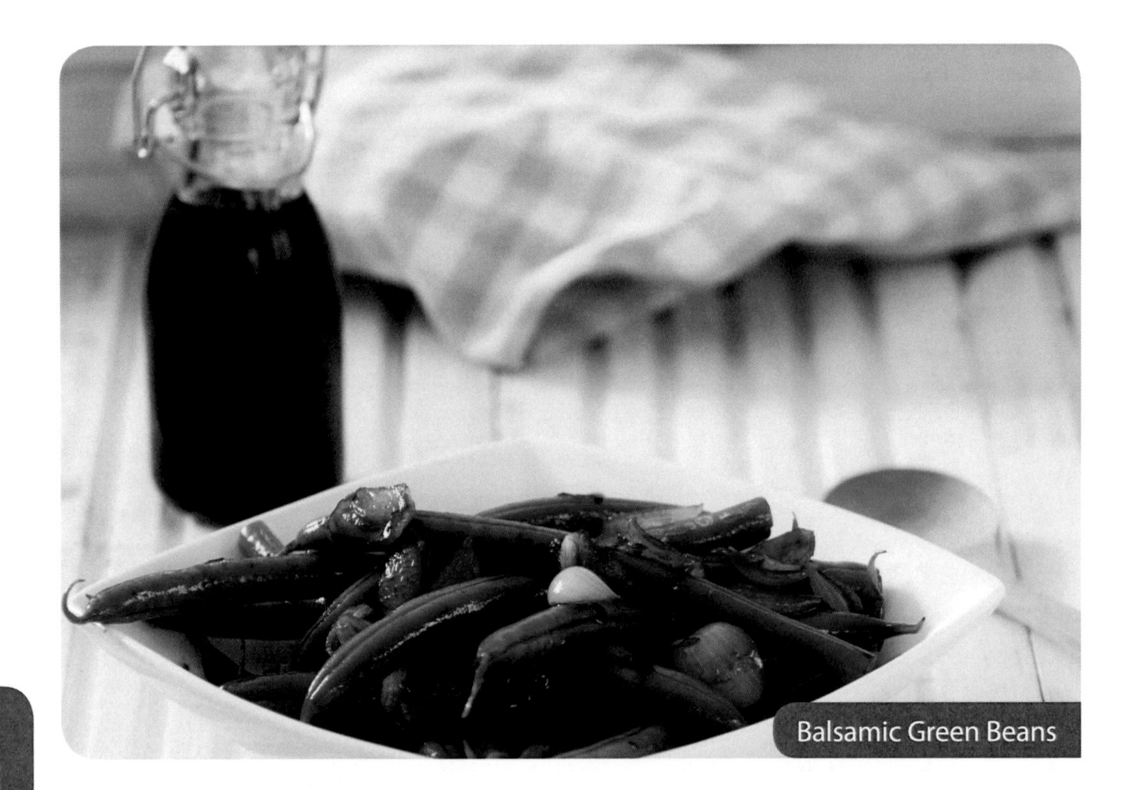
Balsamic Green Beans

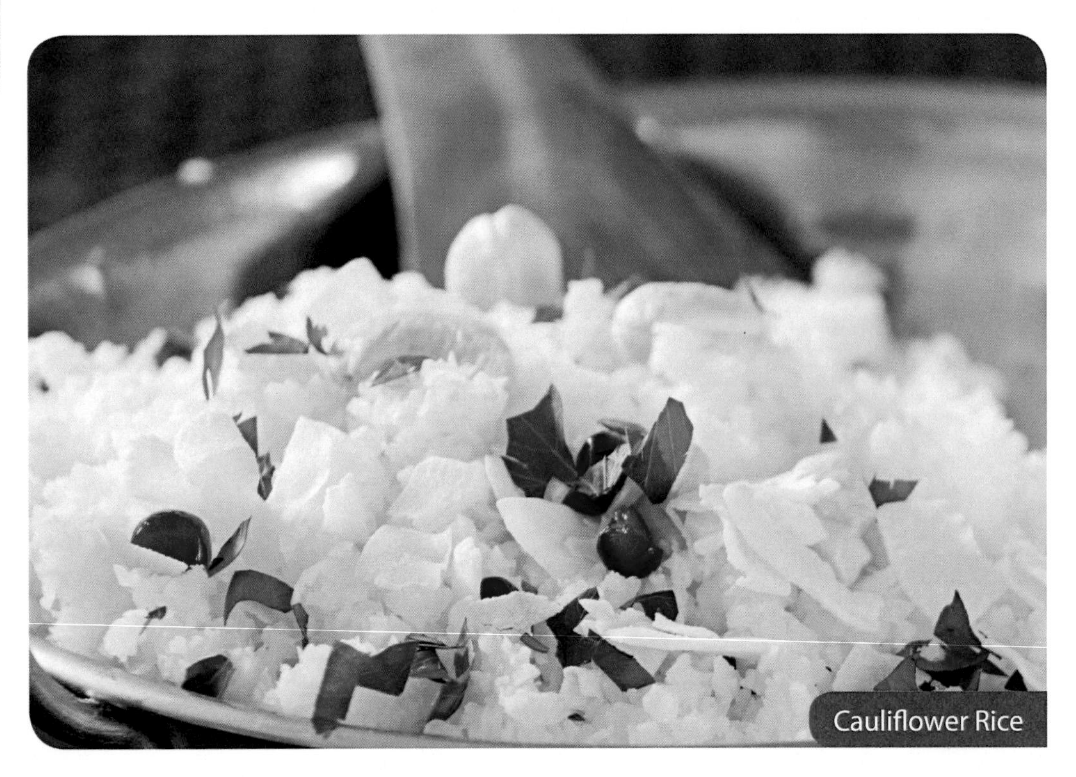
Cauliflower Rice

CAULIFLOWER RICE

 *Servings: 2*

 *Preparation Time: 10 minutes*

 *Cooking Time: 10 minutes*

 *Total Time: 20 minutes*

Ingredients

1 medium head cauliflower

1 tbsp coconut oil

1 pinch sea salt

Preparation

1. Blitz the cauliflower in a food processor or grate it so it resembles small grains.
2. Remove any large uneven bits.
3. Heat the coconut oil in a large frying pan and add the cauliflower with a good pinch of salt.
4. Stir fry slowly until the cauliflower is tender; about 8-10 minutes.
5. Serve hot and add some flaked almonds and pomegranate seeds for added texture if you wish.

BROCCOLI WITH CASHEW NUTS

 *Servings: 2*

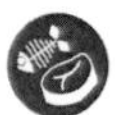 *Preparation Time: 5 minutes*

 *Cooking Time: 5 minutes*

 *Total Time: 10 minutes*

Ingredients

2 heads broccoli, in florets

1 pinch sea salt

1 lemon, zest only

30g raw cashew nuts

Preparation

1. Bring a large pan of water to the boil and add salt.
2. Add the broccoli and blanch for about 3-5 minutes or until tender crisp
3. Drain thoroughly and then toss the broccoli with the lemon zest and cashew nuts to serve.

BROCCOLI WITH MUSTARD SEEDS

 *Servings: 2*

 *Preparation Time: 10 minutes*

 *Cooking Time: 10 minutes*

 *Total Time: 20 minutes*

Ingredients

2 heads broccoli, in florets

1 tbsp lard

1 tbsp mustard seeds

1 pinch sea salt

1 squeeze lemon juice, freshly squeezed

Preparation

1. Bring a large pan of water to the boil and add salt.
2. Add the broccoli and blanch for about 3-5 minutes or until tender and crisp.
3. Drain, cool in ice cold water and drain again.
4. Melt the lard in a large frying pan and when hot throw in the mustard seeds.
5. Add the broccoli to the pan, stir, and squeeze over a small drop of lemon juice.
6. Serve hot.

GREEN BEANS WITH LEMON

 *Servings: 2*

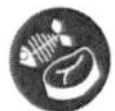 *Preparation Time: 5 minutes*

 *Cooking Time: 10 minutes*

 *Total Time: 15 minutes*

Ingredients

200g green beans

Sea salt

1 lemon, zest and juice

Preparation

1. Cook the beans in boiling salted water for about 8-10 minutes.
2. Drain and then toss the warm beans with the lemon juice and zest.
3. Season with plenty of black pepper and serve.

GREENS WITH CHILLI AND WALNUT

 *Servings: 2*

 *Preparation Time: 10 minutes*

 *Cooking Time: 10 minutes*

 *Total Time: 20 minutes*

Ingredients

½ head Savoy cabbage, shredded

2 tbsp walnuts, chopped

1 pinch sea salt

2 red chillies, finely chopped

1 tbsp olive oil

1 pinch freshly ground black pepper

Preparation

1. Prepare the cabbage, chillies and walnuts.
2. Place a large pan of water on to boil and add a good pinch of salt.
3. Add the cabbage and blanch for 5-10 minutes depending your taste.
4. Drain and add the oil, walnuts and chillies to the cabbage.
5. Toss together to coat and serve hot.

GREENS WITH LEMON, OLIVE OIL AND GARLIC

 *Servings: 2*

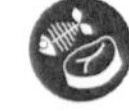 *Preparation Time: 20 minutes*

 *Cooking Time: 10 minutes*

 *Total Time: 30 minutes*

Ingredients

½ head Savoy cabbage, shredded

1 garlic clove, crushed

1 tbsp olive oil

1 tbsp lemon juice, freshly squeezed

1 pinch sea salt

1 pinch freshly ground black pepper

Preparation

1. Prepare the cabbage and garlic.
2. Place a large pan of water on to boil and add a good pinch of salt.
3. Once the water is boiling add the shredded cabbage.
4. Blanch for about 5-10 minutes depending on how well cooked you prefer it.
5. Drain the cabbage and add the oil, lemon and crushed garlic.
6. Toss everything together to coat and serve hot.

PAN STEAMED BROCCOLI

 *Servings: 2*

 *Preparation Time: 5 minutes*

 *Cooking Time: 10 minutes*

 *Total Time: 15 minutes*

Ingredients

1 head broccoli, florets

1 tbsp lard, dripping or goose fat

1 pinch sea salt

50ml water

1 pinch black pepper

Preparation

1. Place a saucepan over a medium heat and add the lard to melt.
2. Break the broccoli into florets and fry lightly for a few minutes.
3. Add the salt and a splash of boiling water.
4. Place the lid on the saucepan and cook for 5 minutes or until tender crisp.
5. Season with black pepper and serve.

PAN STEAMED CARROTS

 *Servings: 2*

 *Preparation Time: 5 minutes*

 *Cooking Time: 10 minutes*

 *Total Time: 15 minutes*

Ingredients

4 large carrots, cut into batons

1 tbsp lard, dripping or goose fat

1 pinch sea salt

1 tbsp fresh parsley, chopped

50ml water

Preparation

1 Place a saucepan over a medium heat and melt the fat.

2 Cut the carrots into batons and add to the saucepan.

3 Stir fry gently for a few minutes.

4 Add the salt and a splash of boiling water.

5 Cover and cook for about 5 minutes or until tender crisp.

6 Toss with parsley before serving.

PEAS WITH ARTICHOKES

 *Servings: 2*

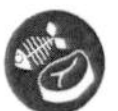 *Preparation Time: 10 minutes*

 *Cooking Time: 5 minutes*

 *Total Time: 15 minutes*

Ingredients

300g frozen peas

1 tbsp olive oil

300g ready prepared artichokes, drained

1 tbsp parsley, finely chopped

Preparation

1. Cook the peas until tender and stir in the artichokes, oil and parsley.
2. Serve hot.

ROASTED CAULIFLOWER WITH MINT

 *Servings: 2*

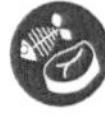 *Preparation Time: 5 minutes*

 *Cooking Time: 30 minutes*

 *Total Time: 35 minutes*

Ingredients

1 medium head cauliflower, in florets

1 tsp turmeric

2 tbsp fresh mint leaves, chopped

1 tbsp olive oil

1 pinch salt

Preparation

1. Preheat your oven to 200C.
2. Toss the cauliflower florets in the oil, salt and spices.
3. Place in the oven and bake for about 30 minutes.
4. Remove from the oven and scatter with fresh mint.
5. Delicious served hot or cold.

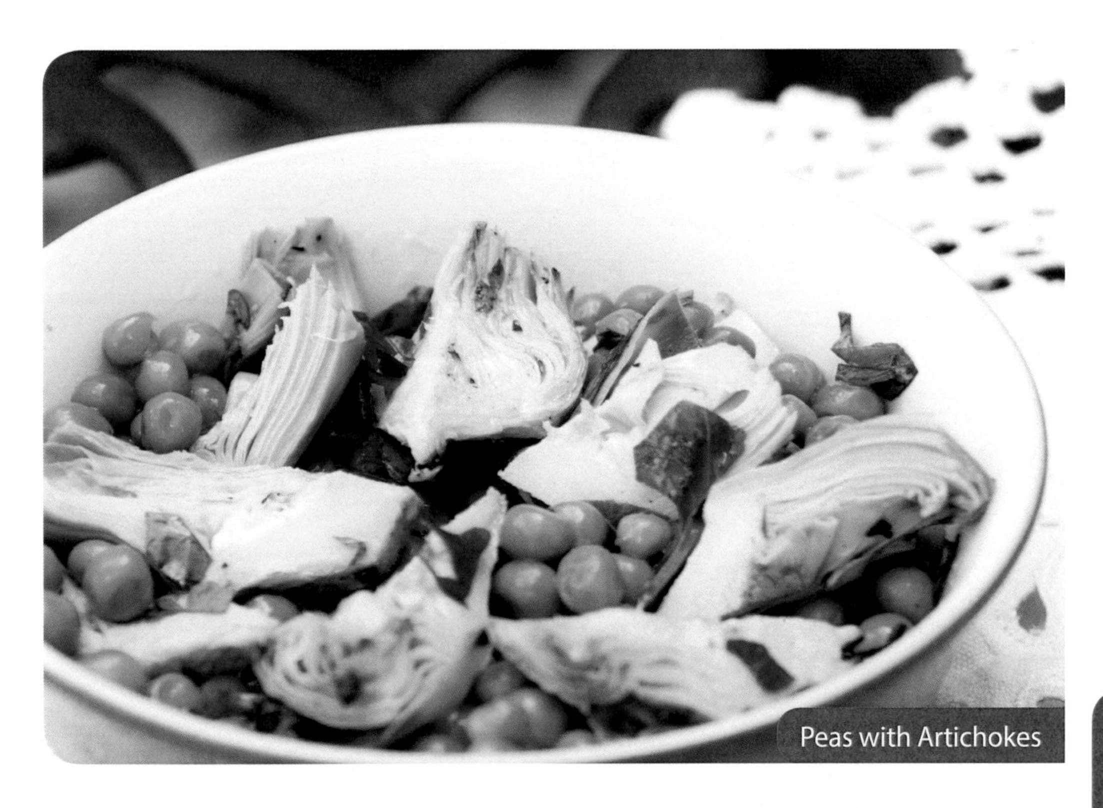
Peas with Artichokes

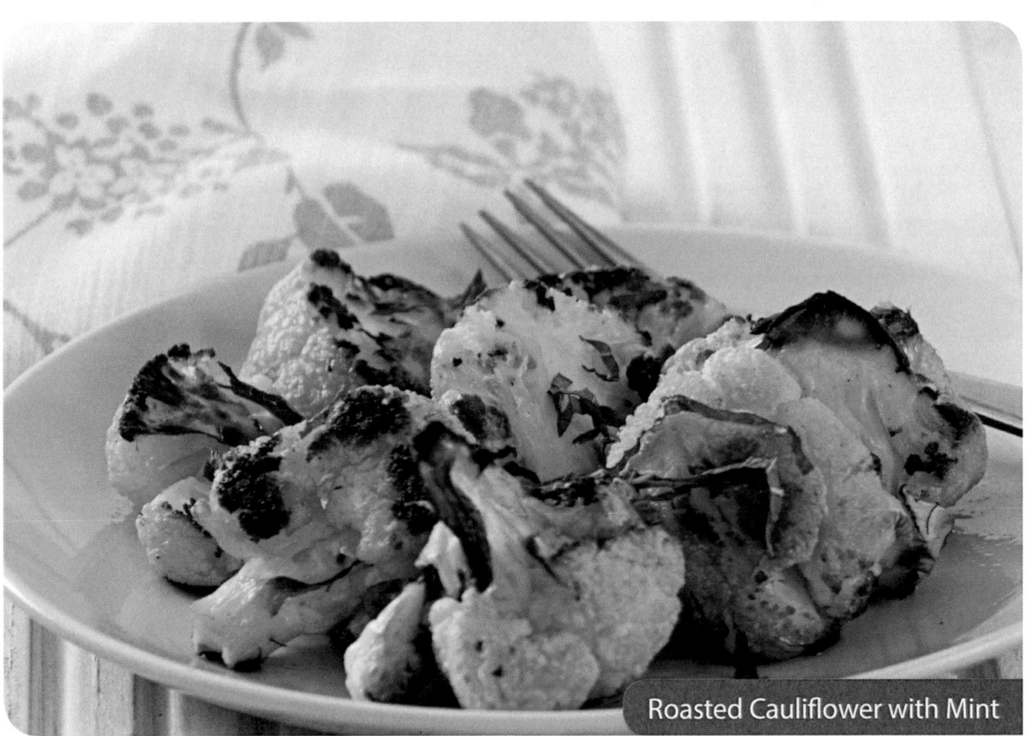
Roasted Cauliflower with Mint

PEAS WITH ONIONS AND BACON

 *Servings: 2*

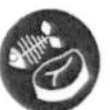 *Preparation Time: 10 minutes*

 *Cooking Time: 10 minutes*

 *Total Time: 20 minutes*

Ingredients

200g frozen peas

2 onions, sliced

6 rashers streaky bacon, chopped
2 tbsp lard, dripping or goose fat

Preparation

1. Heat the fat in a frying pan and add the onions.
2. Cook slowly, stirring occasionally until melting and golden.
3. Add the chopped bacon and stir for a few minutes until cooked through.
4. Add the peas and cook until defrosted.
5. You may need to use a drop of water or chicken stock to keep it moist.
6. Serve hot as a side dish; especially good with fish.

ROAST CAULIFLOWER WITH TURMERIC

 *Servings: 2*

 *Preparation Time: 5 minutes*

 *Cooking Time: 30 minutes*

 *Total Time: 35 minutes*

Ingredients

1 medium head cauliflower

2 tbsp lard, dripping or goose fat

Sea salt

1 tsp turmeric

Preparation

1. Preheat the oven to 200C
2. Break the cauliflower into florets and toss with the turmeric.
3. Place in a baking dish with the fat and sprinkle with salt.
4. Roast until tender, this will be about 30 minutes.
5. Serve hot or cold.

ROAST CINNAMON APPLES AND SQUASH

 *Servings: 2*

 *Preparation Time: 10 minutes*

 *Cooking Time: 30 minutes*

 *Total Time: 40 minutes*

Ingredients

1 butternut squash peeled and cut into 1inch cubes

2 apples, cored and chopped into large chunks

1 tsp ground cinnamon

Sea salt

2 tbsp lard, dripping or goose fat

SIDES
VEGETABLES

Preparation

1. Preheat the oven to 180C.
2. Prepare the butternut squash and the apples and place in a baking dish.
3. Sprinkle with cinnamon and salt, and add the fat.
4. Bake in the oven for about 30 minutes until the squash is tender.
5. Serve hot as a side dish; especially good with pork.

ROASTED MEDITERRANEAN VEGETABLES

This dish keeps well so can be made in bulk to keep in the fridge for other meals.

 *Servings: 4*

 *Preparation Time: 20 minutes*

 *Cooking Time: 30 minutes*

 *Total Time: 50 minutes*

Ingredients

- 2 courgettes, cut into large chunks
- 2 red onion, quartered with root intact
- 2 tbsp extra virgin olive oil
- 1 tsp freshly-ground black pepper
- 2 bulbs young fennel, cut into 6 with root intact
- 1 aubergine, cut in 1 inch cubes
- 1 red pepper, cut into 1 inch squares
- 1 pinch sea salt
- 2 sprigs fresh thyme
- 6 garlic cloves, still in skins

Preparation

1. Preheat the oven to 200C.
2. Prepare the courgettes, aubergine, onion, pepper and fennel.
3. Place all the ingredients on a large baking tray and toss to coat thoroughly in oil.
4. Cook in the oven for 30 minutes, turning occasionally with a spatula so that they cook evenly.
5. Cook until the vegetables are tender and brown but not too soft.
6. Remove from the oven and serve hot or cold.

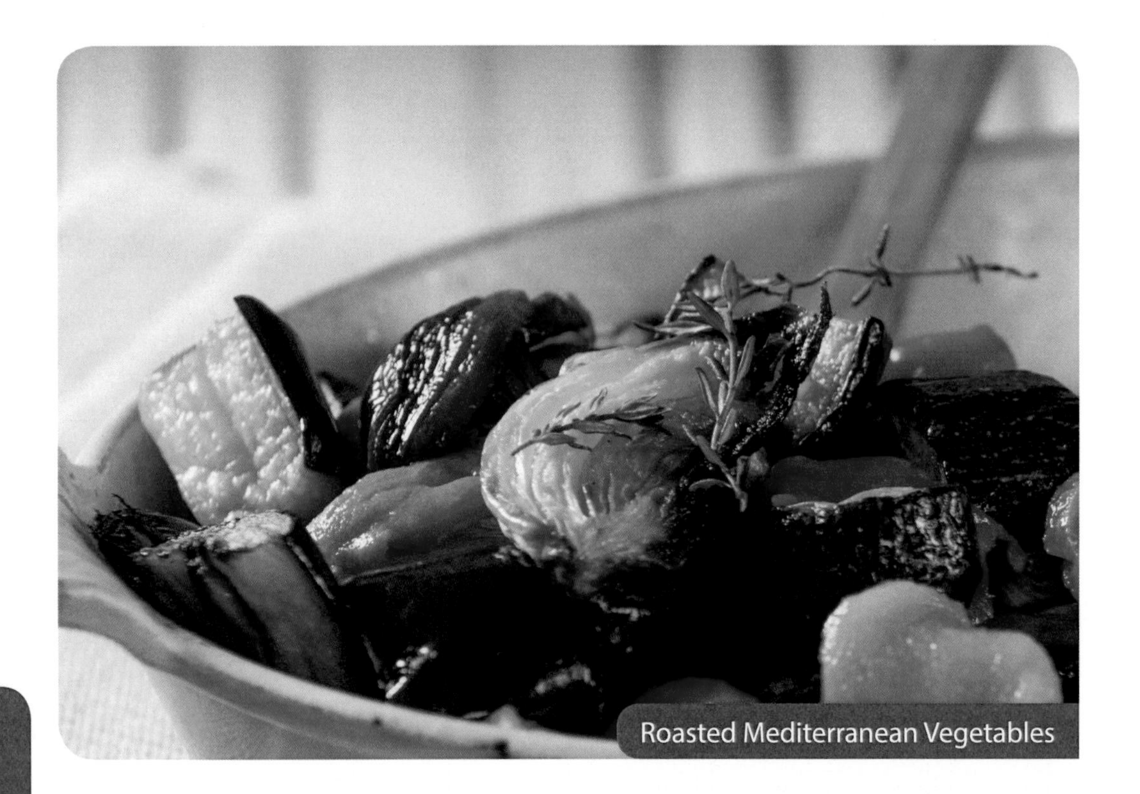
Roasted Mediterranean Vegetables

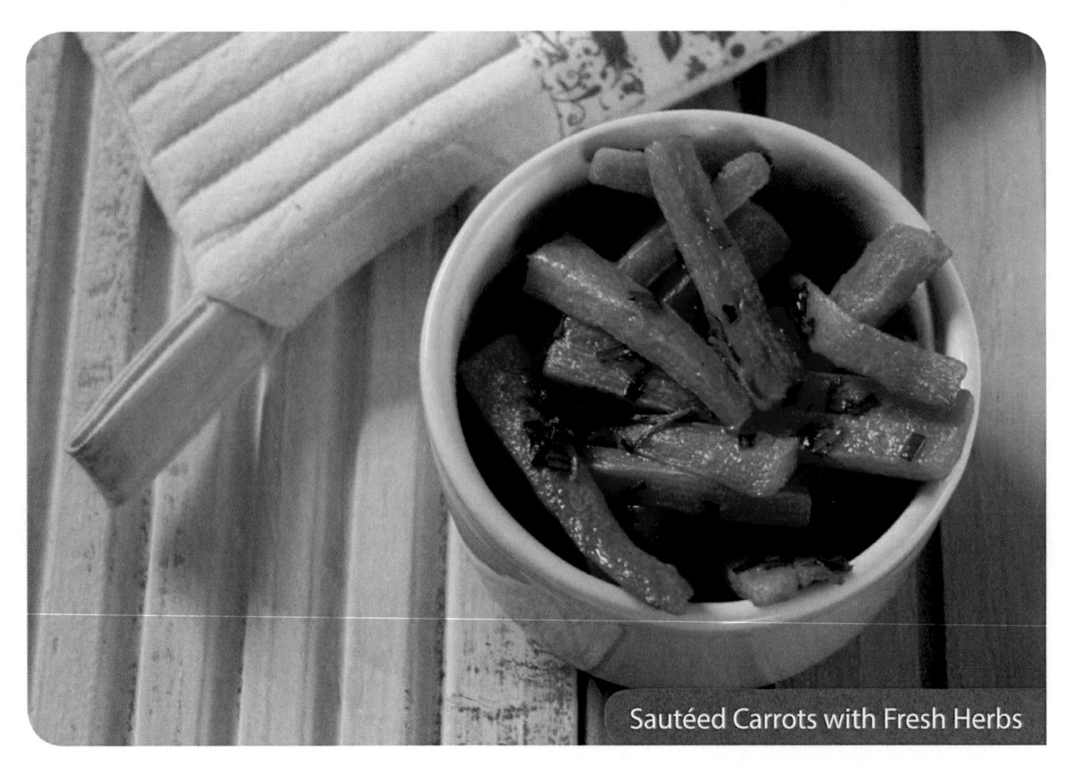
Sautéed Carrots with Fresh Herbs

SAUTÉED CARROTS WITH FRESH HERBS

 *Servings: 2*

 *Preparation Time: 10 minutes*

 *Cooking Time: 20 minutes*

 *Total Time: 30 minutes*

Ingredients

300g carrots, cut into batons

Sea salt

1 tbsp fresh chives, chopped

2 tbsp lard, dripping or goose fat

½ orange, juice only

1 tbsp fresh parsley, chopped

Preparation

1. Prepare the carrots and the herbs.
2. Heat the fat in a frying pan and sauté the carrots for about 5 minutes.
3. Add the orange juice with the seasoning to the pan.
4. Cook until all of the orange has evaporated.
5. The carrots should be tender and the edges browned.
6. Season to taste and stir through the herbs.
7. Serve hot.

SAUTÉED COURGETTES WITH LEMON

 *Servings: 2*

 *Preparation Time: 10 minutes*

 *Cooking Time: 10 minutes*

 *Total Time: 20 minutes*

Ingredients

4 small courgettes, thinly sliced

2 tbsp lard, dripping or oil

Sea salt

Freshly ground black pepper

1 pinch dried oregano

1 lemon, juice and zest

Preparation

1. Prepare the courgettes.
2. Heat the fat in a frying pan and add the courgettes.
3. Fry quickly, tossing occasionally, until starting to soften.
4. Season with salt, pepper and oregano then remove from the heat.
5. Toss the courgettes in the lemon and serve hot.

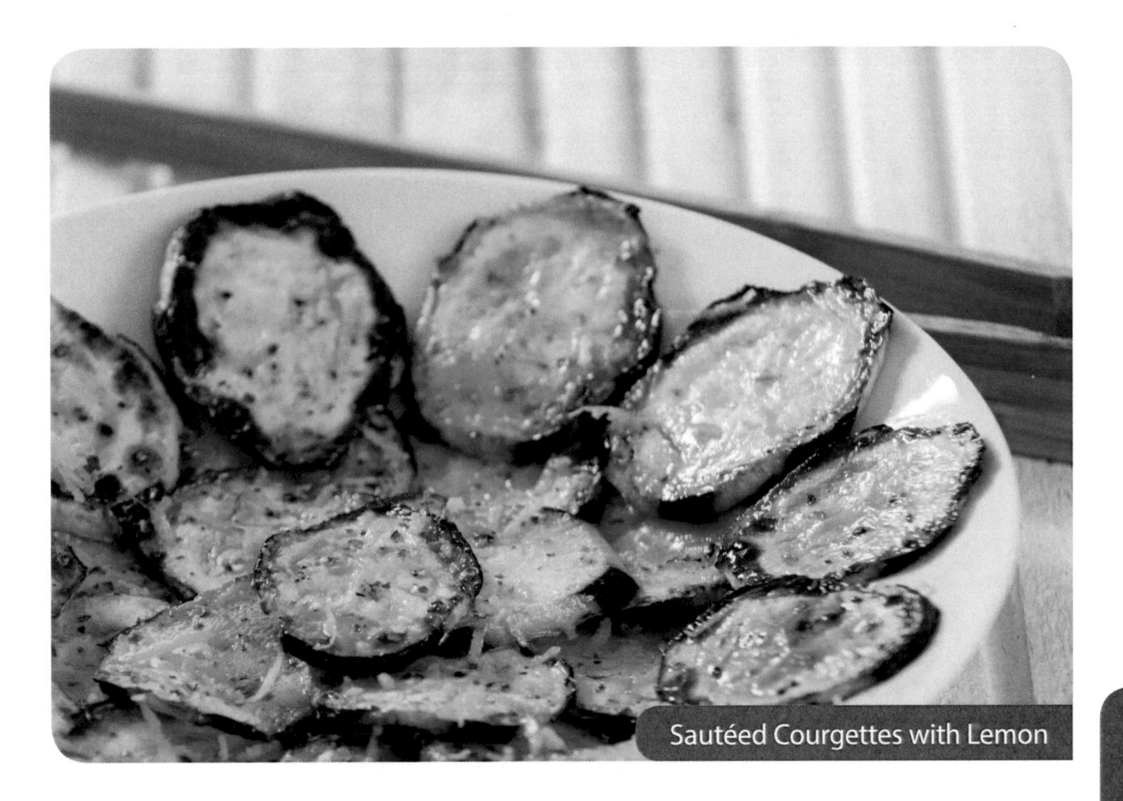
Sautéed Courgettes with Lemon

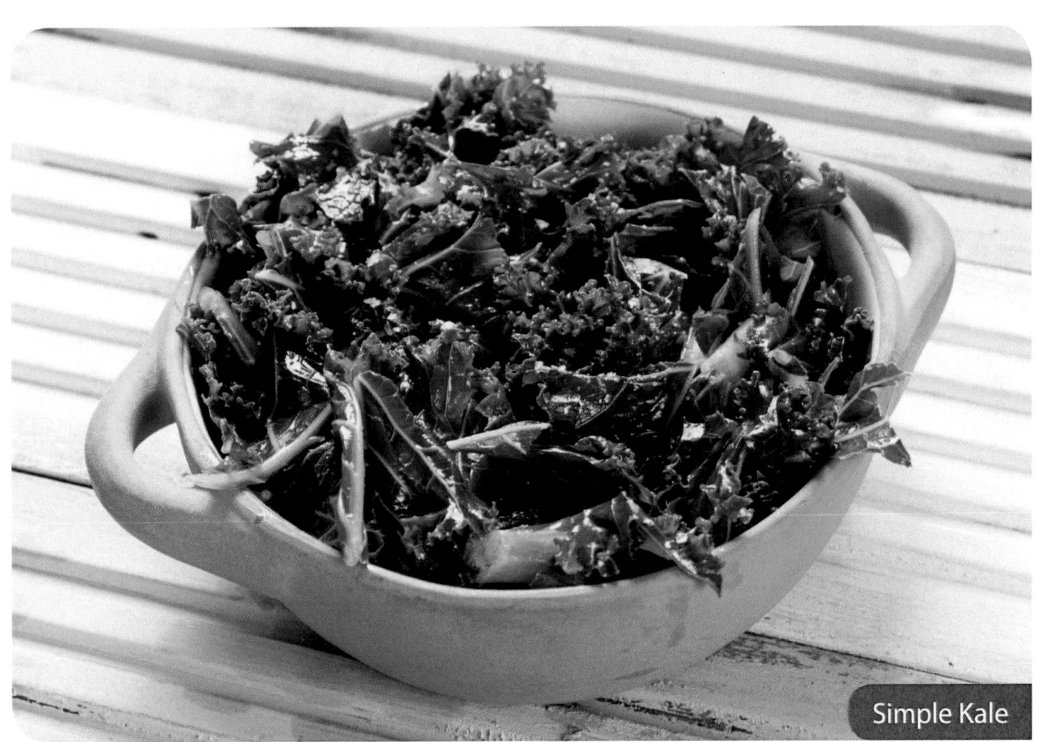
Simple Kale

SPINACH WITH GARLIC AND RAISINS

 *Servings: 2*

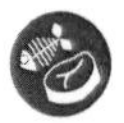 *Preparation Time: 5 minutes*

 *Cooking Time: 5 minutes*

 *Total Time: 10 minutes*

Ingredients

1 tbsp lard, dripping or goose fat

1 garlic clove, crushed

Sea salt

2 tbsp raisins

100g baby spinach leaves

1 lemon, juice only

Freshly ground black pepper

Preparation

1. Heat the fat in a frying pan and add the spinach.
2. Keep stirring until the spinach wilts.
3. Add the garlic, seasoning, lemon juice and raisins and stir for a couple of minutes.
4. Serve hot.

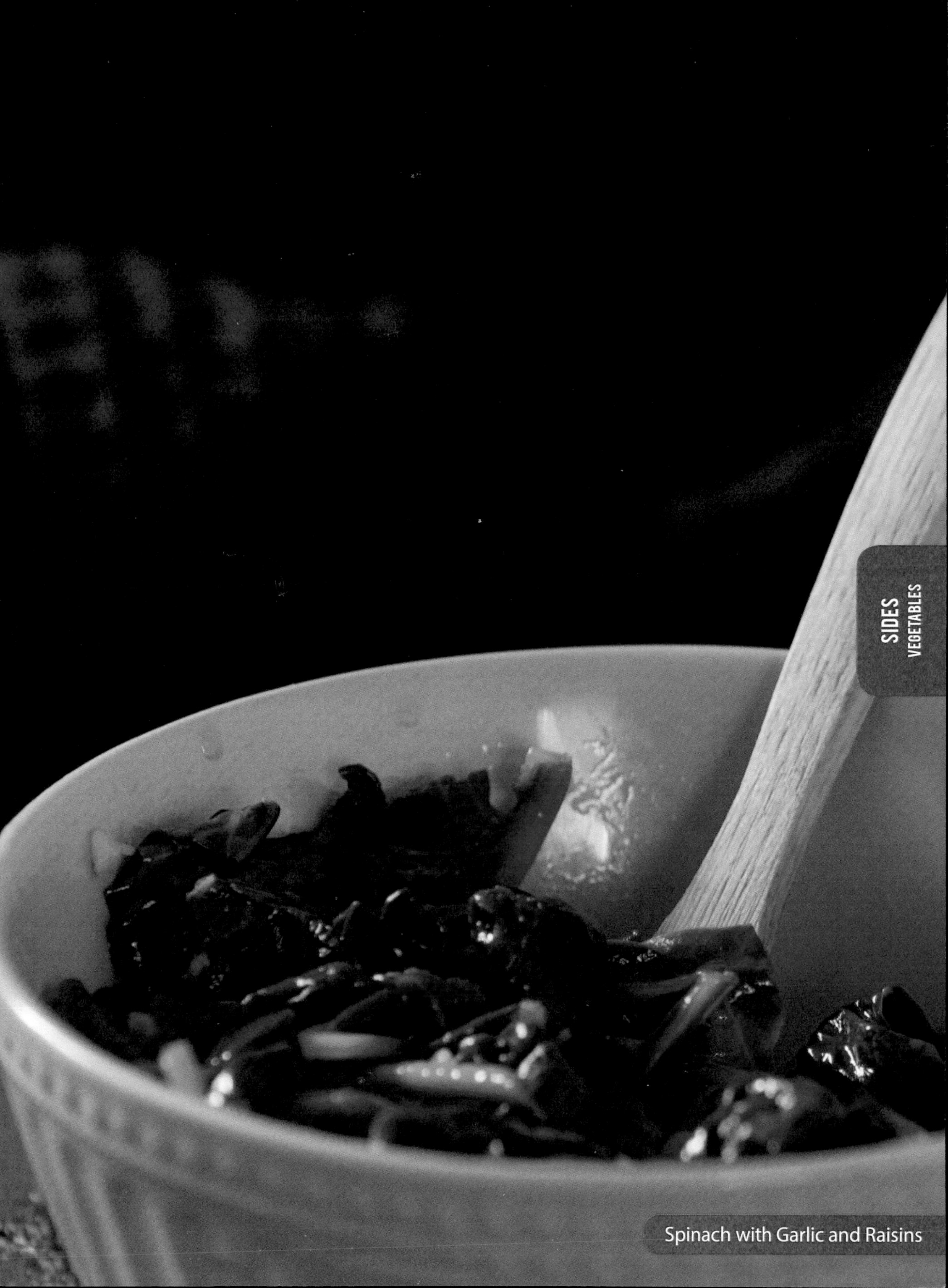

Spinach with Garlic and Raisins

SIMPLE KALE

 *Servings: 2*

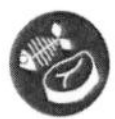 *Preparation Time: 15 minutes*

 *Cooking Time: 10 minutes*

 *Total Time: 25 minutes*

Ingredients

200g kale, shredded

Sea salt

1 squeeze lemon juice

Preparation

1. Bring a large pan of water to the boil.
2. Salt generously and add the kale.
3. Cook, covered, for roughly 8-10 minutes until the kale is tender.
4. Drain and squeeze over a little lemon juice before serving hot.
5. Save any leftover kale for bubble and squeak on Sunday.

WILTED SPINACH

 *Servings: 2*

 *Preparation Time: 5 minutes*

 *Cooking Time: 5 minutes*

 *Total Time: 10 minutes*

Ingredients

1 tbsp lard, dripping or goose fat

100g baby spinach leaves

Freshly grated nutmeg

Sea salt

Freshly ground black pepper

Preparation

1. Heat the fat in a frying pan and add the spinach.
2. Keep stirring until the spinach wilts.
3. Season generously with salt, pepper and nutmeg.
4. Serve hot.

STARCHY VEGETABLES

BAKED SWEET POTATO

As an alternative to whole baked sweet potatoes, try cutting into wedges. This will also help to reduce cooking times when you are in a hurry. Sweet potatoes do not take as long as white potatoes so take care not to overdo them.

 *Servings: 2*

 *Preparation Time: 10 minutes*

 *Cooking Time: 30 minutes*

 *Total Time: 40 minutes*

Ingredients

2 large sweet potatoes

1tbsp olive oil

Sea salt

Preparation

1. Preheat the oven to 200C.
2. Prick the sweet potatoes with a fork and rub all over with the oil and salt.
3. Place directly on the oven shelf and bake for about 30 minutes until cooked through (if doing wedges, cook on a baking sheet and reduce time to 20 minutes).

FRIED SWEET POTATOES

 *Servings: 2*

 *Preparation Time: 10 minutes*

 *Cooking Time: 15 minutes*

 *Total Time: 25 minutes*

Ingredients

2 large sweet potatoes, cubed

Lard, dripping or goose fat for shallow frying

Sea salt

4 garlic cloves, smashed

2 sprigs rosemary

Preparation

1. Heat an inch of fat in a frying pan.
2. Add the sweet potato, garlic and rosemary.
3. Fry the sweet potatoes for about 10-15 minutes.
4. They should be golden brown and cooked right through.
5. Drain on kitchen paper and season with sea salt before serving hot.

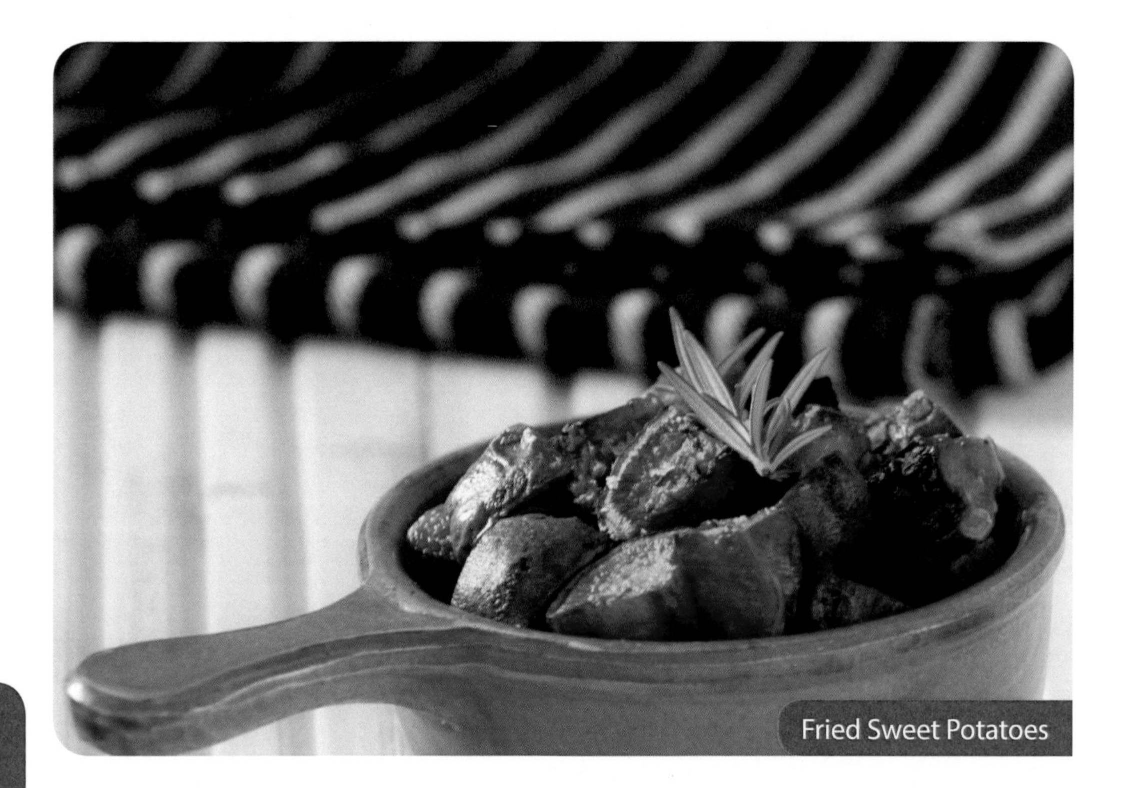

Fried Sweet Potatoes

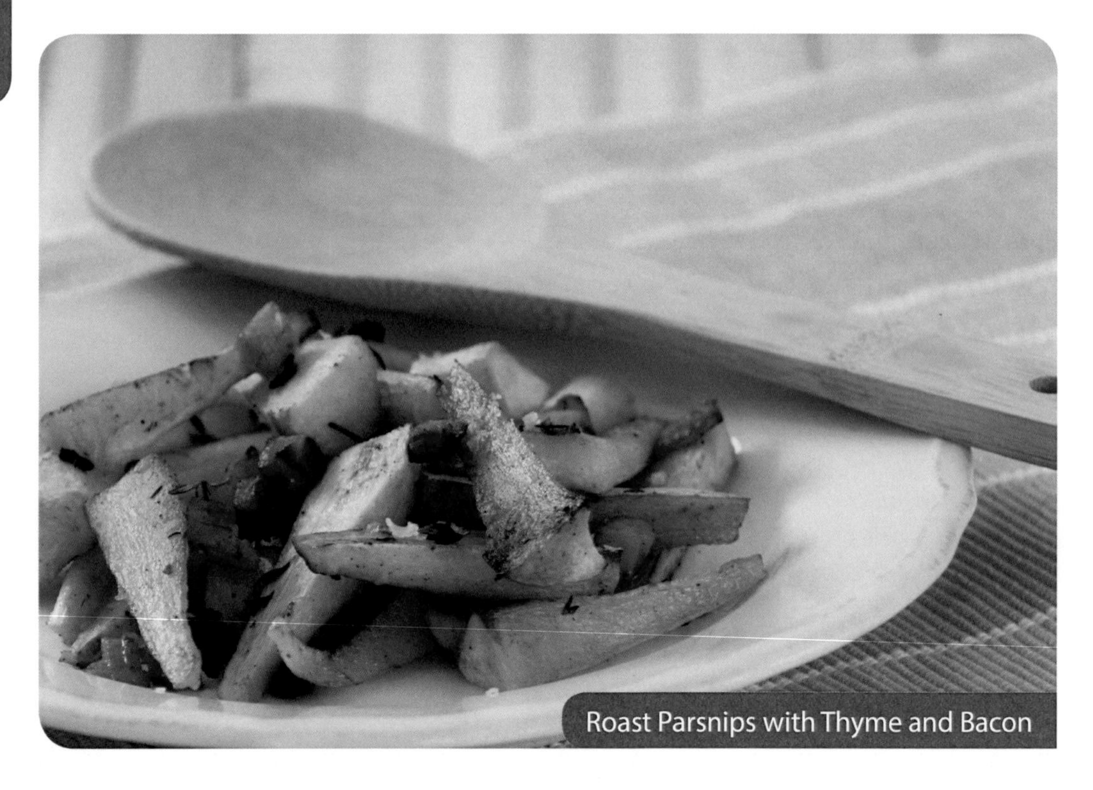

Roast Parsnips with Thyme and Bacon

ROAST PARSNIPS WITH THYME AND BACON

 *Servings: 2*

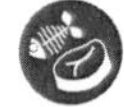 *Preparation Time: 10 minutes*

 *Cooking Time: 30 minutes*

 *Total Time: 40 minutes*

Ingredients

4 parsnips, cut into wedges

2 rashers streaky bacon, chopped

2 tbsp lard, dripping or goose fat

2 sprigs fresh thyme

Preparation

1. Preheat the oven to 200C.
2. Prepare the parsnips and bacon and then place all ingredients in a roasting dish.
3. Bake for around 30 minutes or until the parsnips are browned and crisp.
4. Serve hot.

ROASTED ROOTS

 *Servings: 2*

 *Preparation Time: 20 minutes*

 *Cooking Time: 40 minutes*

 *Total Time: 1 hour*

Ingredients

2 tbsp lard, dripping or goose fat

4 parsnips, cut into wedges

2 fresh thyme sprigs

4 carrots, cut into wedges

2 red onions, quartered with root intact

Sea salt

Preparation

1. Preheat the oven to 200C.
2. Heat the fat on a baking tray and then add the vegetables with the thyme, garlic and sea salt.
3. Roast for about 30 - 40 minutes until soft and browned, turning occasionally.
4. Serve hot.

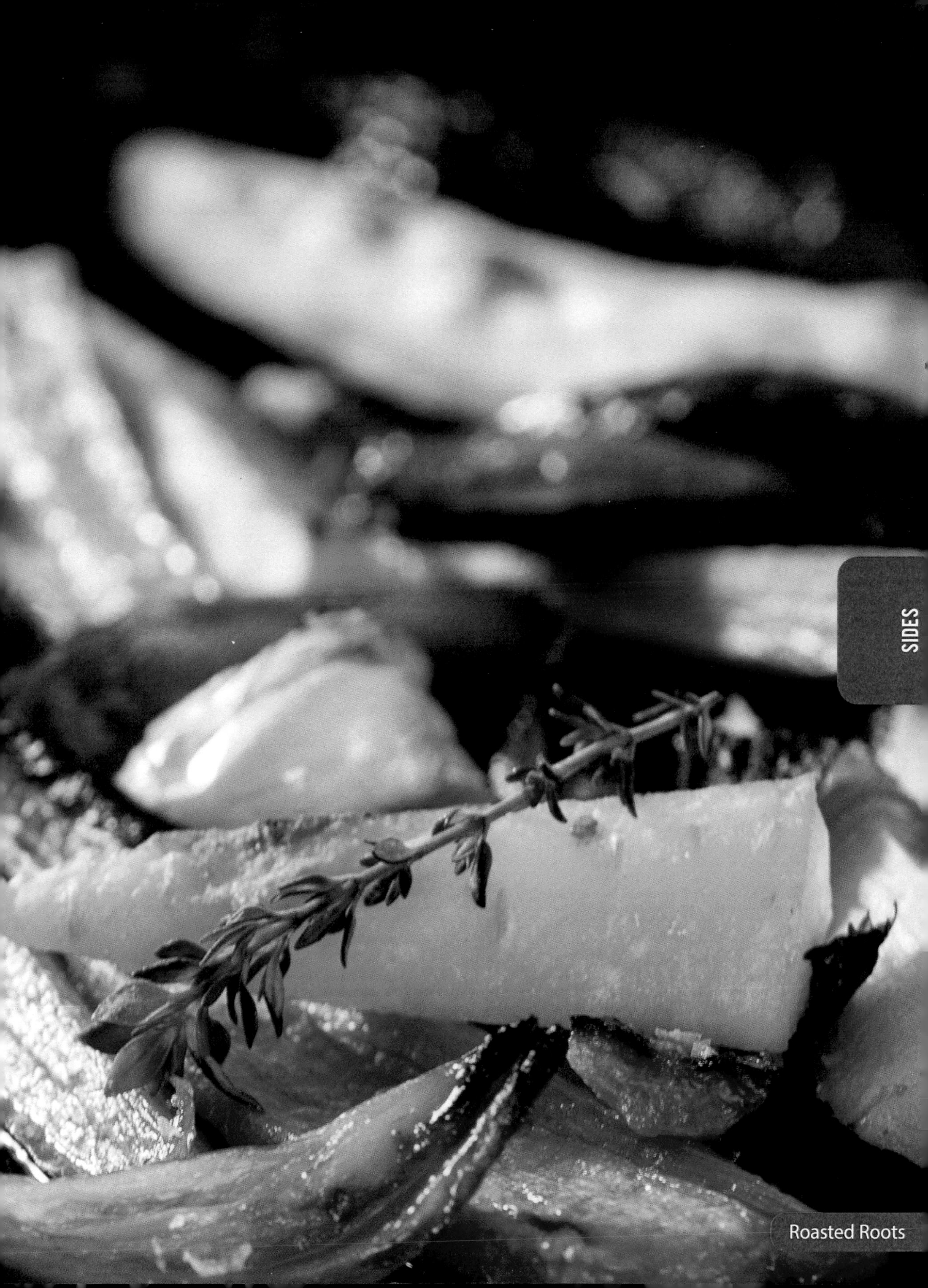
SIDES
Roasted Roots

ROOT MASH

A great alternative to potatoes, full of sweet earthy flavours and far more goodness. Choose whichever varieties of roots are available and try to get as broad a range as possible. You can also serve single root mash, or sweet potato mash. Try often overlooked ingredients such as celeriac and salsify.

 *Servings: 2*

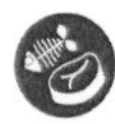 *Preparation Time: 10 minutes*

 *Cooking Time: 20 minutes*

 *Total Time: 30 minutes*

Ingredients

150g carrots, diced

150g parsnip, diced

150g swede, diced

1 tsp sea salt

Procedure

1. Place all the roots in a pan of salted water and bring to the boil.
2. Cook for about 20 minutes or until the roots are soft.
3. Drain, put the roots back into the pan and cover with a piece of kitchen paper to absorb excess water.
4. Mash the roots until soft and fluffy and serve hot.

SWEET POTATO FRIES

 *Servings: 2*

 *Preparation Time: 10 minutes*

 *Cooking Time: 20 minutes*

 *Total Time: 30 minutes*

Ingredients

2 large sweet potatoes

4 tbsp lard, dripping or goose fat

Sea salt

Preparation

1. Preheat the oven to 200C.
2. Cut the potatoes into fries, fairly skinny ones, leaving skins on.
3. Heat the fat on a baking tray and when hot add the fries.
4. Shake or stir around to coat and put back in the oven.
5. Cook for about 20 minutes, turning as needed, until the fries are browned all over.
6. Drain on kitchen roll and serve piping hot with a good pinch of sea salt.

SAUCES & STOCK

BASIC TOMATO SAUCE

This basic recipe is best cooked for a few hours to create a slick and glossy tomato sauce full of flavour. Used as the base of other recipes it is a good way to inject flavour into a midweek supper without resorting to ready-made jars. Fresh herbs work best, especially if you have a few woody herbs growing outside, but dried will be just fine if it is all that you have. Woody herbs such as thyme, rosemary and bay freeze particularly well so if you buy a large bag just pop it straight into the freezer and use as required.

 *Servings: 6*

 *Preparation Time: 5 minutes*

 *Cooking Time: 2 hours*

 *Total Time: 2 hours, 5 minutes*

Ingredients

800g chopped tinned tomatoes

1 tsp sea salt

2 sprigs thyme

1 head garlic, cut in half horizontally

4 tbsp olive oil

1 bay leaf

1 sprig rosemary

Preparation

1. Place a large saucepan over a low heat and add all of the ingredients.
2. Using the empty tin, measure out the same amount of water and add to the pan.
3. Leave the sauce alone, giving it the occasional stir, until it is thick and glossy. The lower and slower it cooks, the better it will be.
4. Once done, fish out the stalks and bits before leaving to cool and using as required. You may wish to blend for a smoother sauce if preferred.

CHICKEN STOCK

Using the bones from a roast chicken to make stock not only proves value for money in providing the means for another meal, but chicken stock is a great way of adding flavour and nutrients to a meal. Use it for making soup, cooking vegetetables or making sauces; it will liven up your cooking no end.

You don't need to add carrots, onions, bay leaves and their ilk to the stock pot, although you can if you wish. The flavour of the chicken is enough in itself and doesn't muddy other flavours with an overpowering stock. A good stock, made from decent bones, will turn to jelly in the fridge. In fact a cheap chicken from a battery hen will often make stock that refuses to set; a sure sign of immature, mineral deficient bones.

A good tip is to freeze chicken bones until they are needed for a stock in a plastic container. They will last for weeks and ensure you have a ready supply of stock bones for when you need them. No need to defrost when making a stock, just add them straight to the pan and follow the instructions below.

 *Servings: 6*

 *Preparation Time: 10 minutes*

 *Cooking Time: 1 hr, 30 minutes*

 *Total Time: 1 hr, 40 minutes*

Ingredients

2 small leftover chicken carcasses (cooked)

1.5 litres water

Procedure

1. You will get better stock if you chop the carcass and the long bones in half first.
2. Lay them in a large pan, preferably one with more height than girth, and cover with cold water by a few inches.
3. Bring the pot slowly to a simmer, skimming off any scum that appears on top of the liquid.
4. Keep the stock at a gentle simmer; cooking it too rapidly makes a greasy, bitter, cloudy stock.
5. Once reduced by about half, remove all bones (strain if you can) and leave to cool completely before keeping in the fridge for up to 3 days.

DESSERTS

No menu plan would be complete without some desserts for those with a sweet tooth. We all have days where we need to treat ourselves to a dessert – sometimes just nothing else will suffice.

We have created some Paleo friendly desserts that will allow you to satisfy your sweet cravings but without filling your body with refined sugars and preservatives. You will be amazed at how good they taste and you will have your family and friends converting to them in no time. They are all quick to make and use only minimal ingredients. You will even be able to eat ice-cream. Sound good to you?

The desserts should be eaten as a treat and have been included as part of your weekly meal plans. By all means substitute our dessert suggestions for your own recipe or creation, remember there is always the option of a fruit salad for those nights where you just want something light and refreshing. You can make a fantastic fruit salad out of your favourite fruits – why not try adding something a bit more exotic or adding pomegranate seeds for some added texture and taste. The options really are endless.

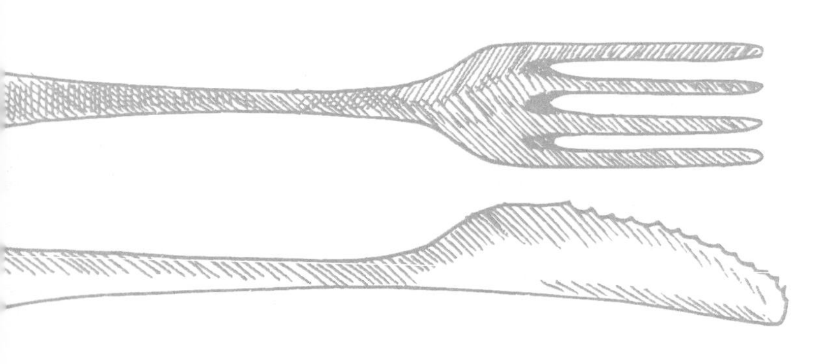

BAKED BANANA SPLIT

 *Servings: 2*

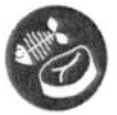 *Preparation Time: 5 minutes*

 *Cooking Time: 15 minutes*

 *Total Time: 20 minutes*

Ingredients

2 banana, unpeeled

50g dark chocolate, chopped

50g raspberries

25g flaked almonds

Preparation

1. Split the banana down the centre and stuff with chocolate.
2. Wrap in foil and bake in a hot oven until the chocolate has melted.
3. Unwrap and top with the raspberries and almonds before eating from the skin with a teaspoon.

COCONUT HOT CHOCOLATE

This is a delicious treat for those cold, wet winter evenings.

 *Servings: 2*

 *Cooking Time: 5 minutes*

Ingredients

50g dark chocolate

200ml coconut milk

Preparation

1. Stir the ingredients together in a small saucepan over a low heat until the chocolate and coconut cream have melted.
2. Pour into mugs and enjoy.

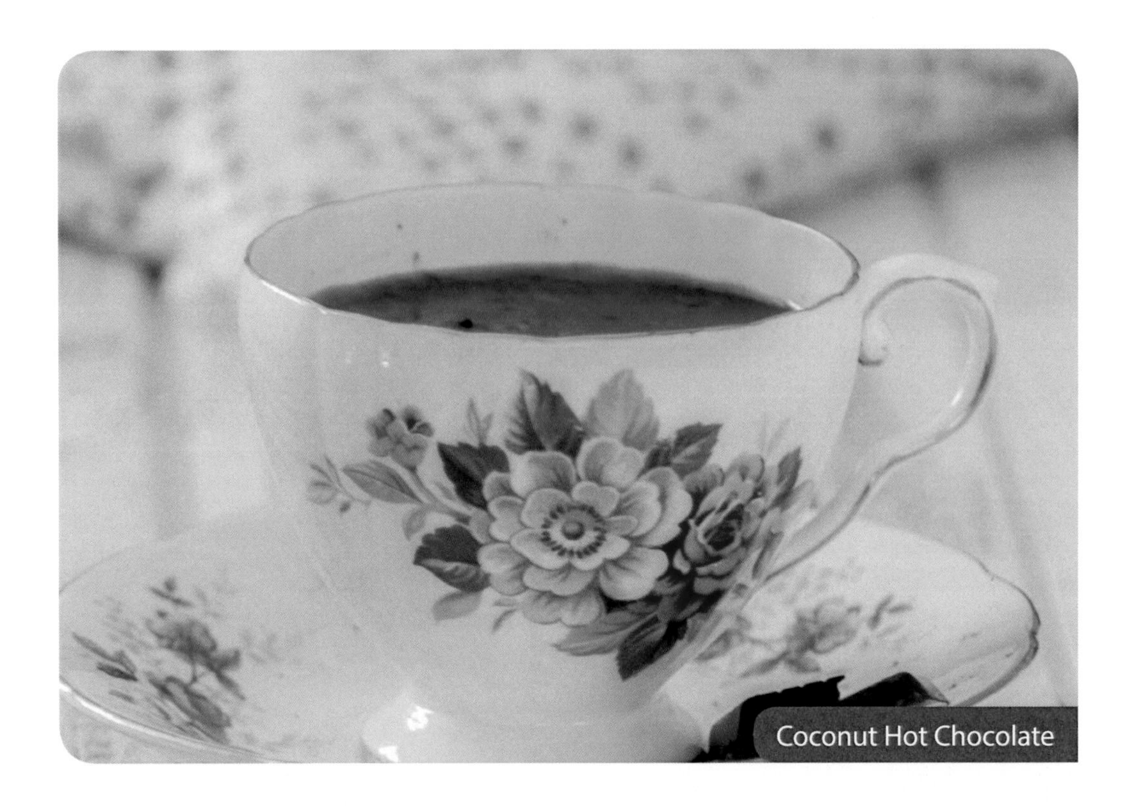

Coconut Hot Chocolate

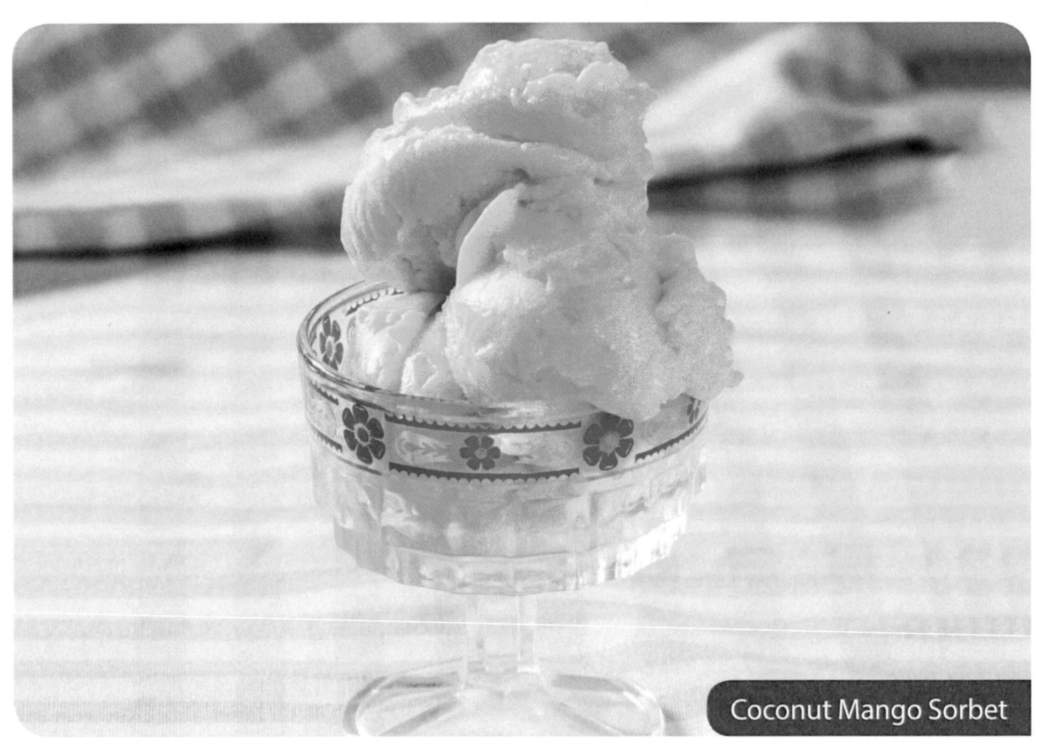

Coconut Mango Sorbet

COCONUT MANGO SORBET

This sweet and flavoursome dish must be prepared and eaten straight away as the sorbet will rapidly melt once made.

 *Servings: 2*

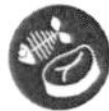 *Preparation Time: 10 minutes*

Ingredients

100ml coconut milk

400g frozen mango cubes

Preparation

1. Blitz together for a smooth frozen dessert.
2. For a thicker result add either more fruit or a few tbsp of ground almonds.

GRILLED PAPAYA WITH LIME

 *Servings: 2*

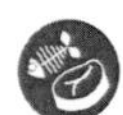 *Preparation Time: 5 minutes*

 *Cooking Time: 10 minutes*

 *Total Time: 15 minutes*

Ingredients

1 large papaya, sliced and peeled

1 tbsp raw honey

1 lime, juice only

Preparation

1. Mix the honey with the lime and drizzle over the fruit slices.
2. Fry or grill to soften and release the flavours, but take care not to overcook or burn.

GRILLED PEACHES WITH CINNAMON

 *Servings: 2*

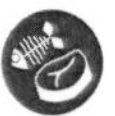 *Preparation Time: 10 minutes*

 *Cooking Time: 5 minutes*

 *Total Time: 15 minutes*

Ingredients

2 peaches, halved

1 tsp coconut oil

1 tsp cinnamon

Preparation

1. Slice peaches in half and remove the stone.
2. Brush with coconut oil and sprinkle with cinnamon.
3. Grill or pan fry for a few minutes just to soften the fruit.

LYCHEE, PINEAPPLE AND COCONUT CREAM

 *Servings: 2*

 *Preparation Time: 10 minutes*

Ingredients

400g tin lychees (or fresh if you can find them)

1 lime, juice and zest

¼ fresh pineapple, chopped

200ml coconut cream

Procedure

1. Arrange the fruit into bowls.
2. Add the lime zest and juice to the coconut cream.
3. Pour the cream over the fruit and serve.

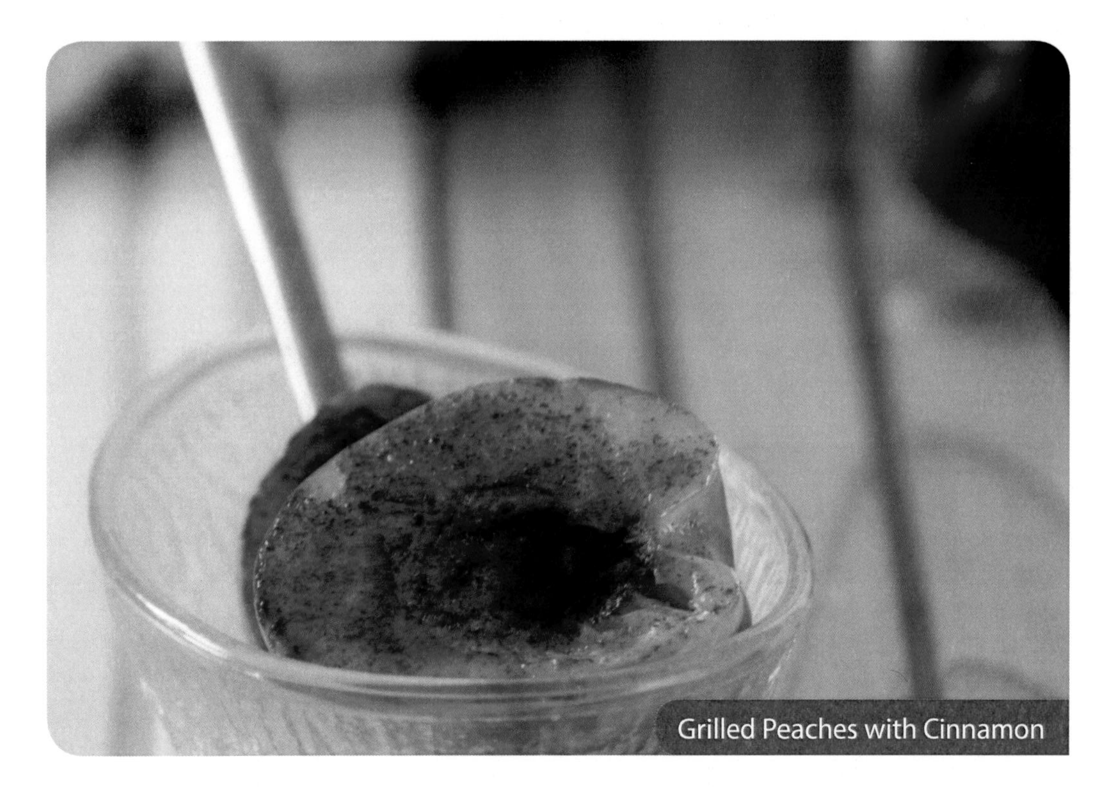
Grilled Peaches with Cinnamon

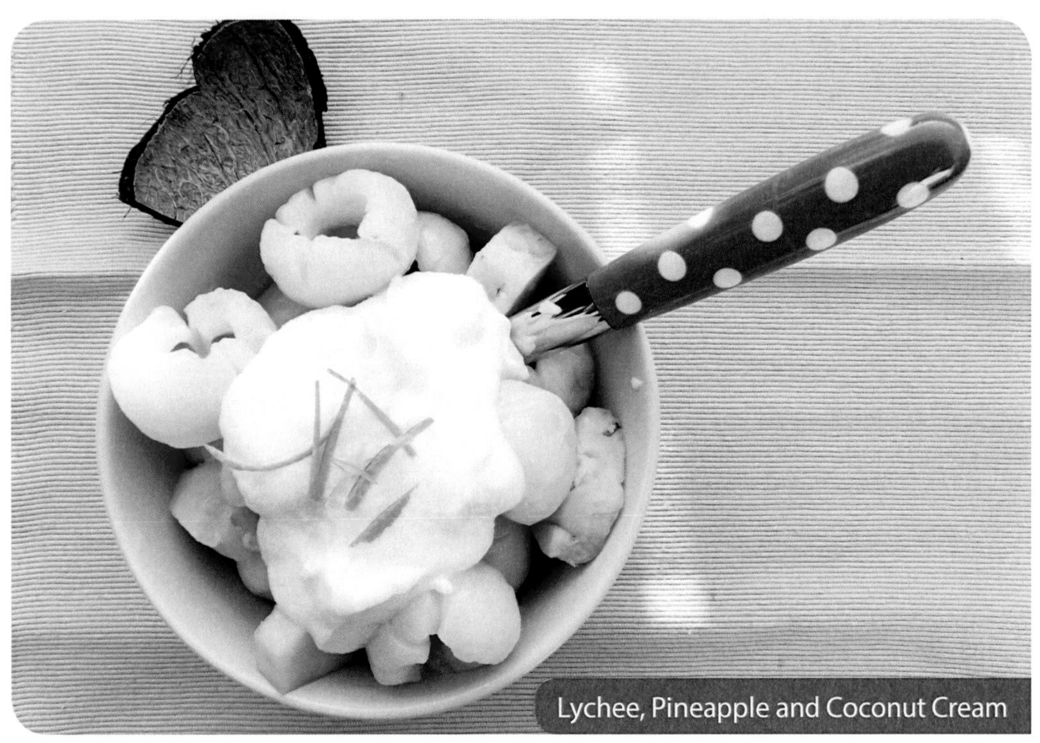
Lychee, Pineapple and Coconut Cream

PAN FRIED APPLES

Choose a firm eating apple that will hold its shape for this dish.

 *Servings: 2*

 *Preparation Time: 10 minutes*

 *Cooking Time: 10 minutes*

 *Total Time: 20 minutes*

Ingredients

4 apples, cored and sliced in thick wedges

2 tbsp coconut oil

1 tsp cinnamon

1 pinch nutmeg

Preparation

1 Coat the apple wedges in the spices.

2 Heat the oil in a frying pan and cook the apples until browned around the edges.

3 Serve warm.

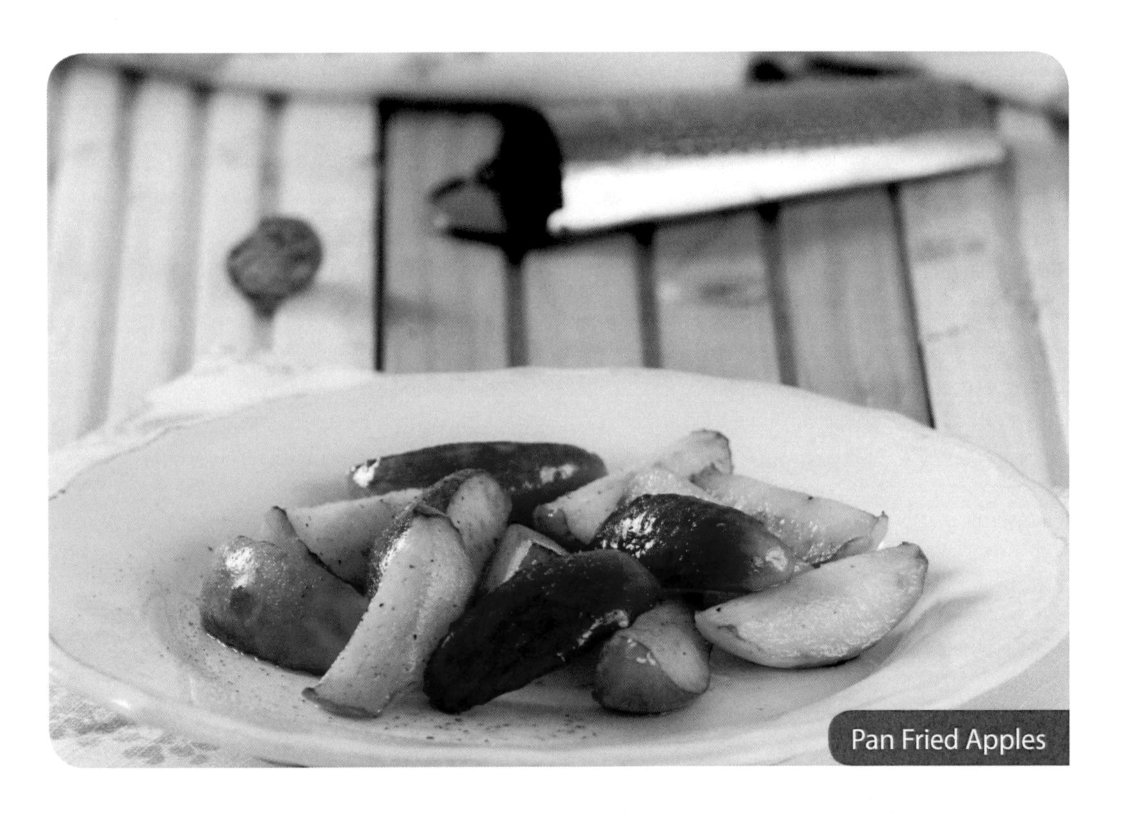
Pan Fried Apples

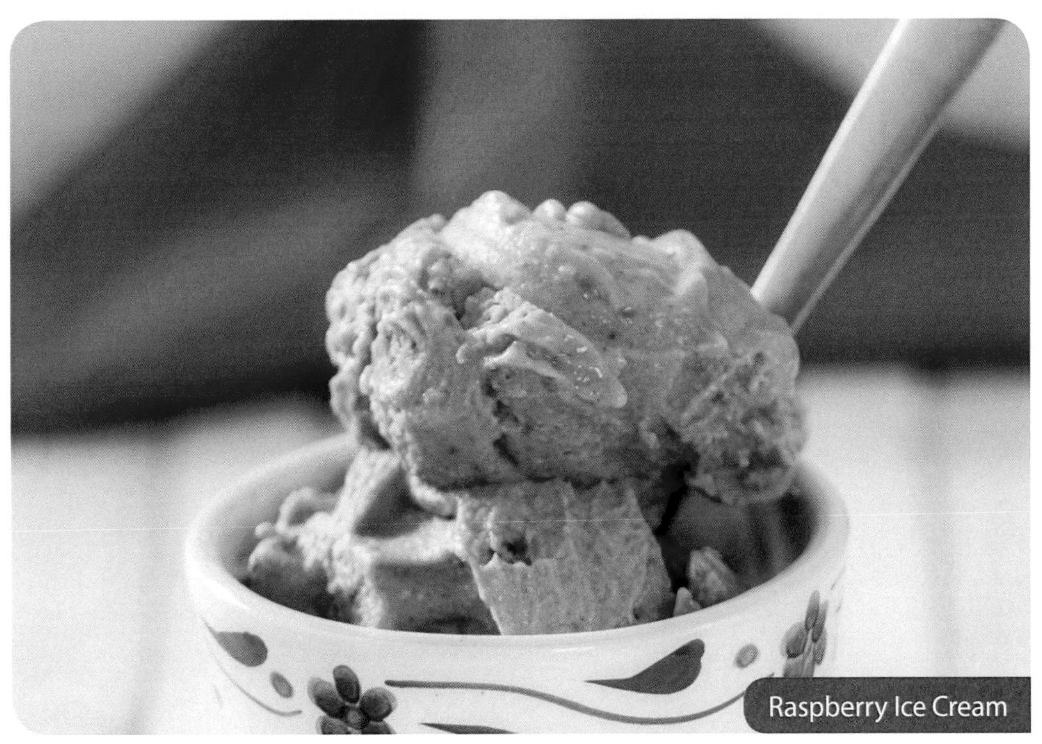
Raspberry Ice Cream

RASPBERRY ICE CREAM

Never throw an old banana away. Peel it and chop into pieces before keeping it in the freezer in a plastic container. The banana can not only be used for ice cream recipes but also for numerous other sweet treats including Paleo brownies.

 *Servings: 2*

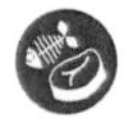 *Preparation Time: 10 minutes*

Ingredients

150g frozen raspberries

1 banana, frozen in chunks

50ml coconut milk

2 tbsp ground almonds

Preparation

1. Place everything into a blender and blitz together to form a soft frozen dessert. Sweeten with a little honey if you feel it needs it.
2. Eat immediately as the ice cream will melt quickly.

ROAST PLUMS WITH STAR ANISE AND CASHEW NUT CREAM

 *Servings: 2*

 *Preparation Time: 10 minutes*

 *Cooking Time: 30 minutes*

 *Total Time: 40 minutes*

Ingredients

8 ripe plums, stoned and halved

1 tbsp coconut oil

2 star anise

FOR THE CASHEW CREAM

100g cashew nuts

100ml water

Preparation

1. Preheat the oven to 200C.
2. Place the plums, star anise and coconut oil in a heat proof dish with a few drops of water; cover with foil.
3. Bake for 30 minutes until soft.
4. Meanwhile, make the cashew cream by blitzing the nuts with the water in a blender until as smooth as you can get it. Any leftovers will last in the fridge for a few days.
5. Serve the hot plums with the cold cashew cream.

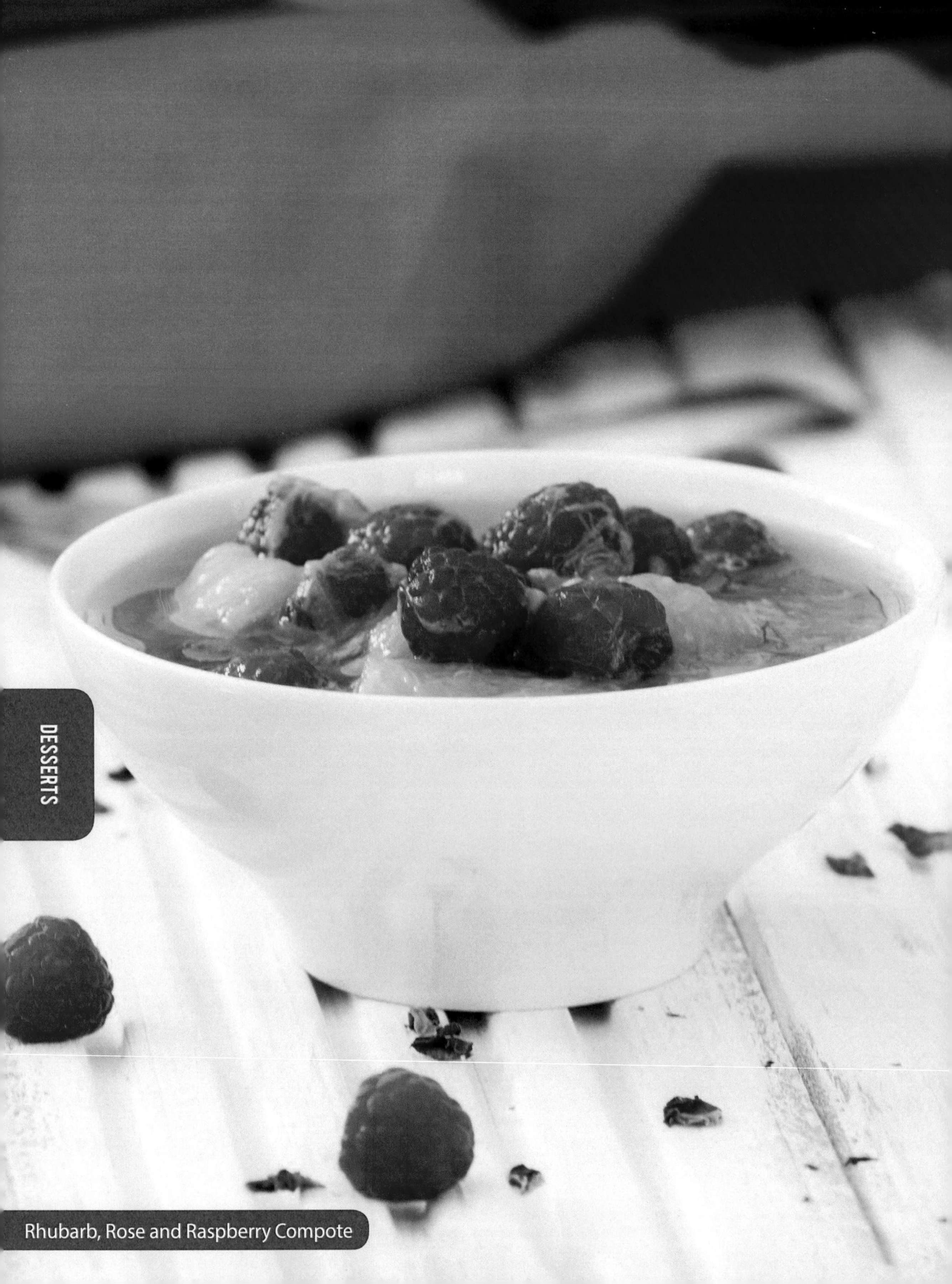

Rhubarb, Rose and Raspberry Compote

RHUBARB, ROSE AND RASPBERRY COMPOTE

 *Servings: 4*

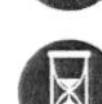 *Preparation Time: 10 minutes*

 *Cooking Time: 10 minutes*

 *Inactive Time: 30 minutes*

Total Time: 50 minutes

Ingredients

500g rhubarb, chopped

150g raspberries

150ml water

1 tbsp honey

1 tbsp rose water

Preparation

1. Place the rhubarb, honey and water in a pan and cook gently for about 10 minutes or until the rhubarb is soft.
2. Add the raspberries and then set aside to cool.
3. Sprinkle with rose water before serving.

VANILLA PEARS

 *Servings: 2*

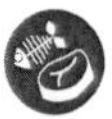 *Preparation Time: 10 minutes*

 *Cooking Time: 20 minutes*

 *Total Time: 30 minutes*

Ingredients

2 soft, sweet pears, peeled and cored

1 vanilla pod, split

FOR THE CASHEW CREAM

100g cashew nuts

100ml water

Preparation

1. Poach the pears in an inch of water, with the vanilla pod, and a lid on the pan so that they steam through as well as poach.
2. Meanwhile, make the cashew cream by blitzing the nuts with the water in a blender until as smooth as you can get it. Any leftovers will last in the fridge for a few days.
3. Eat the pears hot or cold with a spoonful of cashew cream.

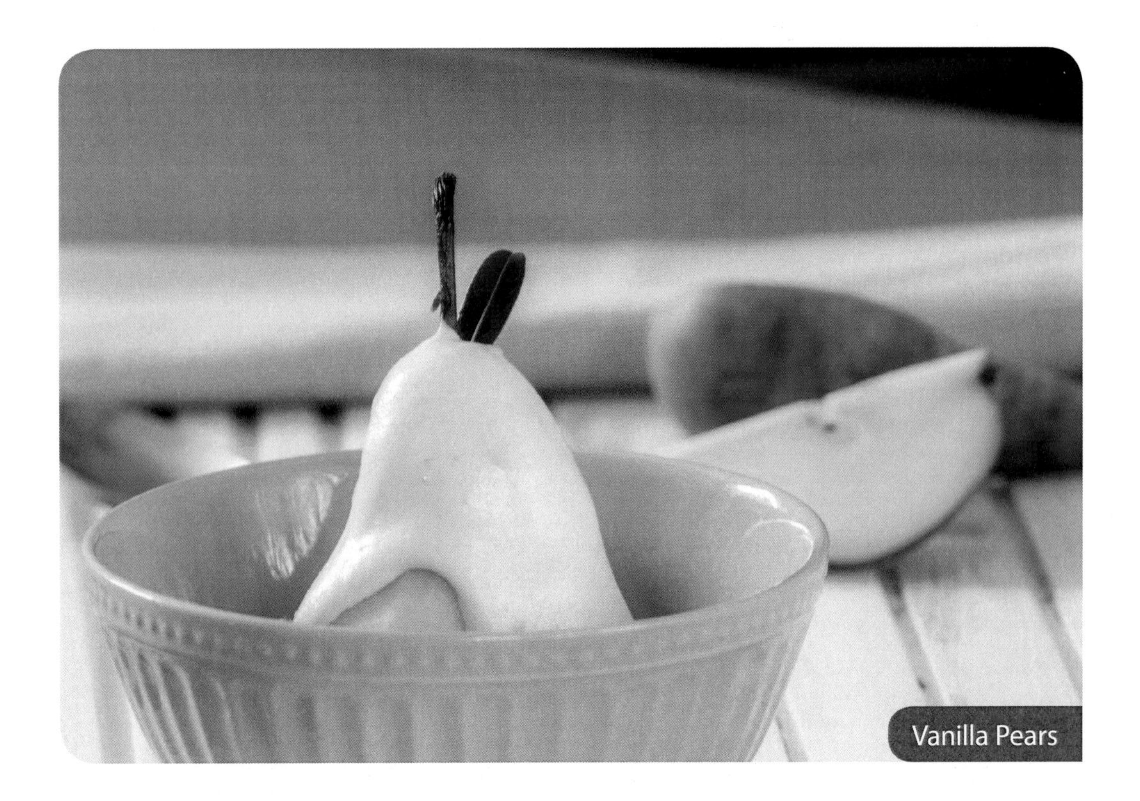
Vanilla Pears

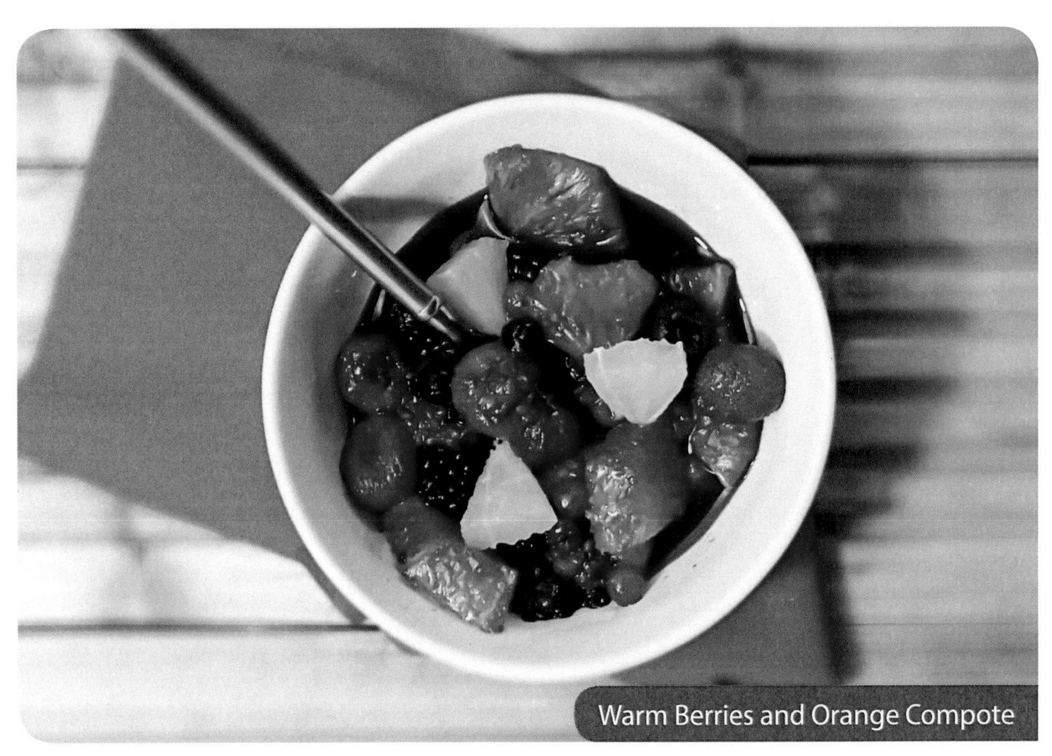
Warm Berries and Orange Compote

WARM BERRIES AND ORANGE COMPOTE

 *Servings: 2*

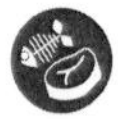 *Preparation Time: 5 minutes*

 *Cooking Time: 10 minutes*

 *Total Time: 15 minutes*

Ingredients

200g frozen berries

1 orange, peeled and segmented

2 tbsp water

1 cinnamon stick

Preparation

1. Prepare the orange by peeling and cutting into segments.
2. Place all of the ingredients in a saucepan over a medium heat.
3. Simmer for about 10 minutes or until the liquid has reduced and the berries are soft.
4. Serve hot or cold.

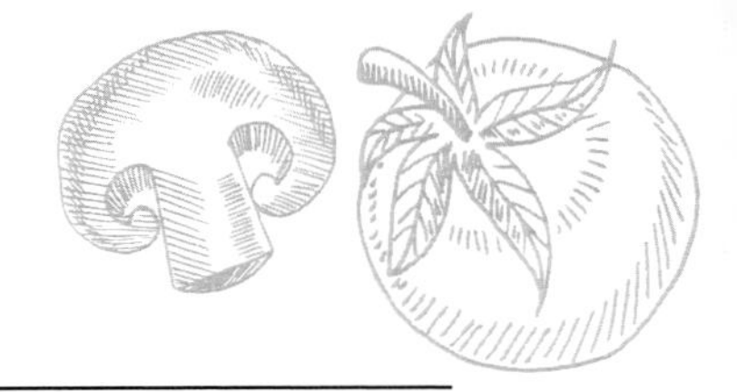

SNACKS

We know that for many people the ability to snack is make or break for the success of a diet. We all love to snack. Whether it is because we are genuinely hungry or we just want to get away from our desk to have a chat in the kitchen at work. Snacking for many is a social activity (think of the cakes you get at work) and is often quite comforting. Many people may not even know that they are snacking as often as they are and it can be a big contributor for many a person's weight gain.

We have therefore created some Paleo friendly snacks that can be used if you are feeling hungry between meals. In the first few weeks of your Paleo transition it is likely that you will need more snacks as your body adjusts to the new routine.

As you progress through the 12 week programme you will find that your appetite levels out and you may not need the snacks as often as you did to start with. You should always remember that this is a snack. It should only be small portion to calm your feelings of hunger and should not develop into a full blown meal in itself as this will impact on your progress.

Our Paleo friendly recipes provide some interesting additions to the usual list of snacks and are useful if you are having friends over and want an alternative to highly processed food options for finger food.

There are also many quick and easy snacks which are easy to pick up when you are out and about from health food stores.

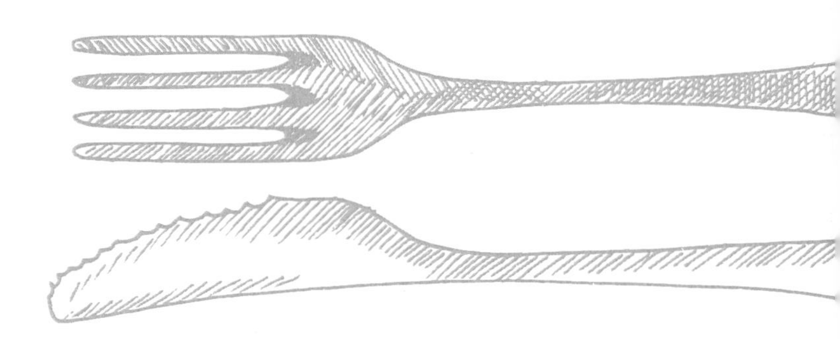

COURGETTE HUMMUS

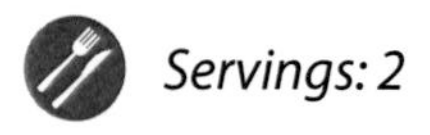
Servings: 2

Preparation Time: 20 minutes

Ingredients

2 medium courgettes, peeled and chopped

1 tsp cumin

1 tbsp lemon juice

2 tbsp olive oil

2 garlic cloves, crushed

1 pinch sea salt

2 tbsp tahini

Preparation

1. Prepare the courgettes and garlic.
2. Use a food processor to blend the courgettes with the garlic, salt and spices.
3. Add the tahini and a little oil with a dash of lemon juice.
4. Depending on the water content of the courgettes you may need to add a little more oil/lemon to taste.
5. The consistency should be similar to that of a dip.
6. You can add a spoonful of ground almonds if you want to make it thicker.
7. Serve cold and store in the fridge.

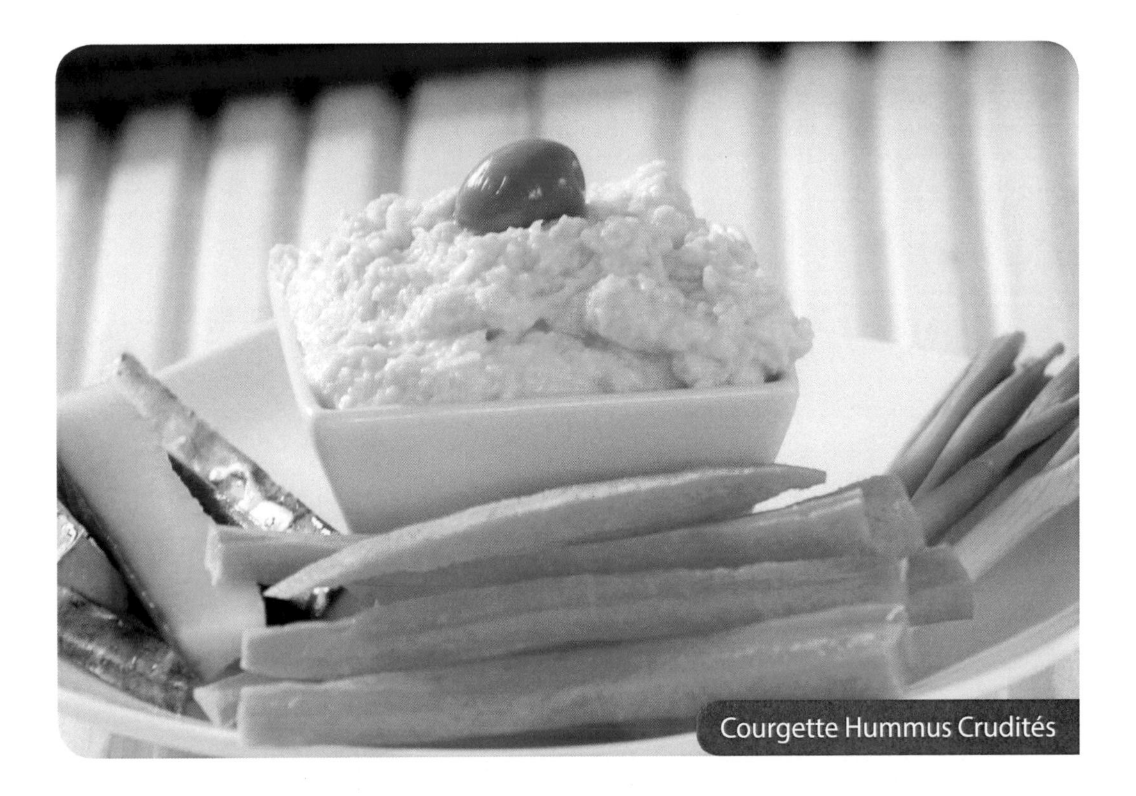

Courgette Hummus Crudités

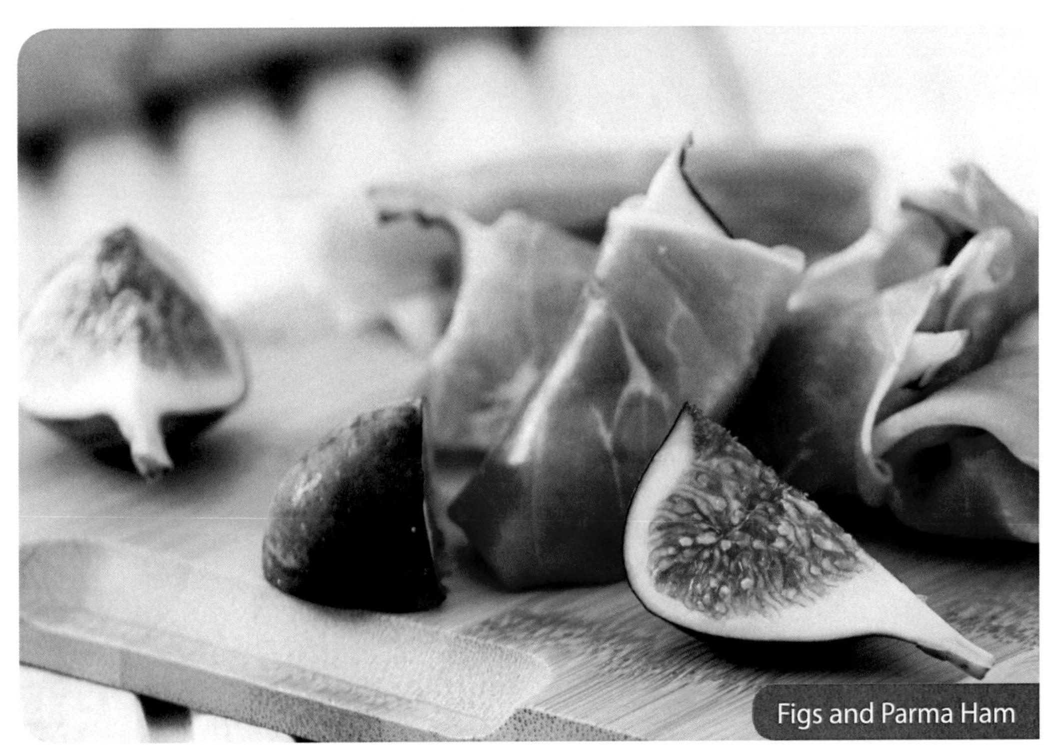

Figs and Parma Ham

CRUDITÉS

These are handy to prepare in advance so that you can keep them in your fridge ready to eat if you get the urge for a snack or need to eat something quickly on the run.

 *Servings: 2*

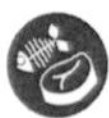 *Preparation Time: 10 minutes*

Ingredients

2 carrots

4 celery sticks

1 cucumber

1 red bell pepper

Preparation

1 Cut the crudités into batons about 5cm in length.

2 Eat with your favourite Paleo dip such as *Guacamole; Fiery Aubergine Dip* or *Avocado, Red Onion and Green Pepper Salsa.*

FIGS AND PARMA HAM

 *Servings: 2*

 *Preparation Time: 5 minutes*

Ingredients

4 ripe figs, quartered

4 large slices Parma ham, torn in quarters

Preparation

1 Wrap the ham around the figs and enjoy the sweet salty flavours.

FLAX CRACKERS

This recipe can take some practice to get the desired thickness. You can change the flavours by using different herbs or spices too. In the UK, flax is often known as linseed although the two terms are now equally widespread. They can be a good accompaniment to the home made Guacamole dip.

 *Servings: 12*

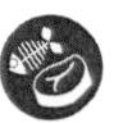 *Preparation Time: 20 minutes*

 *Cooking Time: 20 minutes*

 *Total Time: 40 minutes*

Ingredients

165g flax seeds (or coarse flax meal)
½ tsp fresh rosemary, finely chopped
150-100ml water
40g chia seeds
1 tsp sea salt

Preparation

1. Preheat your oven to 200C.
2. Grind the seeds to a coarse meal (or look for ground flax meal).
3. Stir in the salt with the rosemary.
4. Mix in the water 30-50ml at a time. You are looking for a dry, course dough which won't fully bind on its own, but largely comes together.
5. Line a baking tray with grease proof paper and place the mixture on top.
6. Spread roughly over the baking sheet and cover with another piece of grease proof paper to prevent it sticking. Place another baking try on top and press down hard. You want to get the mixture to spread evenly across the tray to a thickness of about 3mm.
7. Once evenly spread, you can use a knife or pizza cutter to score the mixture. This will help later when breaking into individual pieces. Take care not to cut right through however – you just want to score the mix.
8. Bake in the oven for about 20 minutes until hard.
9. Remove from the oven and place onto a wire rack, allowing the crackers to cool completely.
10. Break into pieces and store in an airtight container for up to 2 weeks.

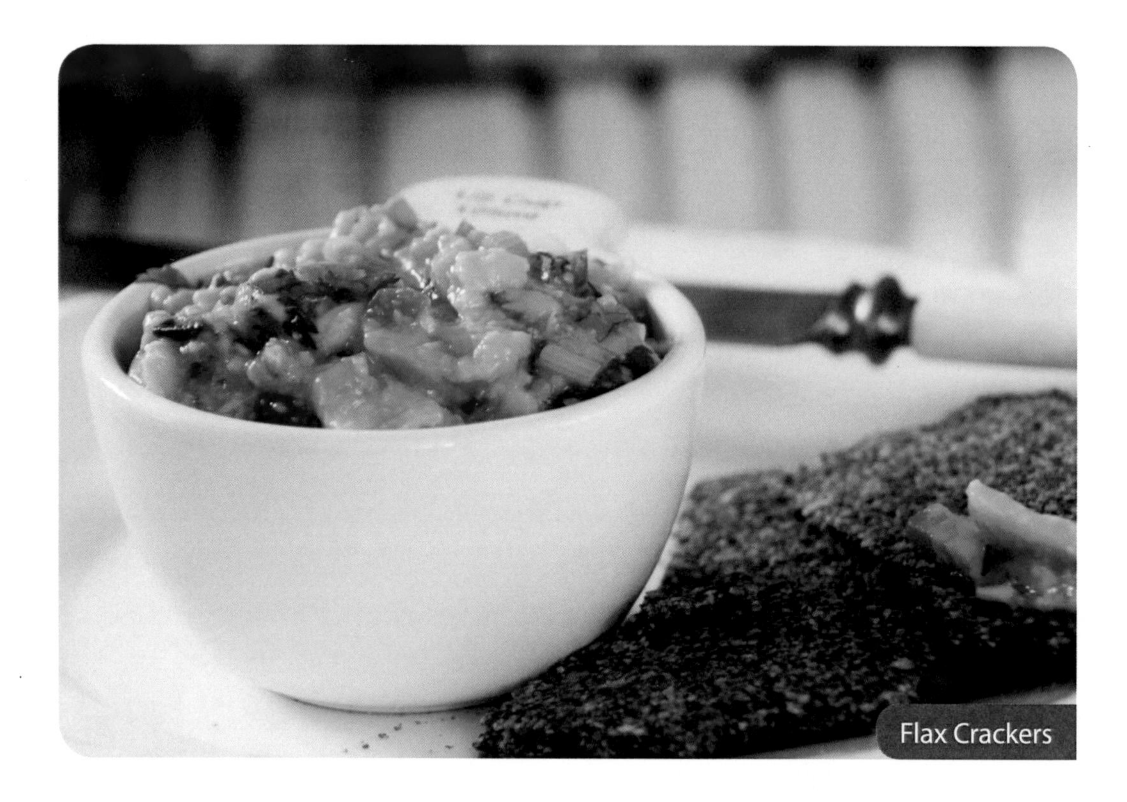

Flax Crackers

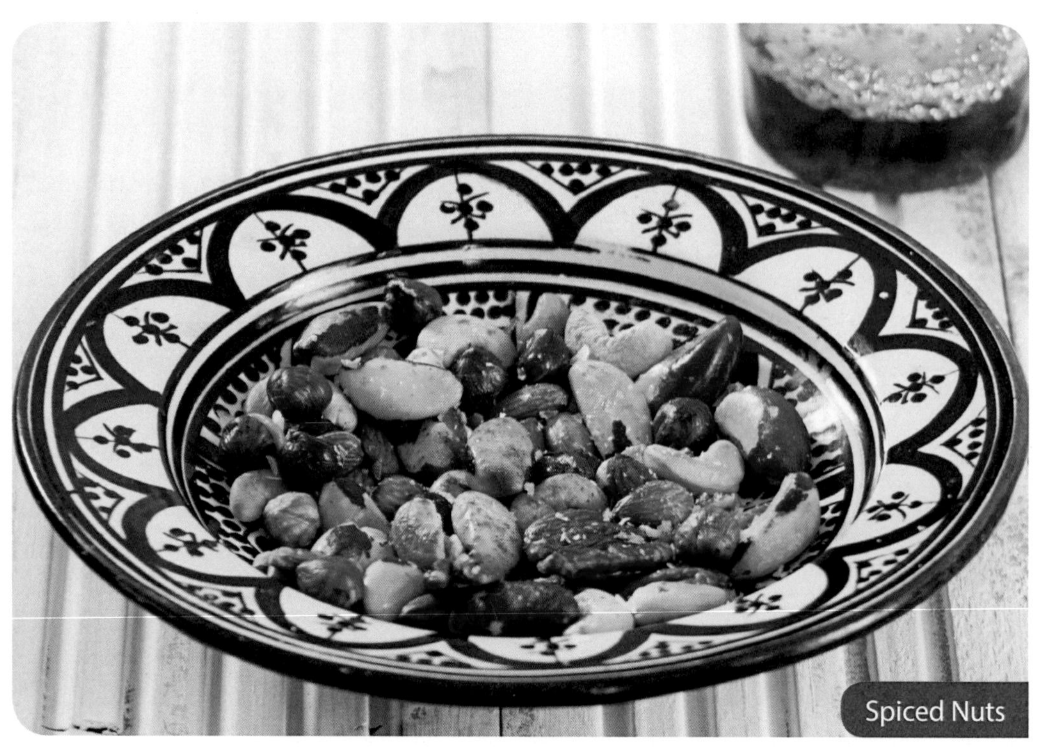

Spiced Nuts

SNACKS

SPICED NUTS

Feel free to select whatever nuts you like for this recipe. We like a good mixture, but that's no reason why you can't use just one type or any other combination you fancy. Try different blends to keep up the variety.

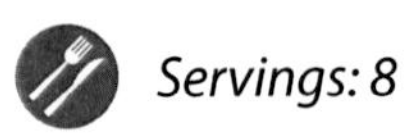

Servings: 8

Cooking Time: 20 minutes

Ingredients

200g mixed unsalted nuts

½ tsp cayenne

½ tsp ground cumin

Sea salt

2 tbsp coconut oil

½ tsp cinnamon

½ tsp ground coriander

Preparation

1. Heat the oil in a large frying pan over a gentle heat and add the nuts.
2. Stir for about 5 minutes so the nuts brown gently.
3. Add the spices with a good pinch of salt.
4. Stir for another minute and remove from the pan to cool.
5. Eat as a snack but make sure it is used as a treat.

KALE CRISPS

 *Servings: 2*

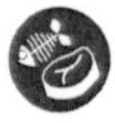 *Preparation Time: 10 minutes*

 *Cooking Time: 40 minutes*

 *Total Time: 50 minutes*

Ingredients

1 bunch kale

2 tbsp lard, dripping or goose fat

1 tbsp lemon juice

Sea salt

Preparation

1. Preheat your oven to 150C.
2. Wash the kale, drain and pat dry.
3. Remove the stems and cut the leaves into even sized pieces.
4. Melt the fat and toss with the kale, coating thoroughly.
5. Season with salt and add the lemon juice.
6. Place the kale in a single layer on a baking tray. You may need 2 or more trays depending on size.
7. Cook for about 40 minutes, turning regularly.
8. Allow to cool and sprinkle with extra sea salt if desired.

MARINATED OLIVES

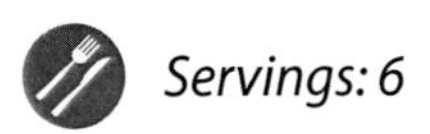 *Servings: 6*

 *Preparation Time: 10 minutes*

Ingredients

300g mixed olives

2 tbsp olive oil

2 tbsp fresh parsley, chopped

2 garlic cloves, finely sliced

1 red chilli, finely sliced

1 tbsp balsamic vinegar

Preparation

1. Mix together and eat as desired.
2. The olives will keep in an airtight jar in the fridge so this is a great snack to prepare at the weekend in advance of the busy week ahead.

SARDINE PATE

 *Servings: 2*

 *Preparation Time: 10 minutes*

Ingredients

1 tin sardines in olive oil

1 lemon, juice only

Freshly ground black pepper

1 small onion, finely chopped

1 tbsp parsley

Preparation

1. Place the sardines and onion in a blender and blitz into a paste (as course as you desire).
2. Add the lemon juice, parsley and a good pinch of freshly ground pepper and mix thoroughly.
3. Serve alone or with our Paleo Flax Crackers.

SMOOTHIES & JUICES

We have provided some juice and smoothie recipes that you can use as an alternative to a snack or if you just feel like you need an extra boost of vitamins. They are quick and easy to make and very satisfying.

Our recipes use both a juicer and blender. If you do not have a juicer we would recommend that you consider getting one. They are a great piece of equipment to have and will ensure that you do not lose any of the great vitamins and minerals from the fruit and vegetables.

As with all our recipes they can be adapted to use your favourite ingredients. Have a play around and see which recipe you like the most. Don't be afraid of the vegetable juices they are really tasty and of course very good for you!

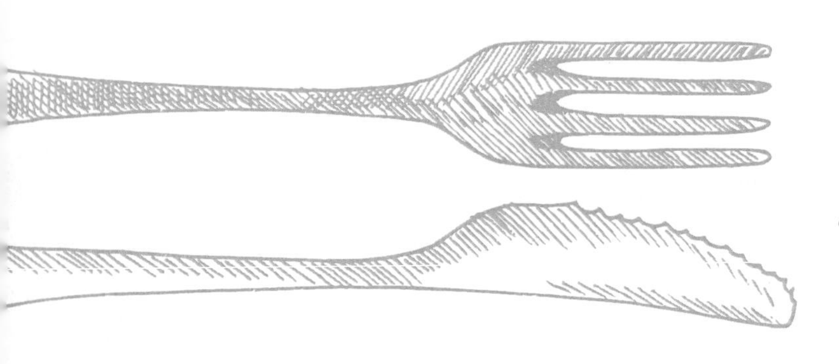

GRAPEFRUIT AND GINGER SHOTS

Grapefruit contains fat burning enzymes and helps keep blood sugar levels stable. It is also a good source of soluble fibre. Ginger stimulates the digestive tract and therefore encourages fat burning.

Knock this shot back for a morning wake-up call and a metabolic boost. Try replacing your morning cup of coffee with this nutritious boost!

 *Servings: 1*

 *Preparation Time: 10 minutes*

Ingredients

1 grapefruit, peeled and halved (depending on your juicer)

1 inch fresh ginger, peeled

Preparation

1. Prepare the grapefruit and ginger.
2. Place the ingredients into your juicer.
3. Knock it straight back.

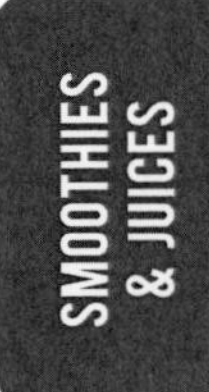

CRANBERRY, STRAWBERRY AND LIME SPRITZER

Cranberries are well known for their antibacterial qualities, whilst limes have an alkalising effect that aids waste elimination. Strawberries not only add sweetness to the sharp fruits but are a good source of soluble fibre; essential for optimal daily detox. This creates a sharp and delicious but detoxifying grown up drink.

 *Servings: 1*

 *Preparation Time: 5 minutes*

Ingredients

10 strawberries, hulled

2 limes, juice only

20 cranberries

250ml fizzy mineral water

Handful of ice cubes

Preparation

1. Blend the strawberries and cranberries together to form a puree.
2. Add the juice of the limes and top up with fizzy mineral water.
3. Serve over ice for a cool and refreshing drink.

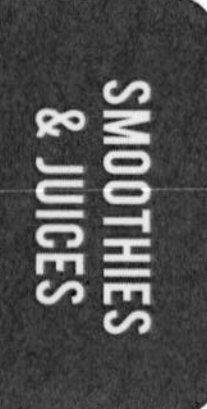

PINEAPPLE, APRICOT AND BANANA

This is a thick satisfying smoothie for those in need of a pick me up, this drink contains pineapple for its sweet flavour and energy boosting manganese as well as dried apricots for much needed potassium and iron. It is boosted with banana for creamy sweetness and a drop of coconut milk to up the comfort stakes. It is a Paleo Pina Colada!

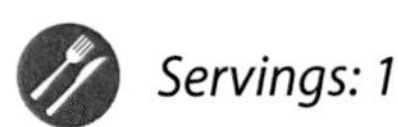

Servings: 1

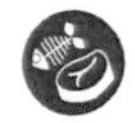

Preparation Time: 5 minutes

Ingredients

½ pineapple, cored and peeled

1 banana, peeled

4 dried apricots

100ml coconut milk

Handful of ice cubes

Preparation

1. Juice the pineapple and then place the juice to a blender.
2. Add the remaining ingredients and blend creating a thick and creamy smoothie.
3. If you find it too thick then you can add some water or coconut water as desired.
4. Serve over ice.

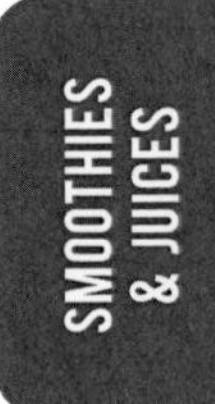

MANGO, PEAR AND GINGER

Pears are one of the greatest ingredients in the fight against colon cancer with a variety of protective benefits. Mango, with its rich soothing texture and silky sweetness, is calming to the stomach as well as an antacid. Finally, no digestive aid would be complete without ginger and its anti-inflammatory properties that soothe the digestion and treat nausea.

 *Servings: 1*

 *Preparation Time: 5 minutes*

Ingredients

2 pears, cored and halved

1 green apple, cored and halved

1 ripe mango, peeled and halved

1 inch fresh ginger, peeled

Handful of ice cubes

Preparation

1. Juice the pears, apple and ginger.
2. Place the juice into a blender.
3. Add the mango and blend.
4. You can either serve over ice or add the ice to the blender with the mango.

GREEN JUICE

This green juice contains a variety of nutrient rich vegetables along with a vitamin packed avocado which will make the juice creamy and satisfying. It is a really useful juice to have as a snack as it is nutrient dense and very filling. It will give you lots of energy and leave you wanting more. You can add any of your favourite green vegetables to this recipe – have some fun trying out different combinations.

 *Servings: 1*

 *Preparation Time: 10 minutes*

Ingredients

2 apples, cored and halved

½ avocado, peeled

Handful of spinach leaves

Handful of ice cubes

1 pear, cored and halved

1 inch of fresh ginger

Half a cucumber, peeled if not organic

Preparation

1. Juice the apples, pear, spinach, cucumber and ginger.
2. Place the juice into a blender.
3. Add the avocado and ice and then blend.
4. Drink straight away.

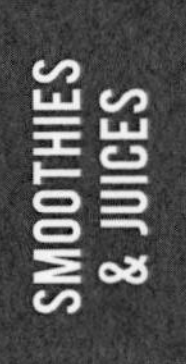

BERRY SCARLET

This juice is a beautiful deep red from the earthy beetroot and vibrant berries. It is a tasty and nutritious juice. The beetroot is full of vitamins and minerals and is packed with powerful antioxidants and the berries are a fantastic source of vitamin C. If you are not keen on the earthy tones of the beetroot then you can amend the levels of beetroot used in the recipe accordingly.

 *Servings: 1*

 *Preparation Time: 5 minutes*

Ingredients

2 apples, cored and halved

2 small fresh beetroot, topped and tailed if still have roots

Handful of mixed berries (fresh or frozen)

Handful of ice cubes

Preparation

1. Juice the apples and the beetroot.
2. Place the juice into a blender.
3. Add the berries and ice (if not using frozen berries) and then blend.
4. Drink this beautiful deep red drink straight away.

BERRY AND BANANA SMOOTHIE

This smoothie is a real comfort drink, full of creaminess and fruitiness it is full of goodness but feels like such a treat. Keeping a bag of frozen berries in the freezer will mean that you can make this smoothie with minimum fuss and also means you do not need to worry about adding extra ice. Try different combinations of berries to find your favourite. You can also use frozen mango in this smoothie.

 *Servings: 1*

 *Preparation Time: 10 minutes*

Ingredients

2 apples, cored and halved

banana, peeled

Handful of mixed berries (fresh or frozen)

tbsp coconut milk

Handful of ice cubes

Preparation

1. Juice the apples and place the juice in blender.
2. Add the banana, berries, coconut milk and ice (if not using frozen berries).
3. Bend all the ingredients together.
4. If you would like a thinner consistency then add a bit more coconut milk.

ICE CREAM MILKSHAKE

Enjoy this thick and creamy milkshake using Paleo friendly ingredients to make sure that you do not miss out on those treats. To make the drink thicker or thinner change the amount of almond milk used until you find your preference. The ice cream will make it creamy and cool with a refreshing fruity flavour.

 *Servings: 1*

 *Preparation Time: 5 minutes*

Ingredients

Handful of strawberries, hulled

½ banana

1 scoop of Paleo Raspberry Ice Cream

150ml almond milk

Preparation

1. Blend all of the ingredients together to create a thick creamy ice-cream milkshake.
2. This is one to save for a treat!

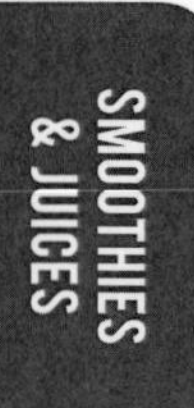

DETOX JUICE

This juice will provide you with a great vitamin boost. It is full of lovely green vegetables that will help to cleanse and detox the system and will leave your skin glowing. To those who are not used to vegetable juices this may be a shock to the system but you can add a bit more fruit if you want to balance out with some sweetness. Try adding apples or pears or some more pineapple.

 *Servings: 1*

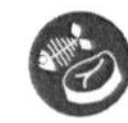 *Preparation Time: 10 minutes*

Ingredients

¼ pineapple, cored and skin removed

Large handful of kale

1 stick of celery

1 inch of fresh ginger, peeled

Large handful of spinach leaves

½ cucumber, peeled if not organic

1 lime, peeled but with pith on

Handful of ice cubes

Preparation

1. Juice all of the ingredients. You may need to place the spinach and kale between other ingredients to help push through the juicer.
2. Pour over ice to serve.

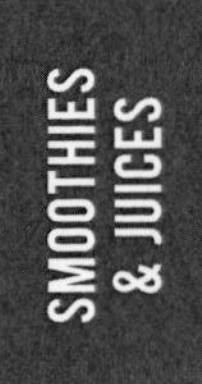

CARROT, GINGER AND APPLE

This juice is nice and simple and is great for aiding digestion. The ginger gives it a nice warming effect and the apples and carrots a lovely sweet flavour. Keep stirring it as it will start to cloud up once made. This is a great juice to have when you feel like you just need a bit of a boost. It is also good for using up the leftover carrots you may have from a shop at the end of the week.

 *Servings: 1*

 *Preparation Time: 5 minutes*

Ingredients

2 green apples, cored and halved

4 carrots, topped and tailed if still have roots

1 inch of fresh ginger, peeled

Handful of ice cubes

Preparation

1. Juice all of the ingredients.
2. Pour over ice to serve.

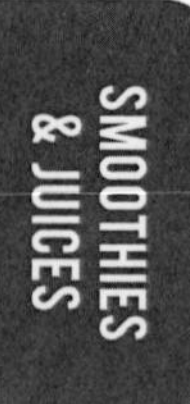

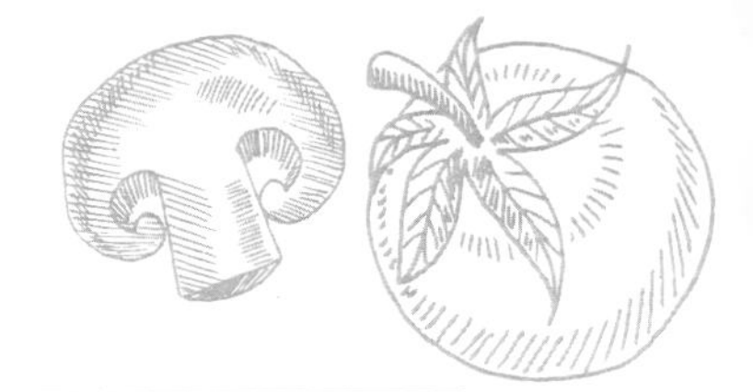

INDEX